Facilitating Learning in Clinical Settings

Edited by

Lindy McAllister
Michelle Lincoln
Sharynne McLeod
Diana Maloney

School of Communication Disorders
The University of Sydney
Australia

First published 1997 by:
Stanley Thornes (Publishers) Ltd

Reprinted in 2001 by:
Nelson Thornes Ltd
Delta Place
27 Bath Road
CHELTENHAM
GL53 7TH
United Kingdom

Transferred to digital printing 2005

A catalogue record for this book is available from the British Library
ISBN 0-7487-3316-7

Every attempt has been made to contact copyright holders, and we apologize if any have been overlooked. Any omissions brought to our attention will be remedied in future editions.

Typeset by Northern Phototypesetting Co Ltd., Bolton

Printed and bound by Antony Rowe Ltd, Eastbourne

Contents

Contributors

Diana Carmody
Student Educator
Department of Social Work
New Children's Hospital, Sydney, Australia

Ellen S. Cohn
Lecturer
Boston School of Occupational Therapy
Tufts University, Medford MA, USA

Vickie Dawson
Project Officer
Department of Speech and Hearing
The University of Queensland, Australia
and
Department of Education
Queensland, Australia

Paul Haglar
Director
Centre for Studies in Clinical Education, Faculty of Rehabilitation Medicine
University of Alberta, Canada

Joy Higgs
Professor, School of Physiotherapy,
Executive Director, Centre for Professional Education Advancement,
Faculty of Health Sciences, The University of Sydney, Australia

Michelle Lincoln
Lecturer, Clinical Educator
School of Communication Disorders, Faculty of Health Sciences
The University of Sydney, Australia

Lindy McAllister
Lecturer, Director of Clinical Education
School of Communication Disorders, Faculty of Health Sciences
The University of Sydney, Australia

Lu-Anne McFarlane
Clinic Coordinator
Department of Speech Pathology and Audiology, Faculty of Rehabilitation Medicine
University of Alberta, Canada

Sharynne McLeod
Lecturer, Clinical Coordinator
School of Communication Disorders, Faculty of Health Sciences
The University of Sydney, Australia

Diana Maloney
Clinical Educator
School of Communication Disorders, Faculty of Health Sciences
The University of Sydney, Australia

Eva Nemeth
Student Educator
Department of Speech Pathology
St Joseph's Hospital, Sydney, Australia

Marisue Pickering
Associate Vice President for Academic Affairs,
Professor of Speech Communication
University of Maine
Orono ME, United States of America

Sandra Robertson
Speech and Language Programme Head
Department of Psychology and Speech Pathology
Manchester Metropolitan University, Elizabeth Gaskell Campus
Manchester, United Kingdom

Judith Romanini
Head
Department of Nursing Therapeutics, Faculty of Nursing
The University of Sydney, Australia

Joan Rosenthal
ProDean, Senior Lecturer (retired)
School of Communication Disorders, Faculty of Health Sciences
The University of Sydney, Australia

Lynette Stockhausen
Senior Lecturer
School of Nursing, Faculty of Health and Behavioural Sciences
Griffith University, Australia

Preface

Although there are many books about facilitating student learning in academic settings, there are few which specifically address the uniqueness of learning in clinical settings. The clinical setting is a unique context in which students experience professional socialization and develop skills which cannot be readily acquired elsewhere. Clinical education provides learning challenges for all students and educators in health and education. Therefore, educators working in this setting require a specialized body of knowledge and skills to successfully help students learn.

The aim of this book is to provide a philosophy and framework in which to ground clinical education practices. This book discusses practical strategies consistent with this framework, which clinical educators can use to empower students to become life-long self-directed autonomous professionals. It provides a perspective on personal and professional growth of students and clinical educators along a continuum towards the goal of interdependent learning in clinical education. Theory-driven practical strategies are presented for students and clinical educators which are directed by principles of adult learning, a client focus and theoretically sound experiential learning. Strategies are presented which the reader can adapt for his or her own setting.

The book contains an overview of how adult learning theory relates to clinical education and practical strategies for implementation. It discusses stages of student growth and development along the continuum toward interdependence, case examples and cautions to using suggested strategies.

The unique features of this book are that it: links theory and strategies in clinical education; grounds clinical education strategies in an adult learning framework; focuses on learning rather than teaching; is multidisciplinary; provides practical strategies for students at different stages on a continuum of independence; discusses learning in a diversity of clinical settings and with a diversity of students; describes clinical education as a triad comprising learner, educator *and* client. The content is based on feedback regarding the effectiveness of strategies from students and clinical educators. The editors have tested the utility of the frameworks and strategies in teaching and learning with clinical educators from many disciplines.

Chapter 1 introduces our philosophies of clinical education and how they link into an adult learning framework. Chapter 2 provides a five-part structure for looking at models of clinical education. A new model, the Teacher–manager model of clinical education is introduced, and roles and responsibilities of the clinical educator are discussed. Chapter 3 discusses professional development of students and clinical educators, covering issues such as motivation for learning, anxiety, professional socialization, learning contracts, ethics, communication skills and feedback. Chapter 4 addresses learning processes in clinical education and explores reflection, self-evaluation, journal writing and peer learning. Chapter 5 covers clinical decision-making and how clinical educators can facilitate their students' development of clinical reasoning in an adult learning framework. Chapter 6 explores the whos, whats, whys and hows of assessment in a clinical education context. Chapter 7 provides theory and practical ideas to clinical educators about students experiencing problems in clinical settings. Chapter 8 provides a summary of the history and current status of research into clinical education and provides support for clinical educators to conduct quantitative and qualitative research. Chapter 9 considers the future of clinical education against the background of change, challenge and creativity. Issues such as gender, race and technological advancement are explored. Each chapter also contains case studies which describe students and situations in the context of theory and practice within the chapters.

Throughout the book the reader gets to know a student called Sally. Sally is on an overseas clinical placement and reflects on her learning as it relates to each chapter. Her postcards to and replies from her clinical educators create a binding theme throughout the book.

Practitioners, researchers, educators and students from many disciplines will be interested in the themes of this book. In particular, doctors, nurses, physiotherapists, speech therapists, occupational therapists, social workers, psychologists, dietitians, diversional therapists, podiatrists, dentists, medical radiation technologists, orthoptists, optometrists and rehabilitation counsellors will find that this book promotes sound clinical education practices in their fields. This book is a potential text for graduate classes in clinical education.

The editors have worked together in the School of Communication Disorders at The University of Sydney for the past six years. Together we have 62 years of experience in clinical education. All four editors have had extensive experience in curriculum development in relation to clinical education and are actively involved in research into student learning. We currently manage a large clinical teaching programme for over 200 allied health science students. We believe that our on-campus speech pathology clinic is one of the largest in the world, accommodating approximately 250 students per semester and 200–300 clients per week. In this environment we have had many opportunities to test our ideas and philosophies on clinical education.

Further, the editors have presented at various conferences and participated in invited teaching seminars. We have taught post-graduate courses in clinical education at The University of Sydney. All four of us regularly provide workshops and seminars for clinical educators in their own disciplines and on a multidisciplinary basis. Much of the content of this book has been presented at clinical education workshops over a number of years and refined through feedback from students and clinical educators.

The editors wish to acknowledge all the students and fellow clinical educators who have contributed to our understanding and thoughts on clinical education. We also wish to thank our families and colleagues who have supported us during the time we have devoted to editing and writing this book.

Lindy McAllister
Michelle Lincoln
Sharynne McLeod
Diana Maloney
Sydney, 1996

An adult learning framework for clinical education

1

Lindy McAllister
School of Communication Disorders,
The University of Sydney, Australia

1.1 CHAPTER OVERVIEW

Some factors which make clinical education such an important and vital part of the preparation of health, education and welfare professionals are explored in this chapter. The chapter considers how clinical education offers unique opportunities to work with student learning styles and to promote deep approaches to learning which result in the development of clinical knowledge/clinical reasoning and the ability to work in complex and changing environments. It considers the goals of clinical education in terms of generic attributes, competence and capability, and discusses reasons why we fail to achieve those goals. The importance of the semantics used in talking about who we are and what we do as clinical educators is considered.

The chapter outlines a philosophical and theoretical approach to clinical education grounded in adult learning, which is more congruent with the broader goals of clinical education. Adult learning theory and approaches are reviewed, and factors which make clinical education a unique context for the application of these theories and approaches are highlighted. Processes of teaching and learning – autonomy, self-directedness, interdependence and peer learning – which are congruent with adult learning are outlined. The characteristics of clinical educators operating effectively within an adult learning framework are discussed.

1.2 LEARNING IN CLINICAL SETTINGS

This is a book which focuses on students' learning, not teachers' instructing or supervisors' supervising. It is about the education of students who will one day be our professional peers, colleagues and co-learners in the clinical settings in which we work. It is a book about clinical education – education for the realities of professional practice in the changing health, education and welfare sectors (see Case Study 1.1).

Case Study 1.1

Sally is an Australian speech therapy student who has just arrived in a developing country in Asia to begin a nine-week period as a volunteer on a project to establish a community-based rehabilitation (CBR) early intervention programme. She will work under the guidance of an Australian paediatrician, who has volunteered for a three-year period to establish community health services in this remote rural area. Sally will work closely on the project with local CBR workers. She doesn't know what will be expected of her by the local or international staff. Because she knows we have a great interest in her and the project, Sally will send us weekly postcards from the project. Her first postcard appears below (see Postcard 1).

Postcard 1

Dear All

Well here I am in ... [the local regional centre]. It was an amazing 11 hour bus trip here from the capital, along narrow roads perched on the edge of the mountains. When I could bear to look down, I could see the flooded rice paddies and the raging rivers – very beautiful. The town has about 5,000 people and I'm staying in the mission guest house half an hour walk from town. The area is very lush at this time of the year and I'm told I'll often walk to work in the heavy monsoonal rain. I was able to buy in the local markets a suitable outfit for work here – light cotton top to the knees, long sleeves, matching trousers. Wait till you see the photos! I start work tomorrow. The Community Based Rehabilitation (CBR) project has been running for about three months. There are four team members all of whom have received six weeks of CBR training in rehab., OT, physio., social work and 2 days on speech therapy (mainly hearing impairment). This is going to be an interesting experience!

love Sally

As we read Postcard 1 from Sally, we shared her excitement and her anxiety. We talked a lot about the personal and professional growth we had witnessed in Sally and how much of a contribution we could claim in that growth. As her clinical educators over the past four and a half years had we provided her with a clinical education that would enable her to meet the challenges she now described? We would look forward to the story which unfolds in the ensuing weekly postcards.

1.2.1 NAMING OURSELVES AND DEFINING WHAT WE DO

In this book we name the process in which we are engaged as *clinical education*; hence we name ourselves as *clinical educators*. We take a broad view of clinical education, which we define as:

a teaching and learning process which is student-focused and may be student-led, which occurs in the context of client care. It involves the translation of theory into the development of clinical knowledge and practical skills, with the incorporation of the affective domain needed for sensitive and ethical client care. Clinical education occurs in an environment supportive of the development of clinical reasoning skills, professional socialization and life-long learning.

Our definition encompasses the acquisition of the knowledge, skills and attributes needed to become a competent professional as well as a competent clinician. Education for professional socialization, the development of moral and ethical positions (see Chapter 3), and the promotion of the attributes of a life-long learner are deemed to be just as important as the development of clinical skills. Our emphasis is on education towards certain goals, not the instruction in certain techniques or supervision of skill acquisition, nor transmission of prescribed information. We believe that the latter are approaches to teaching and learning which do not fit with the current goals of professional preparation. We will return to a discussion of these goals in a later section.

We believe that this naming of ourselves and the work in which we are engaged is vital for clarity of purpose and clarity of communication. In stating our position, we allow an exploration of the meaning attached to our work, and the philosophical and theoretical foundations of our work.

1.2.2 THE SEMANTICS OF CLINICAL EDUCATION

The process of preparing students for work in the health, education and welfare sectors has many names: clinical instruction, fieldwork education, supervision, clinical teaching and clinical education to name a few. Similarly, we find in the literature ourselves referred to as clinical instructors, clinical tutors, clinical supervisors, clinical teachers and clinical or fieldwork educators. These terms are often used interchangeably as if they had the same meaning. We suggest that there is confusion and limitation inherent in the ways currently used in the literature to name and define what we do. Getting the semantics right is important with regard to the perceptions we and others have about the scope and value of our work.

Some of the confusion derives from the historical usage of the terms. Cross (1994) has commented on the change in terminology in physiotherapy clinical education in the United Kingdom. She traces the development of clinicians' roles from the 1960s to the 1990s, from clinical instructor to clinical educator. She describes the *clinical instructor* as a clinician working in a fairly circumscribed environment, who with almost 'amateurish enthusiasm' drilled students to reproduce traditional procedures.

As student numbers increased and curricula broadened in the 1970s, the role became one of *clinical supervisor* of the activities of several students, ensuring that they did not disrupt the normal running of the department. There is an element of controlling and limiting students inherent in this description. The 1980s brought increased professional autonomy and university-based education programmes. 'Training' was transformed into 'education' (Cross, 1994, p. 610). *Clinical teachers* placed a greater emphasis on individual student development.

The enormous changes in the health, education and welfare sectors in the 1990s have required that clinicians develop expertise in a wide range of personal, interpersonal and management skills, in addition to core discipline skills (Cross, 1994). Cross suggests that 'physiotherapy educators … have a responsibility to equip students fully to take up the cause of quality physiotherapy in the future' (p. 610). The role is now one of *clinical educator*, developing in students a breadth of personal, interpersonal and management skills.

Cross makes it clear that the terms used were linked to expectations and roles of the time. These expectations and roles have changed for all professions. The professions have a broader view of who they are and what they do. Terminology must change to reflect these broader visions, roles and expectations.

A definition offered by the *Shorter Oxford English Dictionary* (Onions, 1992) for education is of relevance to our argument. *Education* is defined as 'the process of nourishing or rearing; the process of bringing up' and 'culture or development of powers, formation of [intellectual or moral] character'. This definition strikes the right note with us. It suggests that we are *educating* for the future, sometimes for as yet ill-defined goals in changing professional contexts. It suggests that the education in which we engage is systematic, but also nourishing and developing of the character of future professionals.

The story of Sally powerfully illustrates what it means to be a clinical educator rather than an instructor, supervisor or teacher (see Case Studies 1.2 and 1.3).

Case Study 1.2

It has taken Sally five years to near completion of our four-year speech therapy degree programme. In the early years of the programme she failed academic and clinical subjects. Sally had difficulty applying theory to practice, developing intervention plans and implementing these proficiently with her clients. In part this was because she had a weak theoretical background, in part because she was chronically disorganized. However, Sally had good interpersonal skills and was helpful and considerate to her fellow students and staff of the clinic. Her clients liked her. The willingness with which Sally accepted and acted on feedback and repeated failed subjects demonstrated her commitment to becoming a good therapist.

We, her clinical educators, respected her and believed in her potential to achieve her goal. It would have been easier for us to have continually shown her what to do and told her how to do it. We could have acted always as instructors. Or we could have supervised all her activities and controlled every learning opportunity. Instead we let her learn from her mistakes provided those mistakes did not compromise client care. We had a clear vision of what it meant to us to be educators, operating within an adult learning framework. We helped Sally identify what she already knew and needed to know next, in order to improve. We helped her to identify resources she could utilize to improve her knowledge and skills. We encouraged her to work with her peers to develop her knowledge and skills, and encouraged her peers to give her feedback about the confusion her disorganization engendered in the clinic.

As clinical educators committed to an adult learning approach, we chose not to stop at the stage of developing clinical skills. We respected Sally and affirmed her personal and professional growth and encouraged her to develop further her professional identity. In other words, we functioned as *educators*. We nourished her character and promoted her professional socialization. As her competence grew, we treated her more like a colleague, sharing the responsibility for decision-making about her learning experiences and goals. We encouraged her to pursue her interest in working in the developing world, and acted as sounding boards as she considered various strategies which would enable her to rearrange her programme to take time out to go to the CBR project in Asia and which would enable her to arrive well prepared.

Case Study 1.3

Throughout the negotiations with us about rearranging her final semester's commitments and gathering materials to take with her to the CBR project, Sally showed great maturity, confidence and organizational skill. In conversations she showed that she had considered various possible needs the project might have and tapped into our network of colleagues with CBR and WHO (World Health Organization) experience. She spoke to colleagues about what she might expect culturally, what information, materials and skills might be most appropriate for a CBR project of this type. She interviewed fellow students from other disciplines who had recently returned from CBR project work in India. She photocopied and organized a wide array of information and read widely outside her own discipline area. All this she accomplished while completing coursework and working part-time to fund her trip and living expenses in Asia. We felt like we were interacting with a peer within a rewarding educational relationship.

Cross (1994) notes that educational relationships such as these have a different balance of power to instructing, supervising or teaching relationships. There is power sharing, based on approachability, disclosure and respect. Cross (1994) suggests that 'the linkage between these three elements holds the potential to empower the clinician–student relationship in a way which supports students in their early attempts to develop basic management skills' (p. 611). Sally has finally developed personal and professional management skills. We believe that she has grown into a competent clinician and a life-long learner, as her first postcard suggests.

Sally's story illustrates the importance of clinical education to the development of professionals. The next section discusses this topic in more detail.

1.3 THE IMPORTANCE OF CLINICAL EDUCATION

Clinical education is a vital and irreplaceable component in preparing students for the reality of their professional role (Grahn, 1989; Williams & Webb, 1994). Because it is such an essential component of professional preparation, we have devoted a whole chapter (see Chapter 8) to research needs in clinical education, in the hope that we can inspire a coherent search for a better understanding of the nature, processes and outcomes of clinical education.

Clinical education is about the real world of professional practice, where learning is holistic and involves transfer, reorganization, application, synthesis and evaluation of previously acquired knowledge, along with the acquisition of new knowledge and skills. Clinical education enables the development of skills best learned in the clinical setting, such as clinical decision-making and problem-solving. The clinical setting promotes the integration of theoretical and skills-based components of the curricula, and efficient reorganization of knowledge, so that it may be applied to the problem-solving and clinical decision-making (see Chapter 5) required in real-life client care. The following sections explore aspects of learning in the clinical setting.

1.3.1 THE DEVELOPMENT OF CLINICAL KNOWLEDGE, CLINICAL REASONING AND CLINICAL KNOW-HOW

Lectures, tutorials, seminars, lab or practical sessions all have an important place in the development of cognitive, technical and affective skills which underpin clinical and professional practice. However, outside the clinical setting this knowledge remains at an abstract theoretical level. Polyani (1958) calls this *explicit knowledge* – the objective, public, written knowledge of the world, the type of fact-laden theory which students bring unintegrated to the clinic, unsure of what it might mean and how to apply it.

Students also need to be able to develop *tacit knowledge* about the reality of their professional role, based on experience. Tacit knowledge is demonstrated in action. It becomes the personal practical knowledge (Brown & McIntyre, 1993) of skilled clinicians. The distinction between explicit and tacit knowledge is similar to the distinction between knowing what and knowing how. Knowing how is the clinical knowledge needed for competent professional work.

Benner (1984) has outlined the stages of learners in their movement from novice to expert status. Not all clinicians become expert, and expert status is not a realistic goal for clinical education programmes aiming to produce entry level graduates. However, aspects of expert practice are goals of clinical education which can only be achieved in clinical settings. Skilled professionals develop through thoughtful reflection on their practice rather than longevity or amount of practice (Oldmeadow, 1996). By engaging in reflective practice (Schön, 1987), professionals become competent in what he calls the 'grey areas' of professional practice, those situations which require creative thinking or problem-solving. Highly skilled professionals develop a sense of what is salient in any situation and recognize patterns. They develop common-sense understanding of their clients and contexts, and skilled know-how (see Chapter 4 on reflection). These attributes can only be developed in meaningful, real-life, ongoing interactions with clients – in other words, in the clinical setting.

1.3.2 THE PROMOTION OF DEEP APPROACHES TO LEARNING

This real-life client care also creates a meaningfulness to learning activities, which is intrinsically motivating to students (Scanlan, 1978). This intrinsic motivation is one of the features distinguishing students engaged in deep approaches to learning as opposed to surface approaches to learning (Marton & Säljö, 1984). Deep approaches to learning are found in students who are affectively engaged in searching for personal meaning and understanding (their own personal practical knowledge), seeing the whole picture or person – not just the isolated features or disembodied problems – drawing on their personal experience to make sense of new ideas and experiences, and relating evidence to conclusions. These deep approaches to learning are in marked contrast to surface approaches exhibited by students who seek only to memorize and reproduce information or skills, see only the discrete 'bits', expect the educator to be in control of their learning, and are largely motivated by the external imperative to pass an assessment or gain their qualification. In other words, they are self-focused rather than client-focused (see Chapter 3 for further discussion).

Professional preparation programmes aspire to engage all students in deep learning, to ensure quality of client care, as well as quality of student learning. Certainly, the clinical education setting has been shown effectively to facilitate deep learning (Coles, 1989; 1990). However, some students even in the clinical setting may remain what Ramsden (1984; 1988) and Entwistle and Waterson (1988) have referred to as strategic learners, those that use their personal organization skills to select the 'right' information and approaches needed to pass assessment tasks and achieve high marks (see Chapter 7). This strategic learning tends to occur in overloaded competitive learning environments. Care needs to be taken to ensure that the clinical education environment is conducive to deep learning. This topic will be explore in more depth later in this chapter and in Chapter 2 in the discussion of teacher-as-manager in clinical education.

1.3.3 UTILIZING AND BROADENING STUDENTS' LEARNING STYLES

Clinical settings and professional practice require many different skills from clinicians. Clinics are busy, task-focused places; things have to get done, often by yesterday. Meeting client needs requires the ability to think on one's feet, sometimes to make decisions quickly or expediently, sometimes with much thought and reflection. Some aspects of clinical practice or clinical management require a thorough understanding of the latest theories and issues. Different people will rise to each of these occasions differently, depending on their learning style.

(a) Describing learning styles

A learning style is conceptualized as the 'preference or habitual strategy used by an individual to process information for problem solving' (Katz & Heimann, 1991, p. 239). Researchers have investigated individual differences in learning styles and there is wide acceptance that individuals do develop consistent and distinctive styles to resolve conflict and analyze experience, or in other words, to learn.

The work of Kolb (1976; 1981; 1984; 1986) has been particularly influential in learning styles research. Kolb proposed a four-category model to facilitate the understanding and investigation of human learning styles and tested the Learning Style Inventory (LSI) as a brief self-descriptive inventory to categorize reported learning preferences. Analysis of an individual's responses reveals a preference for one of four styles:

- A person who reports that he or she learns most from abstract conceptualization and reflective observation is classified as an *assimilator*.
- A person who reports that he or she learns most from concrete experience and reflective observation is classified as a *diverger*.
- A person who reports that he or she learns most from abstract conceptualization of events and active experimentation is classified as a *converger*.
- A person who reports that they learn most from concrete experience and active experimentation is classified as an *accommodator*.

Honey and Mumford (1986) developed a Learning Styles Questionnaire (LSQ) which has much in common with Kolb's (1981) Learning Style Inventory (LSI). The LSQ determines individuals' preference between four primary learning styles: reflector, theorist, activist and pragmatist, each of which are different from Kolb's (1981, 1984) reported learning styles. According to Honey and Mumford (1986)

- A *reflector* learns by listening to different perspectives before coming to a conclusion. He or she likes to observe and reflect on experiences. A reflector would be classified as an assimilator or a diverger by Kolb (1984) depending on his or her preference for abstract or concrete conceptualization.
- An *activist* thrives on the challenge of new experiences and learns by active experimentation. Kolb (1984) would classify this learner as an accommodator or a converger depending again on his or her preference for abstract or concrete material.
- A *theorist* analyzes and synthesizes observations into theories, attempting to make pieces of information form a whole.
- A *pragmatist* prefers to experiment with new ideas, theories and techniques and is interested in the practicality and application of information.

People who report that they utilize three or four of Honey and Mumford's learning styles are referred to as 'all rounders'. Learners may also have combinations of two learning styles (for example, activist–reflector).

(b) The learning styles of health science students

Kolb (1984) suggested that learning style is shaped by four forces: early educational experiences, educational specialization, professional career choice and current job role. Predominant learning styles are apparent for people pursuing health science careers (for example, Katz & Heimann, 1991; Lovie-Kitchin, Coonan, Sanderson & Thompson, 1989; McLeod, Lincoln, McAllister, Maloney, Purcell & Eadie, 1995; Vittetoe & Hooker, 1983; Wells & Higgs, 1990). Careers such as medicine consist predominantly of people who display a *converger* learning style, whereas careers such as occupational therapy consist of people who predominantly display an *accommodator* learning style (Kolb, 1984). McLeod *et al.* (1995) found that second- and third-year speech therapy students were predominantly *activists*.

(c) Application of learning styles in clinical education

Learning styles are of interest to clinical educators for two reasons. Firstly, it is thought that by matching learning opportunities to students' reported learning styles more successful and efficient learning will occur (Vittetoe & Hooker, 1983; Svincki & Dixon, 1987). Secondly, it is thought that students who can effectively utilize a variety of learning styles will be able to adapt successfully to any learning situation (Honey & Mumford, 1989; Dixon, 1985). Consequently clinical educators may utilize learning styles either to maximize student learning or to challenge students to adapt their styles to the demands of the learning situation. Identification of learning styles may enable clinical educators to be more sensitive to the differences students bring to their learning experiences. Clinical education experiences can be challenging or comfortable depending on whether or not the learning experience matches students' personal learning styles. Clinical educators can decide whether they wish to support students by providing learning opportunities which utilize their dominant learning styles, or to challenge students by encouraging them to explore learning opportunities using other than their dominant learning styles.

An understanding of their learning style may help students become deep learners, adept at creating their own personal practical knowledge and clinical know-how, as well as the skills necessary for clinical practice (see Chapter 4). Working with students' learning styles may help them better achieve the goals of clinical education.

1.4 GOALS OF CLINICAL EDUCATION

The settings and demands of professional practice are changing (see Chapter 9). So too should the missions of the professional preparation programmes and the goals of clinical education change. Higgs, Glendinning, Dunsford and Panter (1991) surveyed allied health professional education programmes and developed the list of goals for clinical education which is shown below. It is important to note that clinical skills and knowledge relevant to the student's discipline are but two of the 15 goals listed. There is an increasing emphasis on generic goals for clinical education to enable graduates to work in complex, changing environments.

Goals of clinical education for the health science professions
(Higgs *et al.*, 1991)

- Understanding of health, illness and the health care system
- Awareness of own attitudes, values and responses to health and illness
- Ability to cope effectively with the demands of the professional role
- Understanding of the interrelated roles of the health care team
- Clinical competencies relevant to the student's discipline, including clinical reasoning skills, psychomotor competencies, and interpersonal and communication skills
- Ability to provide a sound rationale for interventions/actions
- Skills in the education of relevant people (for example, patients, clients, the community, staff)
- Self-management skills (for example, time and workload management)
- Ability to process, record and use data effectively
- Ability to evaluate critically and develop own performance
- Ability to review and investigate the quality of clinical practice
- Professional accountability commitment to clients/self/employers
- Commitment to maintain and develop professional competence
- Skills necessary for lifelong professional learning
- Ability to respond to changing community health care needs

1.4.1 PREPARING STUDENTS FOR COMPLEX, CHANGING WORK ENVIRONMENTS

Higgs *et al.* (1991) and Engel (1995) have highlighted that graduates of health science education programmes are expected not only to be competent in the practice of their discipline – that is, to be able to apply the basic sciences and applied sciences to the care and management of clients, and to be adept and professional in their interactions with colleagues and clients – they are also expected to develop competence in what Schön (1987) describes as the 'indeterminate zones of practice' (p. 11), those grey areas of 'uncertainty, uniqueness, and value conflict [which] escape the canons of technical rationality' (p. 6). Such situations arise in most professions. For example, in clients whose life-span is limited and where the costs of support services and intervention are high, professionals may face ethical dilemmas in addressing concerns of offering intervention to enhance the quality of remaining life. Clinical education which seeks to promote competence in these grey areas must build on different theories of teaching and learning to those used in instruction and supervision for competent, clear-cut, discipline-specific practice. Schön argues for the development of the reflective practitioner. Strategies for promoting reflection in students are discussed in Chapter 4.

More recently, Engel (1995, p. 29) developed a similar position in his discussion of the need for a 'capability approach' to medical education. He outlined two major tasks for medical schools. He suggested that medical schools should continue to help students acquire the discipline specific competences required to fulfill the responsibilities expected of new graduates under supervision. In addition, he suggested medical schools should seek to provide a general education that focuses on the generally applicable competences, in which he includes the abilities to adapt to change and participate in change, to communicate for a range of purposes (for example, obtain and give information, negotiate, consult and counsel), to collaborate in groups or teams, and to be self-directed life-long learners who can apply critical reasoning and a scientific approach to decision-making in unfamiliar situations (see Chapter 5).

1.4.2 FACILITATING STUDENTS' DEVELOPMENT OF GENERIC ATTRIBUTES

In addition to being prepared to function in complex and uncertain environments, university graduates are expected to develop generic attributes which enable them to function in less uncertain but more diverse settings and roles. These attributes include a variety of knowledge skills, thinking skills, personal skills, attributes and values, and professional and technical skills. There is a lively debate about generic attributes, their relationship to professional competences and the competence movement in general, particularly in the United Kingdom. The place of competences in higher education has been criticized. However, Gonzci (1994) argues that it is possible to develop competency standards for professions which are holistic and integrate cognitive, affective and technical aspects of professional work. It is this holistic integrated view of competence which has been embraced by the professions in Australia for example, and which has allowed the integration of professional competency standards into the university professional preparation programmes (see Chapter 6 for a discussion of competency-based clinical assessment of students).

1.4.3 FACILITATING CAPABILITY IN STUDENTS THROUGH CLINICAL EDUCATION

Stephenson (1996) has moved the debate about competence forward with his discussion of *capability*, which he defines as 'an all-round human quality, and integration of knowledge, skills and personal qualities used effectively and appropriately in response to varied, familiar and unfamiliar circumstances'. He suggests that capability is having justified confidence in one's ability to 'take appropriate and effective action, communicate effectively, collaborate with others and learn from experiences in changing circumstances'.

The work of Schön and Stephenson highlights the need for clinical education to emphasize personal qualities and capability for professional practice in uncertain and changing environments (see Chapter 7). In this book, we would argue that clinical education is ideally and uniquely suited to achieve the development of capability.

With the knowledge explosion in all disciplines, graduates are expected to be critical consumers of information and life-long learners who maintain competence in their discipline, expand and test their own knowledge and skills, and contribute to the expansion of knowledge in the field. Practical and manageable ways in which clinical educators can contribute to the knowledge and practice of clinical education are considered in a later chapter on research (see Chapter 8). Professional practice in the clinical setting requires professionals to be life-long learners (Lincoln & McAllister, 1993). Appropriate clinical education has the potential to set students on the path of life-long learning.

1.4.4 LIFE-LONG LEARNING

The ability to be a life-long learner is a valued attribute and essential component of capability. Candy (1994) has discussed the development of life-long learning through undergraduate education. He has profiled the qualities or characteristics of life-long learners, an adaptation of which appears on page 14.

It is essential to be a life-long learner who is aware of one's learning style and approaches to learning, who has the ability to access learning resources, and who self-directs and self-evaluates one's learning. The ability to collaborate with other professionals in learning, and in service delivery is vital. This collaboration could be called *interdependence*, a concept which will be elaborated in a later section. Employers value such attributes and the changing nature of professional practice demands it.

As Cross (1994) has noted, the goals of clinical education have grown from a training and instruction focus on the drilling of prescribed procedures to include an emphasis on the development of generic attributes essential to professional competence, capability and life-long learning. The changes and challenges discussed in Chapter 9 create a growing imperative to achieve the goals of clinical education.

Profile of the attributes of a life-long learner (Candy, 1994)

- *An inquiring mind:*
  - a love of learning
  - a sense of curiosity and question asking
  - a critical spirit
  - comprehension monitoring and self-evaluation
- *Helicopter vision:*
  - a sense of the interconnectedness of fields
  - an awareness of how knowledge is created in at least one field of study, and an understanding of the methodological and substantive limitations in that field
- *Information literacy:*
  - knowledge of major current resources available in at least one field of study
  - ability to frame researchable questions in at least one field of study

  - ability to locate, evaluate, manage and use information in a range of contexts
  - ability to retrieve information using a variety of media
  - ability to decode information in a variety of forms: written, statistical, graphs, charts, diagrams and tables
  - critical evaluation of information
- *A sense of personal agency:*
  - a positive concept of oneself as capable and autonomous
  - self-organization skills (time management, goal-setting, etc.)
- *A repertoire of learning skills:*
  - knowledge of one's own strengths, weaknesses and preferred learning style
  - range of strategies for learning in whatever context one finds oneself
  - an understanding of the differences between surface and deep learning.

1.5 ARE WE ACHIEVING THE GOALS OF CLINICAL EDUCATION?

The goals for clinical education outlined in previous sections are not new. Over a decade ago, Stritter, Baker and Shahady (1986) outlined their learning vector model (see Chapter 2) which has as goals independent learning and autonomy. Most contemporary clinical education programmes would espouse similar goals and values. One indicator that these values were being enacted and goals achieved would be the nature of the interactions between clinical educators and their students. Such interactions should exemplify the promotion of the broader goals of clinical education.

However, the literature suggests that interactions between clinical educators and students are often counterproductive to the pursuit of the goals of interdependence, autonomy, self-direction and self-evaluation. Research into the communications between clinical educators and students reveals a consistent picture of clinical educators dominating interactions, doing most of the initiating, talking, information-provision and problem-solving (Anderson, 1988) (see Chapter 8). Students take a passive, responsive role even though they say they would like to take greater responsibility for directing the interaction and problem-solving themselves (Kenny & McAllister, 1993). The research literature suggests this pattern to be resistant to change and unresponsive to growth and change in the student (Anderson, 1988).

Another indicator that the goals of clinical education were being met would lie in the content of educational sessions conducted with students in clinical settings. Grahn (1989) studied clinical education situations in radiation therapy and concluded that they were 'capricious endeavours. Anything, good or bad, could be the outcome' (p. 27).

We suggest two of many possible reasons for these incongruities between the goals and processes of clinical education. The interactions with students described above are those of *instructors* acting out of a philosophy of instructing for limited skills, rather than of *educators* facilitating learning and educating for broader goals. Further, it is suggested that clinical education lacks a theory of education which would promote the attainment of the broader goals of clinical education outlined previously. A review of the clinical education literature (Kenny, 1996) revealed, with a few exceptions, a marked lack of any explicit reference to a theory of clinical education. Opacich (1995) alluded to a similar belief in her critique of the lack of a philosophy of clinical education in occupational therapy.

One notable exception to atheoretical discussions of clinical education is the work of Stengelhofen (1993). She does discuss the differences between adult learning (andragogy) and pedagogy and the characteristics of adult learners. Stengelhofen then goes on to discuss the implications of these for the roles clinical educators can adopt with students.

We believe that adult learning theory is congruent with the goals of clinical education and argue that widespread adoption might enable clinical education more successfully to meet the goals to which it aspires. The following section briefly reviews key elements of the adult learning literature.

1.6 ADULT LEARNING

Knowles (1970), in discussing the search for a theory of adult learning, introduced into the English language literature on adult learning the term *andragogy* which he defined as the art and science of helping adults learn. Today this term is used to refer more broadly to an approach to teaching and learning for any age group, which is student-centred and which fosters learner autonomy. This is in contrast to traditional notions of pedagogy, which was initially used to refer to the didactic teaching of children but is now commonly used to indicate teacher-directed learning.

1.6.1 CHARACTERISTICS OF ADULT LEARNERS

There are a number of key assumptions about the characteristics of adult learners upon which Knowles (1980) bases his model of andragogy. These assumptions are that as adults mature:

- they become more self-directing, although they may choose dependence on the teacher in some circumstances
- their life experiences become a rich resource for learning and they tend to learn better through experiential means
- their learning needs are more often determined by life circumstances at the time, for example the need to acquire job-related skills
- their learning becomes more problem-centred for immediate performance in life circumstances.

Although subsequent investigators have refined Knowles' original concepts, there tends to be general agreement in the literature regarding the characteristics of adult learners. Brookfield (1986) concludes that autonomy in the learning programme and the use of one's life experience as a learning resource are the two characteristics of adult learning most frequently reported in the literature on adult learning.

1.6.2 PRINCIPLES OF ADULT LEARNING

Brookfield (1986, p. 31) summarizes the work of several authors who have attempted to specify the principles of adult learning, as follows:

'adults learn throughout their lives, with the negotiations of the transitional stages in the life-span being the immediate causes and motives for much of this learning. They exhibit diverse learning styles – strategies for coding information, cognitive procedures, mental sets – and learn in different ways, at different times, for different purposes. As a rule, however, they like their learning activities to be problem centred and to be meaningful to their life situation, and they want learning outcomes to have immediacy of application. The past experiences of adults effect their current learning, sometimes serving as an enhancement, sometimes as a hindrance. Effective learning is also linked to the adult's subscription to a self-concept of himself or herself as a learner. Finally, adults exhibit a tendency toward self-directedness in their learning.'

The implications for clinical education of these characteristics of adult learners and principles of adult learning will be elaborated throughout this book.

1.7 CLINICAL EDUCATION: A UNIQUE OPPORTUNITY FOR ADULT LEARNING

It can be argued that clinical education is an ideal context in which to adopt an adult learning approach. Clinical education is by its very nature experiential: it involves obtaining experience in working with clients in real contexts. These clients bring to the health, education or welfare setting real problems which they wish to solve. Clients' needs provide the immediacy for problem-solving and clinical decision-making, and the motivation needed for successful learning by adult learners. To be successful, students need to engage in deep learning, as discussed earlier in this chapter. Students learning to be clinicians engage in problem-solving with their clients, their clinical educators and their peers, as they seek to solve the presented problems. They draw not only on what they know, their previous clinical and classroom experiences but also past life experiences. As students are motivated by the need to solve real and immediate problems presented in the clinical and professional environments, they are likely to reflect on their actions and decisions, either during the client contact or after it (see Chapter 4). Students in clinical settings have a real need to make the most of the experience in which they find themselves. The reality of the clinical environment is highly congruent with adult learning theory.

We suggest that adult learning theory provides a strong theoretical foundation for clinical education. The characteristics of adult learners are those demonstrated in students engaged in clinical experiences. The principles of adult learning lend themselves to application in the clinical setting. The characteristics of effective facilitators are congruent with those characteristics needed for effective clinical educators. The goals of adult learning and clinical education are similar in that they both emphasize the need for self-directedness and autonomy. The following section will explore further some of the common themes which arise in adult learning and clinical education. It will discuss ways in which adult learning principles can be incorporated into clinical education programmes to promote the attainment of the goals of clinical education outlined earlier in this chapter.

1.7.1 AUTONOMY AND SELF-DIRECTEDNESS

Autonomy and self-directedness are both processes of learning as well as desired goals of learning. Candy (1991) states that 'a person may be regarded as autonomous to the extent that he or she conceives of goals and plans, exercises freedom of choice, uses the capacity for rational reflection, has willpower to follow through, exercises self-restraint and self-discipline, views himself or herself as autonomous' (p. 125). Four dimensions of self-direction are elaborated by Candy (1991): personal autonomy, self-management in learning, the independent pursuit of learning, and student control of instruction. The implications which these dimensions have for managing clinical education programmes are explored below.

(a) Constraints to autonomy and self-directedness

It is apparent that a clinical education programme wishing to promote the goals of autonomy and self-directedness will need to consider carefully issues of student control, freedom, independence and interdependence within the learning programme. Legal and ethical concerns related to client care dictate that students can not have full control of their learning programme. Their clinical educators are ultimately legally responsible for client care. The gatekeeping function held by universities for the professions also means that clinical education programmes have some basic curricula to be covered and assessed, and need to be able to certify competence in their graduates. There is a potential dilemma for programmes and clinical educators in seeking to enact adult learning principles of student freedom to direct their learning whilst maintaining legally and societally determined controls.

Some guidance on dealing with this dilemma comes from the work of Torbert (1978) on the paradoxical concept of *liberating structures*. Torbert argues that structure for a learning programme comes from its organization and the leadership exercised in implementing the learning programme. The nature of the constraints built into a programme structure can paradoxically free students to achieve more than they could have otherwise. These concepts of liberating programmes, and paradoxical structure and freedom are important in the implications they hold for clinical education programmes and clinical educators.

In applying these concepts Higgs (1993) sees freedom and control as occurring on a continuum. At one end lies clinical educator dominance and control, at the other a *laissez-faire* approach by the clinical educator and control by the student. The balance of these two would be *controlled freedom*, such as that which can occur in *liberating programme structures* defined by Higgs (1993) as 'the dynamic framework ... a complex whole in which numerous environmental, task, social and individual dimensions need to operate congruently to optimize learning opportunities and outcomes' (p. 126).

Higgs recognizes that students need to be ready to undertake the learning task at hand, a concept which she refers to as *learner task maturity* (see Chapter 2). Students need to be prepared and supported in their readiness for a task. The clinical educator needs to structure tasks and control students' access to tasks relative to their readiness for the tasks, in order to enhance the likelihood that the freedom they will have within the task leads to successful learning and, in the context of clinical education, to client care. The clinical educator in a liberating programme structure functions as a manager of the student's learning programme. The application of the Teacher-manager model to clinical education is discussed in Chapter 2.

1.7.2 INTERDEPENDENCE

The promotion of autonomy and self-directedness as goals and processes of a clinical education programme does not imply total independence. That is, independence does not imply that students learn in isolation from each other, and are unable to learn from the experiences of others. Autonomy and self-directedness occur in a social context. True autonomy requires emotional maturity. Students should not continually need approval and reassurance. They should also be technically independent, able to carry on with a task and cope with problems which may arise in a mature, professional way. They should not have to run for help immediately, but should be able to analyze the problem and discuss the decisions they made and the strategies they implemented in later consultations with their clinical educators. Simultaneously, students must operate interdependently, contributing to the social (in this case the clinical and professional) structure in which they find themselves, as well as receiving from it.

This concept of interdependence is vital in clinical education and clinical practice. It provides the key to assuring the ethical and legal demands placed on clinical educators and clinical practitioners with respect to client care are met. Students who have moved through dependence to independence in the task or client problem at hand can be expected to function interdependently with their clinical educators. We interpret this to mean that such students should keep their clinical educators informed of their plans and outcomes, even though these may be developed and executed independently of the clinical educator.

Boud (1988) argues that students pass thorough stages of development from dependence to counterdependence to independence and finally to interdependence. He suggests that in this final stage, students are engaged in mature relationships within their world, interrelating with their world rather than being apart from it. We would suggest that on reaching this stage, students are demonstrating the outcomes of the professional socialization process (see Chapter 3). The stages through which students move on their way to achieving interdependence, as outlined by Boud, are not unlike those of Anderson's (1988) continuum of supervision, discussed in Chapter 2. We would expect that students functioning interdependently would use their clinical educators as a resource and sounding board for discussion or problem-solving, just as they would use their peers in this way. Evidence of these behaviours is a hallmark of student growth.

1.7.3 PEER LEARNING

Health, education and welfare professionals rarely work alone. Their work settings almost always call upon them to work as part of a departmental or multidisciplinary team. Lincoln and McAllister (1993) noted that the major way in which professionals continue to learn, that is to function as life-long learners, is to learn with and from their peers. Therefore, it makes sense to establish the process of peer learning in the clinical education setting. Working with peers is in fact one of the hallmarks of experiential and self-directed programmes, and a goal of clinical education.

The collaborative models of clinical education discussed in Chapter 2 highlight the need for effective peer learning. The ability to learn from and with peers is a characteristic of adult learners (Lincoln & McAllister, 1993). Members of a peer group bring to the group different life and prior clinical learning experiences. Sharing these, participating in each other's ongoing learning, assisting each other with reflection during and after experiences can significantly enhance peers' learning. It can also help reduce the anxiety (see Chapter 3) associated with clinical education (Chan, Carter & McAllister, 1994). Clinical educators who actively utilize the resources that peers bring to a group and create a learning environment in which peer learning can occur are using adult learning theory in their approach to facilitating student learning. Peer learning is discussed in depth in Chapter 4.

(a) Benefits of peer learning

The benefits of peer learning can be enormous for the clinical educator and the clinic, as well as for the students. Clinical educators who regularly use peer teaching or collaborative learning report reduced stress for themselves in that they have fewer competing demands in managing students' clinical education programmes, they have more free time to attend to the non-client aspects of their job and they do not have to play social host to solo students in their facility (Callan, O'Neill & McAllister, 1994).

Economic benefits to the facility have also been identified. Ladyshewsky and Healey (1990), in a Canadian study of physiotherapy students, reported greater efficiency in the planning and orientation phases of students' placements, greater input into problem-solving and more time available for improving the quality of client care. Perhaps more importantly for clinic administrators, after the settling-in phase of a block clinical placement, two senior students were able to carry a caseload greater than that of a solo clinician. This finding has recently been replicated with a study by Ladyshewsky and Barrie (1996) with speech therapy students in Australia.

(b) Pitfalls in peer learning situations

The benefits of peer learning or collaborative learning accrue only through careful management of clinical placements by clinical educators. Best and Rose (1996) have identified some of the challenges in this approach which need to managed. They include the risk of comparison of one student with another, competition between students, personality clashes, dealing with students functioning at different levels, assurance of client safety, dealing with a shortage of client numbers or appropriate clients for student learning, limited physical space for students to work or students working in different areas of the facility. We know from experience that careful planning, skilled monitoring and treating students like adult learners can overcome most of these challenges.

1.7.4 LEARNING FROM EXPERIENCE

Clinical education programmes are by their nature experiential. Students actively engage in experiences with clients, their families and other professionals. These experiences can be enormously satisfying, or very bewildering; they can engender in students great highs and lows of emotional reaction to all aspects and individuals in the clinical setting. Students will almost always report that they learned a lot in clinic. However, learning does not accrue only from experience. What is also required for learning to occur is reflection.

Boud, Keogh and Walker (1985) proposed a model for reflection *following* experience. The key elements of the model are 'returning to the experience', 'attending to feelings' and 're-evaluation of the experience' leading to new learning. This model is discussed in Chapter 2, along with application to the clinical education setting suggested by Mandy (1989). Boud and Walker (1990) have also explored possibilities for promoting reflection *during* experience. A variety of strategies for promoting reflection are discussed in Chapter 4.

The work of Boud and his colleagues has been widely applied in the development of reflective curricula in many professional education programmes. Another major catalyst to the development of reflective curricula has been Schön's (1983, 1987) work on reflective practitioners and their education. Schön's views that reflection on practice is what allows practitioners to work in uncertain and changing environments, the 'grey area' of professional practice as he calls them, have been discussed earlier in this chapter.

This section has outlined a theoretical and philosophical framework for clinical education grounded in adult learning theory. We have suggested that the principles of adult learning and the characteristics of adult learners are highly congruent with the characteristics of students in clinical education settings and with the nature of clinical education. There also needs to be congruence between the characteristics of facilitators of adult learning and the characteristics of clinical educators.

1.8 CHARACTERISTICS OF EFFECTIVE CLINICAL EDUCATORS OPERATING IN AN ADULT LEARNING FRAMEWORK

Heron (1989) has discussed the characteristics of facilitators in adult learning programmes. Many of these characteristics have also been identified by clinical educators and students alike as facilitative of learning in clinical settings.

1.8.1 COMMUNICATION AND INTERPERSONAL SKILLS

The characteristics of clinical educators consistently identified in the literature as most valued by students are communication and interpersonal skills (Emery, 1984; Cupit, 1988; Jarski, Kulig & Olsen, 1990; Neville & French, 1991; Onuoha, 1994; Williams & Webb, 1994) (see Chapter 7). These were rated higher or more frequently mentioned than professional competence or teaching skills. This is the case whether the studies used questionnaire-based methods of data collection with quantitative analysis, or the critical incident technique with subsequent qualitative data analysis, such as was used by Williams and Webb (1994).

Neville and French (1991) listed the following personal attributes desirable for clinical tutors: friendly, helpful, forthcoming with information and approachable. The physiotherapy students surveyed by Cupit (1988) listed as their top three desirable attributes for clinical supervisors: an awareness of the student as a person and future colleague; being inspiring and enthusiastic about work, teaching and student learning; and being encouraging and emotionally supportive. The next two attributes on the list were being a good professional role model and an ability to draw on and extend student knowledge. Even when discussing educative skills, communication and interpersonal skills are given priority. For example, when listing the qualities of effective clinical teachers (as named by Irby, 1978), the qualities listed under group instruction skills are to do with rapport, respect, listening and answering, and questioning skills. To be effective facilitators of student learning, clinical educators need to develop their interpersonal and communication skills. Detailed discussions of these skills in clinical education are found in Chapters 3 and 7.

This value on communication skills and interpersonal skills accorded by both students and clinical educators is of interest, given that Pickering (1984) found that feelings were rarely discussed in interactions between students and clinical educators. The clinical educators in Pickering's study made journal entries in which feelings were noted, and the work by Chan, Carter and McAllister (1994) highlighted the anxiety that students feel about their interactions with clinical educators (as well as about their work with clients). Yet these feelings about relationships with clinical educators, the clinical education process and assessment are apparently rarely raised by either party for discussion.

The work of Boud, Keogh and Walker (1985) and Mandy (1989) stresses the need to deal with feelings in the clinical education process. Clearly this is an area warranting attention from clinical educators who wish to facilitate student learning within an adult learning environment. Providing negative (as well as positive) feedback and assessing students in ways which are congruent with adult learning principles are difficult tasks for clinical educators. These topics are discussed further in Chapters 3 and 6.

1.8.2 PROFESSIONAL AND TEACHING SKILLS

Although the studies discussed in the previous section highlighted the value of communication and interpersonal skills, that is not to imply that students do not also value sound professional and teaching skills. The studies by Onuoha (1994) and Williams and Webb (1994) found that students do value these skills when they are utilized within an adult learning approach, and enacted through the use of good interpersonal and communication skills. Williams and Webb found that students appreciated the characteristics of clinical educators which encouraged active participation in the learning process. The fact that there was a difference in value placed on andragogic skills by students and clinical educators lead Onuoha to suggest that clinical educators need to be educated themselves on teaching and learning within an andragogic (adult learning) framework.

1.9 SUMMARY

This chapter has discussed the nature and goals of clinical education. It has suggested that clinical education lacks a theory and a philosophy, and argued that the adoption of adult learning theory and approaches may make the broader goals of clinical education more achievable. The congruence between adult learning and clinical education processes has been discussed. The final section has highlighted the value placed on facilitating clinical learning within an adult learning framework by students and clinical educators, and the need for more education of clinical educators.

REFERENCES

American Speech and Hearing Association (1978). Current status of supervision of speech-language pathology and audiology. Special Report. *Asha*, **20**, 478–86.

Anderson, J. L. (1988). *The supervisory process in speech-language pathology and audiology*. Boston: College Hill Press.

Benner, P. (1984). *From novice to expert: Excellence and power in clinical nursing practice.* Menlo Park: Addison-Wesley.

Best, D. & Rose, M. (1996). *Quality supervision, theory and practice for clinical supervisors.* London: W. B. Saunders.

Boud, D. (1988). Moving towards autonomy. In D. Boud (Ed.). *Developing student autonomy in learning.* London: Kogan Page.

Boud, D., Keogh, R. & Walker, D. (1985). Promoting reflection in learning: A model. In D. Boud, R. Keogh and D. Walker (Eds), *Reflection: Turning experience into learning,* (pp. 18–40). London: Kogan Page.

Boud, D. & Walker, D. (1990). Making the most of experience. *Studies in Continuing Education,* **12,** 2, 61–80.

Brookfield, S. D. (1986). *Understanding and facilitating adult learning.* Milton Keynes: Open University Press.

Brown, S. & McIntyre, D. (1993). *Making sense of teaching.* Buckingham: Open University Press.

Callan, C., O'Neill, D. & McAllister, L. (1994). Adventures in two to one supervision: Two students can be better than one. *SUPERvision,* **18,** 15–16.

Candy, P. (1991). *Self-direction for lifelong learning: A comprehensive guide to theory and practice.* San Francisco: Jossey Bass.

Candy, P. (1994). *Developing lifelong learners through undergraduate education.* Commissioned Report No. 28. National Board of Employment, Education and Training. Canberra: Australian Government Printing Service.

Chan, J., Carter, S. & McAllister, L. (1994). Sources of anxiety related to clinical education in undergraduate speech-language pathology students. *Australian Journal of Human Communication Disorders,* **22,** 57–73.

Coles, C. (1989). The role of context in elaborated learning. In J. Balla, M. Gibson & A. Chang (Eds). *Learning in medical school: A model for the clinical professions.* Hong Kong: Hong Kong University Press.

Coles, C. (1990). Elaborated learning in undergraduate medical education. *Medical Education,* **24,** 14–22.

Cross, V. (1994). From clinical supervisor to clinical educator: Too much to ask? *Physiotherapy,* **80,** 9, 609–11.

Cupit, R. (1988). Student stress: An approach to coping at the interface between clinical and preclinical. *Australian Journal of Physiotherapy,* **34,** 215–19.

Dixon, N. M. (1985). The implementation of learning style information. *Lifelong Learning,* **913,** 16–20.

Emery, M. (1984). Effectiveness of the clinical instructor: Students' perspectives. *Physical Therapy,* **64,** 1079–82.

Engel, C. E. (1995). Medical education in the 21st century: The need for a capability approach. *Capability,* **1,** 23–30.

Entwistle, N. & Waterson, S. (1988). Approaches to studying and levels of processing in university students. *British Journal of Educational Psychology,* **58,** 258–65.

Gonzci, A. (1994). Competency based assessment in the professions in Australia. *Assessment in Education,* **1,** 27–44.

Goodyear, R. & Bernaud, J. (1992). *Fundamentals of clinical supervision.* Massachusetts: Allyn & Bacon.

Grahn, G. (1989). Educational situations in clinical settings. *Radiography Today,* **55,** 26–7.

Heron, J. (1989). *The facilitators' handbook.* London: Kogan Page.

Higgs, J. (1993). The teacher in self-directed learning: Manager or co-manager. In N. Graves (Ed.). *Learner managed learning: Practice, theory and policy.* World Education Fellowship.

Higgs, J., Glendinning, M., Dunsford, F. & Panter, J. (1991). Goals and components of clinical education in the allied health professions. *Proceedings of the World Confederation for Physical Therapy: 11th International Conference.* London: World Confederation for Physical Therapy.

Honey, P. & Mumford, A. (1986). *The manual of learning styles* (2nd ed.). Berkshire: author.

Honey, P. & Mumford, A. (1989). *Capitalising on your learning style.* King of Prussia, Pennsylvania: Organisation Design and Development Inc.

Irby, D. M. (1978). Clinical teacher effectiveness in medicine. *Journal of Medical Education,* 58, 808–15.

Jarski, R., Kulig, K. & Olsen, R. (1990). Clinical teaching in physical therapy: Student and teacher perceptions. *Physical Therapy,* 70, 173–8.

Katz, N. & Heimann, N. (1991). Learning styles of students and practitioners in five health professions. *The Occupational Therapy Journal of Research,* 11, 238–45.

Kenny, B. & McAllister, L. (1993). An investigation of typical and self-evaluation supervisory conferences in speech pathology. *Proceedings of the annual conference of the Australian Association of Speech and Hearing,* Darwin, Australia.

Kenny, B. (1996). An investigation of students' self-evaluation skills in supervisory conferences. Unpublished master's thesis, University of Sydney, Sydney, New South Wales, Australia.

Knowles, M. (1970). *The modern practice of adult education: Andragogy versus pedagogy.* New York: Association Press.

Knowles, M. (1980). *The modern practice of adult education: From pedagogy to andragogy.* New York: Cambridge, The Adult Education Co.

Kolb, D. (1976). *Learning styles inventory: Technical manual.* Boston, MA: McBer & Co.

Kolb, D. (1981). Learning styles and disciplinary differences. In A.W. Chickering *et al., The Modern American College,* pp 232–55. San Francisco: Jossey-Bass.

Kolb, D. (1984). *Experiential learning: Experience as the source of learning and development.* Englewood Cliffs, NJ: Prentice Hall.

Kolb, D. (1986). *Learning style inventory: Technical manual.* Boston, MA: McBer & Co.

Ladyshewsky, R. & Barrie, S. (1996). Measuring quality and cost of clinical education. Paper presented at the annual conference of the Higher Education Research Development Society of Australia, Perth, July.

Ladyshewsky, R. & Healey, E. (1990). *The 2:1 teaching model in clinical education: A manual for clinical instructors.* Toronto: University of Toronto, Department of Rehabilitation Medicine.

Laschinger, H. & Boss M. (1983). Learning styles of nursing students and career choices. *Journal of Advanced Nursing,* 9, 375–80.

Lincoln, M. & McAllister, L. (1993). Facilitating peer learning in clinical education. *Medical Teacher,* 15, 17–25.

Lovie-Kitchin, J., Coonan, I., Sanderson R. & Thompson, B. (1989). Learning styles across health sciences courses. *Higher Education Research and Development,* 8, 27–37.

Mandy, S. (1989). Facilitating student learning in clinical education. *Australian Journal of Human Communication Disorders,* 17, 83–93.

Marton, F. & Säljö, R. (1984). Approaches to learning. In F. Marton, D. Hounsell & N. Entwhistle (Eds). *The experience of learning.* Edinburgh: Scottish Academic Press.

McLeod, S., Lincoln, M., McAllister, L., Maloney, D., Purcell, A. & Eadie, P. (1995). A longitudinal investigation of the learning styles of speech pathology students, *Australian Journal of Human Communication Disorders*, **23**, 13–25.

Neville, S. & French, S. (1991). Clinical education: Students; and clinical tutors' views. *Physiotherapy*, **77**, 351–3.

Oldmeadow, L. (1996). Developing clinical competence: A mastery pathway. *Australian Physiotherapy*, **42**, 1, 37–44.

Onions, C. T. (Ed.) (1992). *The shorter Oxford English dictionary on historical principles* (3rd ed.). Oxford: Oxford University Press.

Onuoha, A. (1994). Effective clinical teaching behaviours from the perspective of students, supervisors and teachers. *Physiotherapy*, **80**, 208–14.

Opacich, K. (1995). Is an educational philosophy missing from the fieldwork solution? *American Journal of Occupational Therapy*, **49**, 160–4.

Pickering, M. (1984). Interpersonal communication in speech-language pathology supervisory conferences: A qualitative study. *Journal of Speech and Hearing Disorders*, **49**, 189–95.

Polyani, M. (1958). *Personal knowledge*. London: Routledge & Kegan Paul.

Ramsden, P. (1984). The context of learning. In F. Marton, D. Hounsell & N. Entwhistle (Eds). *The experience of learning*. Edinburgh: Scottish Academic Press.

Ramsden, P. (1988). *Improving learning: New perspectives*. London: Kogan Page.

Romanini, J. & Higgs, J. (1991). The teacher as manager in continuing and professional education. *Studies in Continuing Education*, **13**, 41–52.

Scanlan, C. L. (1978). Integrating didactic and clinical education – high patient contact. In C. W. Ford (Ed.). *Clinical education for the allied health professions*. St Louis: C. V. Mosby.

Schön, D. (1983). *The reflective practitioner: How professionals think in action*. London: Temple-Smith.

Schön, D. (1987). *Educating the reflective practitioner*. San Francisco: Jossey Bass.

Stengelhofen, J. (1993). *Teaching students in clinical settings*. London: Chapman & Hall.

Stephenson, J. (1996). *Beyond competence to capability and the learning society*. International Programme of Seminars and Workshops on Higher Education. University of Sydney, April.

Stritter, F. T., Baker, R. M. & Shahady, E. J. (1986). Clinical instruction. In W. C. McGaghie & J. J. Frey (Eds). *Handbook for the academic physician* (pp 99–124). New York: Springer Verlag.

Svincki, M. D. & Dixon, N. M. (1987). The Kolb model modified for classroom activities. *College Teaching*, **35**, 141–6.

Torbert, W. R. (1978). Educating toward shared purpose, self-direction and quality work: The theory and practice of liberating structure. *Journal of Higher Education*, **49**, 109–35.

Vittetoe, M. C. & Hooker, E. (1983). Learning style preferences of allied health practitioners in a teacher education programme. *Journal of Allied Health*, February, 48–55.

Wells, D. & Higgs, Z. A. (1990). Learning styles and learning preferences of first and fourth semester baccalaureate degree nursing students. *Journal of Nursing Education*, **29**, 385–90.

White, R. & Ewan, C. (Eds). (1991). *Clinical teaching in nursing*. London: Chapman & Hall.

Williams, P. L. & Webb, C. (1994). Clinical supervision skills: A delphi and critical incident technique study. *Medical Teacher*, **16**, 139–55.

Models and roles in clinical education

2

Sharynne McLeod
School of Communication Disorders,
The University of Sydney, Australia

Judith Romanini
Department of Nursing Therapeutics,
The University of Sydney, Australia

Ellen S. Cohn
Boston School of Occupational Therapy,
Tufts University, Medford MA, USA

Joy Higgs
School of Physiotherapy,
The University of Sydney, Australia

Note: The Teacher–manager model (section 2.3) is the work of Judith Romanini and Joy Higgs

2.1 CHAPTER OVERVIEW

The clinical environment provides a unique learning opportunity for both students and clinical educators. This environment is rich with opportunity yet difficult to control, stimulating but often confusing, rewarding but sometimes intimidating and, above all, full of surprises. This chapter considers models of clinical education and the roles and responsibilities of clinical educators. Models of clinical education are categorized five ways, as: descriptive models, integration models, developmental models, interactive process models and collaborative models. A new and comprehensive model of clinical education, the Teacher-manager model is presented in detail. The roles and responsibilities of clinical educators provide further insight into perspectives on clinical education. Seven roles are identified and discussed: role model, colleague, teacher, evaluator, administrator/manager, counsellor and researcher.

Postcard 2

Dear All

I've survived the end of my first week! Sometimes I wonder what I've taken on. It's clear to me that the CBR team leader and the doctor here expect me to 'train' the workers to do basic speech therapy-type tasks. After the emphasis we've experienced in the clinic at uni. about **facilitating learning**, not telling, and after facilitating my year 2 student partner last semester, I'm not sure what role to take here that will meet their needs and mine. I'm glad I read a bit before I came about the 'train the trainer' model. As the CBR workers' knowledge and skills is generally fairly low, I guess starting by instructing would be okay. I guess then I'll cycle through observing, giving feedback, and evaluating (not sure how or what) – a bit like a therapy session!

love S.

2.2 MODELS OF CLINICAL EDUCATION

A knowledge and understanding of the models which are available in clinical education empowers clinical educators to work in a way which best suits the needs of themselves, their students and clients. Models have been defined as tools for generating ideas, guiding conceptualization and generating explanation (Reed, 1984). Clinical educators can use models to 'make sense of, order, refine, articulate, and teach the process being experienced' (Pickering, 1987, p. 112). To be successful in communicating with students, clinical educators need to specify their own thinking relative to the reasons, values, philosophies and models of clinical education that they plan to use in the clinical education setting. Discussion with students of the model(s) to be utilized in the clinical setting enables students to know where they stand, to understand what is important to their clinical educator and what is expected of them.

Over the years the term 'model' has been used loosely to describe various models, paradigms, aspects and procedures of clinical education. The various uses of the term model will be accommodated in this chapter in order to provide a comprehensive overview of authors' attempts to clarify just what clinical education is. Numerous models of clinical education have been developed as a result of the diversity of disciplines involved in clinical education, the phases in the historical development of the discipline of clinical education and the various philosophies that underpin the relationship between clinical educator, student and client. When adopting a model, clinical educators not only take into account philosophies such as promoting adult learning, attitudes and preferences of various professions and professionals, but also practicalities of budgeting time, money and space.

Models of clinical education embrace the many different aspects of the complex process of clinical education. In order to clarify the differences between the models, we have categorized them as: descriptive models, integration models, developmental models, interactive process models and collaborative models.

2.2.1 DESCRIPTIVE MODELS

A number of models exist which take a broad view of clinical education and describe its various components.

(a) Trigonal model

Farmer and Farmer (1989) proposed a *Trigonal model* of clinical education. They stated that clinical education has three interrelated components: constituents, concepts, and contexts (see Figure 2.1). The *constituents*, or people, involved in the process of clinical education include the clinical educators, students, clients, families and other clinicians. It is critical to acknowledge the role of clients and their families noted in this model as they are frequently overlooked in discussions of clinical education (Maloney & Sheard, 1992). The *concepts* include the ideas and theories of clinical education. The *contexts* are the settings where clinical education occurs, including universities, hospitals, schools and community-based settings. These three components affect the five domains of clinical education: professional, research, educational, administrative, clinical. The interaction between the three components and the five domains is called the *Pentagonal model* (Farmer & Farmer, 1989).

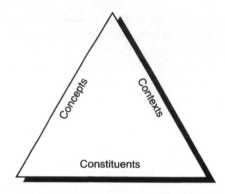

Figure 2.1 Trigonal model of clinical education (Farmer & Farmer, 1989)
Reproduced with permission from S. Farmer & J. Farmer, *Supervision in communicaton disorders*. Copyright © 1989. All rights reserved. Reprinted by permission of Allyn & Bacon.

(b) Open systems in action

Clinical education programmes have also been described as operating like systems (Higgs, 1993). A system comprises interdependent, interconnected elements which form a complex whole (Koontz, O'Donnell & Weihrich, 1982). When viewed from a systems perspective, clinical education programmes are open systems, as they receive and process inputs from the environment and return new products to the environment (Von Bertalanffy, 1969). Further, clinical education programmes are living systems which involve participants in ill-defined problems, complex goals and outcomes that are difficult to predict.

The use of a systems approach to the exploration and management of clinical education programmes provides several advantages (Higgs, 1993). Firstly, as Emery (1969) suggests, the 'gestalten'[1] properties of living systems (such as clinical education programmes) can only be revealed by using an open systems approach to the study of living phenomena. Secondly, systems theory provides the concept of the individual (for example, students and clinical educators) as a purposeful and responsible subsystem within a larger system (for example, a learning programme). This is consistent with adult learning theory where students are viewed as active participants in the learning programme who take increasing amounts of responsibility for their learning. Thirdly, systems and learning programmes are successful if they are congruent within their elements. In educational programmes, congruence between elements such as leadership, goals and programme organization is important (Torbert, 1978). Similarly, congruence between the system's goals, role, procedures and

---

[1] A system is seen as being 'gestalten' when the effects of the whole system are greater than the sum of the effects of parts of the system.

interpersonal factors, promotes effective system operation (Rubin, 1980). Creating congruence between elements of a clinical education programme is highly desirable. It is important that students receive compatible messages from clinical educator behaviour, clinical programme goals, and assessment strategies to promote effective achievement of clinical education goals.

2.2.2 INTEGRATION MODELS

A subset of the descriptive models of clinical education are integration models. Students' learning experiences, particularly between the academic and clinical subjects, may be fragmented (Kent, 1989–1990). As a result of this fragmentation, there has been a recent emphasis on integration of learning experiences across the curriculum. Integration models were developed to provide a framework for coordination between the academic and clinical components, the off-campus and on-campus learning experiences and various disciplines. Two integration models are described.

(a) Conceptual model

The *Conceptual model* (Pickering, Rassi, Hagler & McFarlane, 1992; Rassi & McElroy, 1992b) was developed as a result of the need to integrate components of a large programme at Vanderbilt University. The model assumes that the goal of professional competency is achieved through the development of attitudes, skills and knowledge in the areas of self study, clinic, classroom and laboratory experiences (see Figure 2.2). An example of the application of integration in the conceptual model is that the coordinator of clinical education 'coordinates interaction of academic faculty and clinical professionals through joint cooperative endeavours such as presentations in seminars and conferences, and the design and administration of clinical exams' (Pickering *et al.*, 1992, p. 58).

(b) Integration model

Another example of an integration model of clinical education is the programme at the University of Alberta (Pickering *et al.*, 1992). The model describes the coordination of the clinical and academic experiences within the university setting, and the integration of the clinical experiences which occur in locations which are external to the university. An example of the application of the integration model is that clinical practicum programmes in occupational therapy, physiotherapy, speech therapy and audiology are integrated through joint continuing education for clinical educators from external sites. Another example of integration is that clinical education staff mix with full-time academic staff in formal and informal activities. An additional example is found in Case Study 2.1.

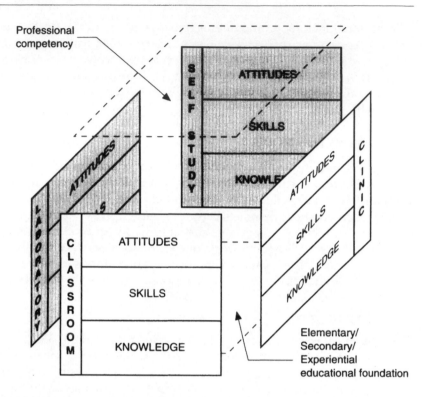

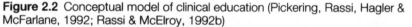

Figure 2.2 Conceptual model of clinical education (Pickering, Rassi, Hagler & McFarlane, 1992; Rassi & McElroy, 1992b)

Reproduced with permission from J. A. Rassi & M. D. McElroy, *The education of audiologists and speech-language pathologists*; published by York Press, 1992.

Case Study 2.1 Application of integration models to a clinical education programme in a health sciences faculty

The Faculty of Health Sciences at The University of Sydney has aimed to integrate clinical and academic staff, a number of health science disciplines and rural and city clinical experiences in a clinical education innovation. An academic staff member has been based in Tamworth (hundreds of kilometres from the university) to coordinate clinical education experiences for students in disciplines such as occupational therapy, physiotherapy, speech therapy, orthoptics, medical radiation technology and diversional therapy. The academic liaises between the university and the rural clinicians, facilitates the development of rural clinical educators and coordinates clinical education placements and resources.

2.2.3 DEVELOPMENTAL MODELS

Cognitive developmental theory provides clinical educators with a useful perspective to understand the various developmental needs and capabilities of a diverse student population (Lognabill, Hardy & Delworth, 1982). Understanding students' developmental needs enables clinical educators to design clinical education experiences which address the unique needs of individual students. Developmental models assume that students progress through hierarchical stages and that development occurs through the interaction between students and their environment (Sprinthall & Thies-Sprinthall, 1983). As students progress from one stage to the next they develop qualitatively different ways of thinking about the same problem and ascribe different meaning to the learning experience itself (see Chapter 5). Thus, developmental models are concerned with how students understand or make meaning of the experience as well as the outcome of clinical education (Wittman & Schwartz, 1991). Developmental models often describe the styles of supervision which should be utilized at different stages to facilitate development of competent professionals.

(a) Continuum of supervision

Anderson (1988) proposed a *Continuum of supervision* in which the aim is to develop independent clinicians who are capable of self-supervision. The model describes changes over time in the amount and type of involvement of both clinical educators and students in the supervisory process. As participation by students increases, the degree of involvement of clinical educators decreases. Anderson's continuum of supervision involves three developmental stages: evaluation-feedback, transition, and self-supervision. Initially, in the evaluation-feedback stage, students are passive, requiring a significant amount of direction from their clinical educator. Beginning students, students who are working with a new type of client or students who have entered a new setting are likely to be in the evaluation-feedback stage. As students move into the self-supervision stage, the balance changes to a more equal peer interaction. Thus, the clinical educator's role is to assist the student to reach a level of independence where the relationship is one of peer-consultation rather than dependency. Joint involvement and active participation of both the clinical educator and the student are unique and critical factors of this model (see Figure 2.3 and Case Study 2.2).

Anderson contends that both time and experience are factors in determining the student's transition along this continuum and that students may require different supervision styles at the same time depending on their experience and expertise with the given learning task.

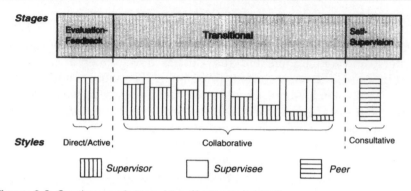

Figure 2.3 Continuum of supervision (Anderson, 1988)

Source: J.L. Anderson, *The supervisory process in speech-language pathology and audiology*; published by College Hill Press, 1988.

Case Study 2.2 Application of the Continuum of supervision (Anderson, 1988) to beginning, intermediate and advanced students

(a) Evaluation-feedback stage

Alison is in the first few weeks of her first clinical placement. She has negotiated with George, her clinical educator that he will write goals for clinical sessions for the first few weeks. Alison has to use the resources in the clinic to generate application of these goals to her clients. Discussion in their conferences is often focused on the clinical process. The aim is to move to the transitional stage as quickly as possible.

(b) Transitional stage

Robert has reached some level of competency and knowledge in his clinical skills. He collaborates with his clinical educator in a process of shared deliberation and joint problem-solving. He participates to varying degrees in decision-making. He is not yet able to operate independently but is moving along the continuum in that direction. He is learning to analyze his clinical actions and plans future strategies on the basis of that analysis. He can make modifications during his clinical sessions, solve problems, assumes some responsibility and collaborates within the supervisory conference. His supervisory conferences are not exclusively focused on the clinical process, but time is spent on the supervisory process as well.

(c) Self-supervision stage

Kate is commencing her final clinical placement. She has been a consistently excellent student, academically and clinically. She has the ability to accurately self-analyze her clinical behaviour and to alter it, based on that analysis. She has a level of clinical independence in problem-solving such that she is no longer dependent on her clinical educator for observation, analysis and feedback about her clinical work. Nevertheless, she still desires and needs peer interaction and a consultative style of supervision. She has negotiated with her clinical educator that she is primarily responsible for her own supervision. She accurately self-evaluates and will call on her clinical educator when appropriate. She has a peer relationship with her clinical educator.

(b) Integrative task maturity model of supervision

The *Integrative task maturity model of supervision* (ITMMS) (Mawdsley & Scudder, 1989) provides an alternative developmental model of clinical education focusing on student independence, maturity and supervisory style. Four levels of relationship between the student and clinical educator are described (see Table 2.1). Students may initially be described as M1: not competent, not confident, not willing. The ultimate goal is level M4: to be competent, confident and willing. The Integrative task maturity model of supervision draws on the work of the *Situational leadership model* of Hersey and Blanchard (1982) to describe supervisory style, task maturity and power bases; the *Wisconsin procedure for appraisal of clinical competence* (W-PACC) (Shriberg *et al.*, 1975) to assess maturity levels of the students; and the *Cycle of clinical supervision* (Cogan, 1973) to describe the process of students maturing. This model is prescriptive, even to the extent of the number of clients seen each week and the seating arrangements during conferences for students at different maturity levels. However, it is useful and able to be adapted to many situations without adhering to the prescriptive detail.

(c) Liberating programme systems (Higgs, 1993)

A model of *Liberating programme systems* (Higgs, 1993) has been developed to incorporate three key concepts: sharing responsibility (between the clinical educator and student) as co-managers of the learning programme, adapting teaching and learning to the student's task maturity and creating a learning environment of 'controlled freedom'.

In this model, the role of the clinical educator is to assess the student's task maturity for the given learning situation and to create (with the student) a learning system in which the student can achieve optimal learning experiences and outcomes. To promote students' self-directed learning, clinical educators need to encourage students to act as co-managers of the learning programme. As part of this process the clinical educator needs to determine the level of readiness of the student for the responsibilities and autonomy involved in the co-manager's role. The term 'learner task maturity' (Higgs, 1993) refers to the student's readiness for the specific task in hand. Such maturity varies with the experience of students as independent learners, with their ability to employ effective approaches to learning and with their previous experience and success with similar learning tasks.

Table 2.1 A summary of the Integrative task maturity model of supervision (Mawdsley & Scudder, 1989)

Student independence	Specific direction from the clinical educator does not alter the student's unsatisfactory performance and inability to make changes	The student needs specific direction and/or demonstration from the clinical educator to perform satisfactorily	The student needs general direction from the clinical educator to perform effectively	The student is effective and demonstrates by taking initiative, and making changes where appropriate
Maturity level	M1 Not competent Not confident Not willing	M2 Not competent Confident Willing	M3 Competent Not confident Willing	M4 Competent Confident Willing
Supervisory style	S1 Telling	S2 Selling	S3 Participating	S4 Delegating

Where the student's task maturity is low, for instance due to unfamiliarity with the learning task or environment, or due to limited advanced learning abilities, then a more structured learning programme is appropriate. However, emphasis on liberation of the student to develop as a learner is central. Where the student's task maturity is high, the student and clinical educator can act as co-managers in the resultant liberating programme system (Higgs, 1993).

A realistic assessment by students of their own task maturity will enable students to redress gaps in their learning, to set appropriate learning goals and to seek assistance from others especially their clinical educators. Also, students need to identify what level of autonomy they desire in learning and in clinical practice. It is important to discuss this with students to avoid an over-confident approach which may be hazardous to clients or an under-confident, cautious approach which could limit the scope for learning. Students need to develop confidence and a base of experience which will help them know how far to experiment and take risks in their learning without compromising their clients' well-being. They also need to be able to trust their clinical educators to guide and facilitate them in this endeavour (see Case Study 2.3).

Case Study 2.3 A clinical educator's application of the Liberating programme systems model

Larry, a clinical educator, has identified a high level of competence and task maturity in two of his students: Jane and Sarah. He has negotiated with them which learning goals and activities will best enhance their development and experience. Larry has enabled a higher level of freedom and risk-taking in learning for these students, while at the same time maintains supervisory responsibility for the health and well-being of these students and their clients.

(d) Learning vector model

The *Learning vector model* of Stritter, Baker and Shahady (1986) also describes the development of students' independence in the clinical setting by describing the stages of interaction between the clinical educator and students (see Figure 2.4).

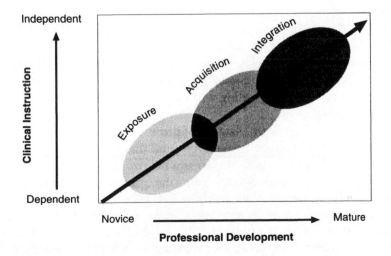

Figure 2.4 Learning vector model (Stritter, Baker & Shahady, 1986)
Source: Stritter, F. T., Baker, R. M. & Shahady, E. J. Clinical instruction. In W. C. McGaghie & J. J. Frey (Eds) *Handbook for the academic physician;* published by Springer Verlag, 1986.

On the vertical axis of the Learning vector model is *clinical instruction* showing students' development from dependence to independence. The horizontal axis shows *professional development*, from novice to mature. These axes intersect to create three stages relevant to professional development: *exposure, acquisition* and *integration*. In the exposure stage, exposure to basic facts and concepts occurs in a highly structured environment where the clinical educator acts as a role model, setting learning objectives and providing feedback. In the acquisition stage, the learner applies clinical skills and focuses on decision-making and reasoning. During the integration phase students develop professional identity utilizing their clinical educator as a consultant.

Stritter *et al.* (1986) suggest five characteristics which comprise *clinical instruction*:

- *Orientation* – students decide what and how much to learn
- *Learner practice* – students master knowledge
- *Evaluation* – students judge the quality or worth of the completed task
- *Feedback* – students decide how successful they were in completing the task
- *Closure* – clinical educators conclude the interaction and plan new learning.

Stritter *et al.* (1986) suggest six characteristics which comprise *professional development*:

- *Cognitive* – use of knowledge base by intuitive and analytical reasoning
- *Technical* – use of procedural skills to ascertain information regarding clients or to conduct procedures
- *Attitudinal* – 'the interests, values and ethics that guide resolution of moral problems, action, choice, argument, and rationalisation' (p. 103)
- *Psychosocial* – communicating with sensitivity to clients and other professionals
- *Socialization* – 'the internalization of professional values, the commitment to the professional role, and the acquisition of norms typical of the fully qualified professional' (pp 103–4)
- *Independent learning* – 'which enables the (physician) to keep abreast of the changing science of his field' (p. 104).

This model is of value in assisting clinical educators to integrate their desired goals for their students. Clinical educators can offer students many opportunities to be exposed to, acquire and integrate; valuing both the clinical instruction aspects and the professional development aspects of clinical education. This model recognizes the multifaceted and complex nature of clinical education.

2.2.4 INTERACTIVE PROCESS MODELS

There are a number of models which describe the interactive process of clinical education. That is, what actually happens in the day-to-day exchange between clinical educator and student. Some of these models also include the interaction with the client. These models are usually represented with arrows or flow charts to indicate a cycle or sequence of events.

(a) Foundational models

Two authors have been influential in the development of clinical education as a profession: Goldhammer and Cogan. Although their models focused on teacher education, they have been widely adopted in the health science professions (for example, Brasseur, 1989; Mandy, 1989; Mawdsley & Scudder, 1989). The relationship between the clinical educator and the student is viewed as a critical element of the supervisory process. Based on the interaction process, both Goldhammer and Cogan formalized the notion of conferences between students and clinical educators.

Goldhammer (1969) proposed five stages in the sequence of clinical supervision: pre-observation conference, observation, analysis and strategy, supervision conference, post-conference analysis. A collection of these sequences is called a *Cycle of supervision*.

Cogan (1973) proposed the *Cycle of clinical supervision* which has eight phases: establishing the supervisory style, planning, planning observation, observing, analyzing the teaching learning process, planning the conference, the conference and renewed planning.

Many subsequent models of clinical education in the fields of education and health sciences have drawn heavily on the philosophy and methodology of Cogan (1973) and Goldhammer (1969). Some examples will be presented.

(b) Supervision process in the practicum experience

Turney *et al.* (1982) proposed a six-stage interactive process of the practicum experience for student teachers that is relevant to health science students. The six stages are: pre-observation conference, observation, analysis, post-observation conference, training, evaluation and closure.

Turney *et al.*'s model described what the clinical educator should do at each stage in each clinical education encounter. Despite placing the student at the centre of this model, they do not provide a concurrent description of what the student should be doing at each stage. Furthermore, although Turney *et al.* recognize that there are many other people involved in the process of clinical education (for example, school principals and school pupils) they are not placed into the model.

(c) Molar model

An early example of an interactive process model in the health sciences literature was the *Molar model* presented by Oratio (1977). He described the elements of an 'integrated supervisory process' within speech therapy (p. 130). He viewed clinical education as an 'intensive series of training experiences': observation-analysis, didactic teaching, live demonstration, post-therapy conferencing, clinical practice, and micro-therapy (or simulations and role plays). Supervision was the central component to these training experiences. The objectives of this model were to change student behaviour in order to change client behaviour (via developing professional independence and clinical autonomy) and to enable effective clinical performance (via technical knowledge, clinical skill and self-exploration).

In his Molar model, Oratio did not indicate the order in which students should undergo each 'training experience'. Thus, he did not provide a view of clinical education as a cyclical or developmental process. Instead, he suggested that students are able to undertake these experiences in any order to develop their clinical performance. This model focuses on the interaction with the client and each part of the model is based on the clinical session. The development of clinical skills is the focus; other aspects of professional development, such as professional socialization, are not included in this model. There is limited recognition of the varying needs of students with different skill levels within this model.

(d) Supervisory process model

Anderson (1988) and Brasseur (1989) have described a five-phased process of supervision which is based on the work of Cogan (1973) and Goldhammer (1969). The stages are: understanding the supervisory process (the objectives of supervision and the roles of the student and clinical educator); planning (for the client, student and clinical educator); observing (the clinical session); analyzing (data in the clinical and supervisory process); and integrating (this usually occurs during a conference). This model is unique in that it acknowledges the value of facilitating growth of the client, student *and* clinical educator in the supervisory process.

(e) Reflective learning model

Mandy (1989) expanded the work of Goldhammer (Goldhammer, Anderson & Krajewski, 1980) to provide a model for facilitating a deep learning approach in clinical education by integrating it with the reflective learning model of Boud, Keogh and Walker (1985). Mandy's model utilizes the same phases as Goldhammer's sequence of clinical supervision, yet identifies different purposes in each. In particular, the fourth phase, the supervision conference, provides the vehicle for the application of the reflective process. Students are asked to (a) return to the experience, (b) recall emotions related to particular events, and (c) re-evaluate the experience via association (connecting new ideas and feelings with existing knowledge and attitudes), integration (processing the associations to see if they are meaningful), validation (looking for internal consistency between new and existing beliefs) and appropriation (making new knowledge a part of how we act and feel). The advantage of this model is that it addresses the affective domain by encouraging students to reflect on their emotions during clinical interactions.

2.2.5 COLLABORATIVE MODELS

Historically a number of professions have utilized a one-to-one or individualized model of clinical education where clinical educators model expected behaviours and competencies and then gradually transfer client care responsibilities to their students (Kolodner, Weiner & Frum, 1989). Within the past decade, there has been a paradigm shift in thinking about education. Traditionally, students have learned in a competitive atmosphere, passively accepting knowledge from their clinical educators. There has been a shift from a 'received knowledge' perspective in which students are taught isolated skills by an expert, to a process-oriented perspective where students construct and reflect on knowledge related to the context (Belenky, Clinchy, Goldberger & Tarule, 1986). In the current view, knowledge is seen as contextual and relative. Table 2.2 highlights the differences between traditional and collaborative approaches to clinical education.

The context in which students learn professional behaviours has also shifted. The current health care environment emphasizes cost containment and realistic functional outcomes (O'Neil, 1993). Intervention must go beyond the diagnosis and understanding of disease to considering clients as active collaborators in the care process. As a result, clinical educators need to prepare future clinicians successfully to provide services in a rapidly changing health care environment (see Chapter 9) and work effectively as collaborative team members with other professionals, clients and their families (Cohn & Crist, 1995).

Due to these shifts in education and health care, there has been increasing interest in collaborative learning (Bruffee, 1987; Crist, 1993; DeClute & Ladyshewsky, 1993; Horger, 1994; Ladyshewsky, 1993; Ladyshewsky & Healy, 1990; Lincoln & McAllister, 1993; Stern, 1994; Tiberius & Gaiptman, 1985) (see Chapter 4). Collaborative learning is a form of indirect teaching in which the instructor states the problem and organizes the students to work it out in peer groups. This interest in collaborative learning is likewise motivated by recent challenges to our understanding of what knowledge is and how health care practitioners reason in clinical practice (Benner, 1984; Cohn & Czycholl, 1991; Higgs & Jones, 1995; Mattingly & Fleming, 1993) (see Chapter 5). Clinicians must recognize the unique conditions presented by each client and make careful observations and interpretations to find the best strategies for resolving each client's particular concerns.

Table 2.2 Differences between traditional and collaborative approaches to clinical education

Traditional/Product-oriented	Collaborative/Process-oriented
• Competitive	• Cooperative
• Clinical educator is held as expert by student	• Clinical educator is co-learner in group
• Clinical educator is in control of time and response	• Group membership shares timing and response
• Clinical educator is in control of content and transfers knowledge to students	• Group decides content and sequence, knowledge is jointly constructed and modified by the group process
• Clinical educator establishes structure of learning experience	• Group shares responsibility for structure
• Clinical educator is an autonomous individual	• Group is interdependent. Roles are shared
• Students are passive learners	• Students are active learners
• Students work on their own with little interaction, impersonal transaction among students	• Prolonged interaction, sharing and helping, oral rehearsal of material being studied, peer tutoring/learning and general support
• Predictable learning objectives	• Objectives are formed by group members
• Traditional assignments	• Multi-dimensional activities

The most compelling theoretical rationale for collaborative learning comes from the Russian psychologist, Vygotsky (Miller, 1993). Mental functioning, in his view, is based on the assumption that it is through social interaction that one learns. If we embrace this social constructionist perspective that knowledge is constructed through interaction with people, we can see the value of learning among peers.

(a) Conceptual approach to collaborative learning

Johnson and Johnson (1990) designed a conceptual approach to collaborative learning. They have identified five basic elements of a collaborative learning situation: positive interdependence, face-to-face interaction, individual accountability, cooperative skills and group processing.

Positive interdependence is a recognition by group members that they are linked together in a way that none of them can be successful unless they all are. Students must believe they sink or swim together. Within every cooperative task, students develop mutual learning goals. During *face-to-face interaction* group members have access to each other's talents and resources and promote each other's success. Students interact to help each other accomplish a task. *Individual accountability* requires each group member to be active, learn, and be able to do the things that they learned in the group. Students team together so they can subsequently perform at a higher level as individuals. Students are held individually accountable for their share of the work. *Cooperative skills* need to be encouraged and taught as carefully as the subject matter. Finally, the term *group processing* infers that students in cooperative relationships need to process their experiences on an on-going basis to become more skillful in working as a group. Clinical educators need to ensure that members of the group discuss how well they are achieving goals and maintaining effective working relationships. Group members need to identify what is helpful or non-helpful.

These concepts of cooperative relationships define the difference between just putting students in groups to learn and collaborative learning. The importance of peer learning which is enhanced by a collaborative/social constructionist perspective is discussed in detail in Chapter 4.

(b) Teaching clinic

Dowling (1979) described a collaborative approach in health sciences as an alternative to one-to-one conventional supervision called a *Teaching clinic*. The teaching clinic approach describes peer group supervision where one participant brings a video of him/herself conducting a session with a client to a peer learning group. The students discuss and critique the video. Dowling suggested six phases in the group supervisory approach: review previous clinic, planning, observation, critique preparation, critique and strategy development, and clinic review.

(c) Clinical teams

Another example of the successful use of the collaborative model is the use of *Clinical teams* in the School of Communication Disorders at The University of Sydney (Rosenthal, 1986). In this model, beginning students are paired with final-year students for their initial clinical placement. The beginning student observes and participates in clinical sessions conducted by the final-year student, and both are under the supervision of a clinical educator. As the semester progresses the beginning student assumes more responsibility and performs a larger portion of the session activities consulting with the final-year student.

2.3 TEACHER-MANAGER MODEL

The Teacher-manager model is a relatively new model and has not been widely discussed in the literature. Unlike the previously described models it has not been categorized as it embraces aspects from all five categories of models, namely: descriptive models, integration models, developmental models, interactive process models and collaborative models.

Clinical educators are not only facilitators of students' learning within an adult learning environment, but they are also managers of the clinical learning programme. This role of manager of learning is compatible with many different clinical education models and with a variety of levels of learner readiness and teacher direction (for example, Anderson, 1988). This section will examine the clinical educator's role as manager of the learning programme and will present a *Teacher-manager model* (Romanini & Higgs, 1991) which provides a useful framework for the implementation of the teacher-manager roles of the clinical educator.

The model was developed as a tool to facilitate the design, implementation and evaluation of learning programmes in a variety of educational contexts (Romanini & Higgs, 1991). In keeping with the learning and management principles discussed above, the special features of the model are its emphasis on:

- clinical educators as overall managers of the learning programme as opposed to directors of students' behaviour. Students are seen as contributors to the learning programmes and as co-learners, not as subordinates
- the importance of interaction between all participants in the learning programme (clinical educators, students and clients) and the value of interdependence between clinical educators and students in particular. The concept is one of a learning group or community
- self-directed learning, with each student acting as an autonomous learner as well as being an integral part of the group. Clinical educators encourage students to develop increasing levels of self-direction and responsibility for their own learning
- the many managerial roles clinical educators play in order to effectively manage the learning programme
- the different phases of a learning programme and the need for clinical educators' roles to change over time in relation to these phases and in response to the student's needs and capabilities.

In the Teacher-manager model, clinical educators are seen as being proactive facilitators of the overall learning programme. This involves a number of management roles including management of the learning environment, student participation in the learning task, group process and individual student development. Students are encouraged to act independently as well as interdependently (with other students and the clinical educator) and to take an increasing level of responsibility for their own learning (Higgs, 1991). Each of these roles is employed in the various stages of the learning programme, that is planning, implementation and evaluation.

2.3.1 THE STAGES IN THE LEARNING PROGRAMME

The first part of the model, the stages in the learning programme, follows a systems model of input, process and output and feedback. It consists of three major stages: preparation, implementation and evaluation (each with sub-stages) and a feedback loop (see Figure 2.5). The three broad stages are typical of many models in the literature. However, the sub-stages are specific to interactive learning programmes which foster adult and self-directed learning. There is an emphasis on cooperative decision-making and the progressive development and clarification of programme goals to meet the students' needs and goals.

(a) The preparation stage

The preparation stage includes those functions of a teacher-manager which are associated with preparing for a learning task. The different sub-stages of preparation are:

1 *Clinical educators' prior planning and preparation*
   Prior to meeting the students, clinical educators are involved in a number of preparatory tasks. These tasks include identifying the clinical educator's own knowledge and skills (strengths and limitations) and as needed addressing these; designing a preliminary and flexible general format for the learning programme in consideration of learning goals, individual differences and resources; identifying possible teaching and learning activities considering students' anticipated prior learning experiences and available opportunities; preparing resources; and planning for the development of a favourable learning environment. Variety and flexibility are vital factors in the model at this stage.
2 *Initial encounter of clinical educators and students*
   This represents the first meeting of clinical educators and students. An important aspect of this sub-stage is the development of the learning climate which should ideally be open, trusting and stimulating to encourage students to broaden their horizons and explore their ways of thinking and learning.
3 *Preliminary exploration of learning goals and strategies*
   This could be viewed as an exploration of 'where we are now' as a

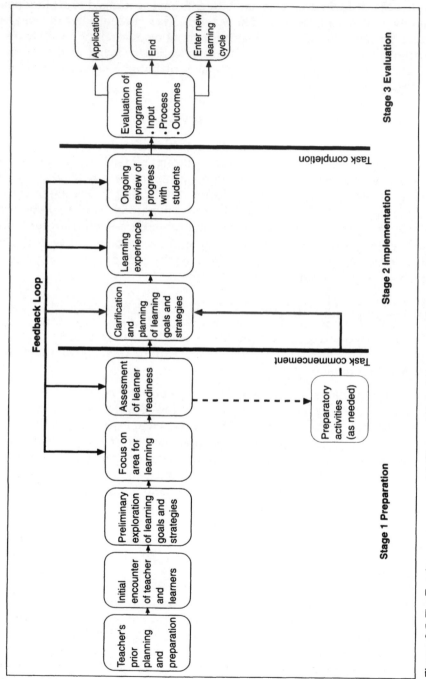

Figure 2.5 The Teacher-manager model: Stages in learning programme management

basis for planning for change (learning). At this stage students' needs, difficulties and wishes are identified. Strategies to address the learning goals are planned. Clinical educators may ask students to identify areas within their learning which they perceive as requiring improvement in order to encourage them to identify specific learning needs related to the overall goals of the programme.

4 *Focus on area for learning*
This sub-phase deals with selecting the general area of learning to be pursued and involves identifying learning needs common to the group.[2] These areas would become the focus for revision or for the main learning programme. The model allows for student choice of content within boundaries set by the clinical educator (based upon the curriculum content and the scope of the clinical educator's expertise). Unlimited choice, by comparison, could result in dissatisfaction among students, difficulty in agreeing upon a topic and lack of capacity of the clinical educator to help participants fulfil their learning needs. Watts (1990) notes that the choice of area for learning may be influenced by factors within the clinical facility such as availability of resources, competing demands of clinicians' time and administrative constraints.

5 *Assessment of learner readiness*
After students have completed a preliminary exploration of their learning needs and set the focus for learning, they should then work with the clinical educator to assess whether they possess the prerequisite knowledge and skills to pursue the various learning tasks. (This is an assessment of learner task maturity, as previously discussed.) This sub-stage of the model suggests a collaborative process between clinical educators and students. While the students can assess their current level of knowledge and skills, they may not adequately understand the prerequisite knowledge and skills required to commence the learning task, because they are insufficiently initiated into the current learning programme. Clinical educators can act as a guide to identification of the task needs. Clinical educators may find differing levels of learner readiness or task maturity within a group of students and within individual students, depending on the task. This will require adaptation of teaching behaviour and as necessary specific revision or remediation.

6 *Preparatory activities (as needed)*
This sub-stage is aimed at assisting the students to gain any specific

[2] This discussion refers to both group and individual learning. In some models learning may occur in a one-to-one situation. Clinical educators may either relate these sections to an individual learner model or where the advantages presented are significant, consider ways of creating a group for the student to learn with (for example, with students from other disciplines).

knowledge and skills they require prior to commencing the learning task. Such activities could include general orientation (for example, via group discussion), or participation in a learning skills development exercise.

(b) The implementation stage

The implementation stage occurs when students are ready to commence the learning task. This involves activities by clinical educators and students which are related to completion of the learning task. It includes the following sub-stages:

1 *Clarification and planning of learning goals and strategies*
Once students have completed the preparation stage they are ready to commence the learning task. Promoting adult learning skills implies commencing with the students' needs and interests, and adjusting the curriculum content and method to adapt to the students' situation and changing needs. Most importantly, the students' experience should play an important role in learning. Clinical educators should assist students to develop specific learning goals within the general topic or task area identified in the preparation stage and to plan learning strategies to achieve these goals. This sub-stage could involve students confronting a pertinent situation or problem, and designing a learning experience based on this problem area.

In group situations this sub-stage also entails clarifying and planning the roles of individuals in the learning task as well as defining the group's learning goals and resolving issues related to the purpose of the group. Students should clarify and agree what they can expect from each other. While they should be aware of each other's roles, it should be noted that these roles may vary during the learning experience. This is more likely to occur when students possess resources or specialized skills relevant to the learning task. The roles of group leader and group member may change according to which students possess the required resources.

2 *Learning experience*
This sub-stage involves the implementation of the planned activities and goals. Clinical educators broadly coordinate activities, act as troubleshooters in relation to problem areas they perceive or anticipate, and respond to students' requests for help. The level of clinical educator facilitation depends on the capabilities of the students to be both self-directed and interdependent. The role of the clinical educator may also be viewed as a change agent or catalyst. There may be a need to commence the students on the learning task by challenging them with alternative ways of interpreting their experience.

3 *Ongoing review of progress with students*
Clinical educators assist students to assess their progress towards
achievement of the learning goals, and to diagnose any difficulties or
problems which may have arisen. As needed the clinical educator may
encourage students to return to a preceding sub-stage of the learning
programme (for example, to take time out for further development of
undetected or emerging pre-requisite knowledge and skills). This is
indicated in Figure 2.5 by the *feedback loop*.

(c) The evaluation stage

The evaluation stage involves clinical educators and students in evaluating the learning programme and its outcomes and determining any subsequent action. It is divided into the following sub-stages:

1 *Evaluation of programme input, process and outcomes*
Here clinical educators and students evaluate the learning programme
to assess how effectively the learning task has been accomplished,
how well individual learning and development has been achieved and
how well the clinical educator has managed the process.
2 *Application*
This refers to the students' application of what they have learned
during the programme, to other areas of their life, learning or work.
3 *The end*
With some students completion of a cycle of a learning programme
will mean the end (or temporary end) to their intentional or formal
learning in the particular area. It is anticipated that these students will
carry their new learning into other areas or consolidate this learning
prior to entering new learning activities. For other students the
learning experience may have been a negative one and they may feel
disinclined to participate in further learning. The processes of
consultation, guidance and feedback advocated by this model are
aimed at avoiding this undesirable outcome.
4 *Entering a new learning cycle*
Students' learning experiences may result in the identification of
further areas to explore and the commencement of new learning
cycles. Students may also develop a general desire to continue
learning which stimulates them to become life-long learners.

2.3.2 THE TEACHER-MANAGER'S ROLES

The Teacher-manager has a number of roles to fulfil during each sub-stage
of the model. These roles may occur either simultaneously, or at different
sub-stages of the learning programme.

(a) Overall programme manager

In the role of overall programme manager, the teacher-manager monitors the whole learning programme and where it relates to the broader educational picture (for example, where a clinical practicum fits in with the total academic experience). To achieve this end, it is advisable for clinical educators to be aware of the general goals of the institution or the educational programme of which the current session is a part, so that they can ensure compatibility between the current clinical experience and these broader goals. In addition, the overall programme manager identifies when a more specific role or action is required, coordinates the programme's activities and participants, and acts as a guide, facilitator or troubleshooter as needed.

(b) Task manager

This role involves the promotion of effective student participation in the learning task and successful achievement of the programme's goals. It involves, for instance, the preparation of appropriate learning resources and adaptation of learning tasks to individual students' needs and learner task maturity.

(c) Group manager

Clinical educators have the role of promoting effective group development and performance throughout the learning programme. This can be achieved through activities such as enabling students to adopt effective group leadership and membership roles, providing leadership where necessary, role modelling and managing conflicts.

(d) Individual development manager

In this role clinical educators promote the development of each student's ability and effectiveness as a learner and assists individual students to achieve their assigned tasks and goals within the learning programme.

(e) Environment manager

This role involves managing the physical, social and individual or personal environmental variables to promote achievement of the learning programme's goals.

2.3.3 USING THE TEACHER-MANAGER MODEL IN CLINICAL EDUCATION

Figure 2.6 illustrates how Parts A and B of the model can be combined as a tool to plan, implement and evaluate clinical education. Experienced clinical educators could use these guidelines simply as a prompt to remind them of the clinical programme sub-stages and the roles which have relevance to each. Beginning clinical educators could benefit from trying out these ideas in their teaching or from using the table (proforma) headings and filling in each of the boxes in relation to their particular learning programme's needs and situation. That is, they could plan their goals and actions for each sub-stage of the learning programme (Part A), in relation to each of the teacher-manager's roles (Part B). A completed proforma could also be of value in team teaching situations to enable effective communication between colleagues.

The Teacher-manager model has been used effectively within clinical education contexts with beginning and more experienced health science educators (Romanini, 1995; White & Ewan, 1991). This experience has led to the conclusion that the model succeeds in clinical education contexts for the following reasons:

• The model values students' individuality and past experience. Application of the model encourages independent learning and the development of skills of self-direction in learning and work.
• The model entails interaction which promotes the development of skills of communication, leadership, group participation and conflict management. Such skills are integral to effective teamwork and professional interaction.
• Active involvement of students in each stage of the learning programme encourages a greater commitment to the learning programme, than if the programme had been directed by the clinical educator.

It is also important to remember in using this model that some people come to the model with very differing concepts of the term 'manager'. For some, this term implies a supervisory role where the manager is the decision-maker and the followers are directed. Clear explanation is needed to orientate clinical educators to the democratic manager concept which is central to the model. In addition, clinical educators using the model need to develop an understanding of the potential areas of overlap between the various manager's roles and they need to become skilled in playing several roles at once and knowing when to switch between roles. Finally, some clinical educators may have difficulty in giving away control and allowing students to experience autonomy. Both students and clinical educators will need to learn how to be co-managers.

2.3.4 SUMMARY OF THE TEACHER-MANAGER MODEL

Clinical educators can be viewed as managers of learning. The Teacher-manager model provides a framework for enabling clinical educators to achieve a number of the major goals of clinical education programmes

PART B: ROLES OF THE TEACHER	Teacher's Prior Planning and Preparation	Initial Encounter of Teacher and Learners	Preliminary Exploration of Learning Goals and Strategies	Focus on Areas for Learning	Assessment of Learner Readiness	Preparatory Activities (as needed)	Clarification and Planning of Learning Goals and Strategies	Learning Experience	Ongoing Review of Progress with Students	Evaluation of Programme Input Process Outcomes	Enter New Learning Cycle	Application	End
	STAGE 1 PREPARATION					PART C: TEACHER'S GOALS AND ACTIONS — STAGE 2 IMPLEMENTATION					STAGE 3 EVALUATION		
TASK MANAGER	investigate availability of experiences	explore students' perspectives of possible tasks	examine appropriate tasks & objectives	collaborative exploration of identified tasks	readiness to perform identified tasks	involve relevant students in preparatory activities	identify specific strategies for tasks	teacher-manager coordinates task	collaborative assessment of progress of task	collaborative evaluation of learning task	performance of task encouraged continued learning	students are able to transfer learning	completion of task may signify end of learning
GROUP MANAGER	explore possible groupings of students	observe group dynamics	note group similarities and differences	be aware of group norms and difficulties	identify group difficulty in learning	students with prerequisites to assist others	students clarify group's goals, roles, procedures	promote group performance to enhance learning	collaborative assessment of group performance	collaborative evaluation of how well the group performed	group process has promoted continued learning	students are able to apply group processes	may signify no further group participation for a time
INDIVIDUAL DEVELOPMENT MANAGER	examine attainable goals for students	introduce concept of individual development	explore areas of individual development	encourage individual differences in area for learning	be cognisant of arising individual differences	encourage individuals to achieve preparatory activities	encourage individuals to clarify specific goals	promote individual's performance of learning experience	encourage individuals to review own progress	collaborative evaluation of individual development	individual development promoted continued learning	students are able to apply individual development	may signify end to individual's learning for a time
ENVIRONMENT MANAGER	select appropriate setting for initial meeting	manipulate environment for group development	promote environment to enhance brainstorming	encourage climate to facilitate sub-stage e.g. culture	manipulate environment to promote goals	promote environment for preparatory activities	manage environment to promote planning goals	promote environment for successful learning	manage environment for ongoing review of progress	collaborative evaluation of environment and influence on learning	environment has enhanced continued learning	environment has promoted transfer of learning	some may not immediately enroll in further programmes
OVERALL PROGRAMME MANAGER	explore fit of placement with overall programme	investigate role of teacher-manager with students	encourage brainstorming within goals of clinical placement	be cognisant of legal and academic requirements	understand assessment process of overall programme	be cognisant of overall programme goals	understand fit of identified learning with overall programme	understand congruence of learning experience with overall programme	be cognisant of overall programme goals	collaborative evaluation of overall placement	clinical & programme goals promote new learning	specific experience able to be applied in the overall programme	some students consolidate experience prior to new learning

Figure 2.6 Teacher-manager's goals and actions

including: fostering student autonomy, promoting effective learning outcomes, helping students develop skills in problem-solving and coping with change, and developing life-long learning skills for self-directed and small group learning. The model advocates the development of skills of independence, self-direction, interaction, communication, leadership, group membership and conflict resolution. These skills can be transferred to the workplace to enable health science graduates to accomplish their tasks effectively, achieve their goals, work cooperatively in teams as leaders and members and take greater responsibility for their work and continuing learning, without constant supervision.

The roles of the clinical educator form an integral part of the Teacher-manager model. All models previously discussed assume certain roles and responsibilites for the clinical educator.

2.4 ROLES AND RESPONSIBILITIES OF THE CLINICAL EDUCATOR

Delineating roles and expectations of clinical educators is an important first step in a number of the models of clinical education (for example, Goldhammer, 1969; Mandy, 1989). The role of clinical educators is crucial to the success of the clinical education programme. Most clinical educators will agree that they play many roles during a clinical placement, and that they often play multiple roles within a single clinical teaching episode (White & Ewan, 1991).

Attempts to delineate the essential roles of clinical educators within the multi-faceted and complex environment of a clinical education programme or system has challenged many educators and researchers (Conohan, Rubeck & Anderson, 1981; Dowling, 1992; Irby, 1978; Stritter, Hain & Grimes, 1975; Wellington & Romanini, 1993). In order to synthesize the range of perspectives on the essential roles of the clinical educator, seven major overarching functions will be described: role model (cf., Farmer & Farmer, 1989; Rassi & McElroy, 1992a), colleague (cf., Hagler & McFarlane, 1991; Rassi & McElroy, 1992a), teacher (cf., Farmer & Farmer, 1989; Hagler & McFarlane, 1991; Rassi & McElroy, 1992a; Turney *et al.*, 1982), evaluator (cf., Turney *et al.*, 1982), administrator-manager (cf., Farmer & Farmer, 1989), counsellor (cf., Hagler & McFarlane, 1991; Rassi & McElroy, 1992a; Turney *et al.*, 1982), and researcher (cf., Farmer & Farmer, 1989; Rassi & McElroy, 1992a). Some of these roles are essential to clinical education, such as teacher and role model. Other roles, such as researcher, may not be fulfilled by all clinical educators.

2.4.1 ROLE MODEL

Clinical educators model professional conduct in everything students observe. Whether clinical educators are having a discussion with the clinic secretary, making a phonecall to a colleague, dealing with a client complaint, presenting a public seminar, or discussing a student's performance, they are always modelling professional behaviour. Being a role model is widely recognized as critical in shaping, teaching, coaching and assisting future clinicians, as it is the most powerful teaching strategy available to clinical educators (Rogers, 1982; Sabari, 1985; Schön, 1987). Students learn most from observing the actions and understanding the reasoning processes of their role models (see Chapter 3 on professional socialization).

(a) Clinician

Prior to assuming the role of clinical educator, most clinical educators were clinicians. Most clinical educators originally trained as a clinician in a specific health science discipline and have spent some time as a practising professional working with clients. As a clinician, the clients' welfare is their primary role.

The shift from being solely a clinician to a duel role of clinician and clinical educator means that the clinical educator has responsibility to clients *and* to students (McLeod, 1989). Sometimes these simultaneous roles may come into conflict. Clinical educators have a professional and ethical responsibility to ensure appropriate services for their clients (American Speech-Language-Hearing Association, 1991; Higgs & Mackey, 1989). However, they also need to provide safe learning environments for their students. Clinical educators may need to be client advocates, ensuring optimal and appropriate services from students and the hospital, university, or other setting. It is the responsibility of clinical educators to model professional conduct and to share information regarding ethical and legal aspects of professional practice with their students (American Speech-Language-Hearing Association, 1985) (see Chapter 3 on ethics).

(b) Life-long learner versus expert clinician

Rassi and McElroy have suggested that a clinical educator should be an expert or master clinician in order to model, demonstrate and instruct students effectively in the process of clinical practice (Rassi & McElroy, 1992a). They suggest that discrepancies between what is taught in lectures and what is practised in the clinical setting are confusing to students. Therefore, the clinical educator should be familiar with the latest research and theoretical frameworks. Utilization of the integration models (for example, Rassi & McElroy, 1992b) where concepts between academic and clinical teaching are integrated (presented earlier in this chapter) may help alleviate the discrepancies between theory and practice. However, the burgeoning knowledge base makes it difficult for clinical educators to be an expert in every area of practice that they encounter. Consequently, today's clinicians need to be life-long learners willing to explore new ideas as the need arises (see Chapter 1). Thus, the role of clinical educators should be to model how they learn and attempt to keep abreast of new ideas. In this role, clinical educators can be open to learning from students who present alternative techniques that they may have learnt recently in lectures and self-study. Furthermore, by framing the role of clinical educator as a life-long learner, it legitimizes the value of searching for solutions together with students. Such modelling encourages development of the notion of interdependence on one another. Thus, the role of expert clinician may not be essential to being an excellent clinical educator.

2.4.2 COLLEAGUE

(a) Establishing and maintaining a collegial relationship

Establishing and maintaining collegial relationships with students is central to the learning process. Christie, Joyce and Moller (1985), in their study of 65 occupational therapy clinical education settings, confirmed the long-standing belief that the relationship between students and their clinical educators is the most powerful component of the clinical education experience. In this study, both students and clinical educators perceived the supervisory relationship as the most critical element in distinguishing good from poor clinical education experiences. Furthermore, communication and interpersonal skills were identified as distinguishing characteristics of effective supervision.

These beliefs are likewise noted in many other fields (for example, American Speech-Language-Hearing Association, 1985; McCrea, 1980; Wellington & Romanini, 1993). The first task of supervision described by the American Speech-Language-Hearing Association (1985) in their list of 13 competencies for effective clinical supervision is 'establishing and maintaining an effective working relationship with the supervisee'. McCrea (1980) investigated the effects of clinical educators' empathic understanding, respect, facilitative genuineness, and concreteness on students' self-exploratory behaviours. Empathic understanding and respect from clinical educators were significant predictors of student self-exploration.

(b) Colleague versus friend

The relationship between students and clinical educators is the beginning of a life-long professional relationship. Former students may become colleagues within a clinical educator's department, a clinical educator's postgraduate student or a friendly face at conferences and workshops. Beginning the friendly interaction of professionals, when in the role of student and clinical educator, provides the foundation for ongoing professional relationships. Working with students as future colleagues is more readily accommodated within the andragogical (adult learning) approach than the pedagogical approach.

Although the image of clinical educators as friends is useful for conveying the empathic caring attitude students desire from their clinical educators, it would be misleading to portray this relationship as that of a social friendship. As Kadushin (1968) noted, establishing a friendship with a student mitigates the clinical educator's authority and ability to evaluate the student's performance. When people develop a close relationship, such as a social friendship it is then difficult to provide objective feedback. Furthermore, unlike a social friendship, students and clinical educators usually meet and grow to know one another because the clinical educator is expected to facilitate the student's growth as a competent practitioner. Thus, it is important to view the relationship as one in which students and clinical educators mutually influence one another, rather than a social friendship.

2.4.3 TEACHER

As a teacher or educator, the clinical educator has many roles including: instructor, demonstrator, person who maximizes learning opportunities, resource person, facilitator, observer, learner, provider of feedback, appraiser/evaluator and curriculum planner.

The educational role of clinical educators is not just one of observing sessions then providing feedback, it is a proactive role in developing students' learning strategies, ensuring quality care for clients and giving priority to students' learning needs (Borders, 1992). Learning in a clinical setting is often dependent on which clients present themselves and what range of problems, issues and challenges need to be dealt with. Thus, it is the role of clinical educators to maximize the learning experience as each opportunity presents itself. In this role, clinical educators are supportive, non-judgemental facilitators of learning, sometimes referred to as a coach (Hagler & McFarlane, 1991; Schön, 1987).

Some of the educational roles of the clinical educator as teacher have been identified by the American Speech-Language-Hearing Association (1985). These are: demonstrating or participating with students in the clinical process; assisting students in developing and refining clinical goals and objectives, assessment and management skills; assisting students in observing and analyzing clinical sessions; assisting students in the development and maintenance of clinical records; and assisting students in developing skills of verbal reporting, writing and editing.

2.4.4 EVALUATOR/ASSESSOR

The evaluative role of the clinical educator is quite different from the other roles identified, as the evaluative role requires the clinical educator to move out of the supportive teaching or coaching role and objectively evaluate the student's performance. Since successful completion of the clinical education experience is a prerequisite for entry into health science professions, this role is more authoritative.

Students should receive *formative* evaluative feedback regarding their professional development throughout their clinical experience so they can change and grow (see Chapter 3 on feedback). This type of evaluation is an ongoing process that directs students' learning throughout the clinical education experience, while *summative* evaluation documents the level of skill attained at the completion of the clinical education experience (see Chapter 6). Although these two processes are different, they are not mutually exclusive. The formative processes enables students and clinical educators to compare perceptions, review learning objectives, plan new learning opportunities, and make necessary modifications in both behaviours and the learning experience. Students need to be assured of their strengths and have their areas for growth identified so they can strive to improve their skills. The second process, which is cumulative, requires documentation of students' performance after completion of the clinical education experience. Each health science discipline will have its own set of standards and criteria for acceptable professional skills required to enter the profession.

Additionally, it is the role of the clinical educator to assist students in evaluating their own clinical performance (self-evaluation) and to interact with students in planning, executing and analyzing supervisory interactions (American Speech-Language-Hearing Association, 1985). Before self-evaluation can be internalized, the standards and expected behaviour need to be defined in an explicit manner, as is done in the evaluation process. Thus, the formative evaluation process can serve as a model to facilitate students to begin the self-evaluation process (see Chapter 4).

2.4.5 ADMINISTRATOR/MANAGER

In the administrative role the clinical educator must ensure that the viability of the organization is maintained. Central to this role is ensuring that clients receive the highest quality of care at all times. Since client care is always the priority, clinical educators may, on occasion, have to place student learning as second priority to ensure that the optimal client care is provided. It is useful for students to understand this legal, ethical and professional priority.

Moreover, clinical educators are managers of the clinical learning programme. As such, they need to coordinate the needs of clients, students, other professionals and the university. Administrative responsibilities include, but are not limited to, the following (Cohn, 1993):

- collaborating with the university programme in the development of a programme that provides the best opportunity for the implementation of theoretical concepts taught as part of the education preparation
- creating an environment that facilitates learning, clinical inquiry, and reflection on one's practice
- preparing, maintaining, and sending to the university current information about the clinical education setting, including a statement of conceptual models related to both the clinical education programme and the service delivery models
- scheduling students in coordination with the university programme and the clinical education setting's needs
- ensuring that the clinical education programme is cost effective. An understanding of how the clinical education programme will impact on staff productivity is essential for planning and allowing staff members time to address both their clinical and teaching responsibilities
- establishing and periodically reviewing the contractual agreements, which outline liability issues, between the university and clinical education settings.

In this administrative-management role clinical educators can create adult learning environments and facilitate self-directed learning by encouraging students to act as co-managers of their learning programmes (Higgs, 1992). Part of effective adult learning is to promote student autonomy through the involvement of the student in the planning, implementation and evaluation phases of learning programmes.

The manager in adult learning programmes shares programme management, power, control and responsibility for learning with the students, and creates a learning environment which allows this sharing to occur by promoting student self-direction and involving students in negotiating and managing learning experiences. For instance, endeavours such as negotiated learning contracts (see Chapter 3) have been successful in the promotion of independent behaviour, cognitive achievement and autonomous learning (Tompkins & McGraw, 1988).

2.4.6 COUNSELLOR

Clinical education is often a forum in which personal and professional issues are raised for students. Many clinical situations provoke reflection on complex, intense issues of life and death, personal tragedy, disease or disability. Students may be confronted with personal responses to the realities of providing health care, or issues which have occurred during a student's life may resurface (see Case Studies 2.4 and 2.5). In fact, in educating psychotherapists, understanding 'counter-transference' (the feelings evoked in the clinician by the client) is considered essential to becoming an effective clinician (Balsam & Balsam, 1984). To work with clients can be a source of personal stress for students, and sensitivity from the clinical educator is required. Students may benefit from exploring how their personal response to clients and the realities of health care impact on their interactions with clients. However, it is important to note that it is beyond the clinical educator's role to provide formal counselling to students. When formal counselling is indicated, clinical educators should make the necessary referral (see Chapter 7).

Case Study 2.4

Andrea has just commenced her clinical placement with clients who have psychiatric disabilites. She has not encountered people with psychiatric illnesses before and is frightened by them.

Case Study 2.5

Fatima has been asked to assess a teenager who has been hit by a car while riding his bike. When she entered the room she smiled at the boy, then walked straight out. You found her in the corridor, sitting on the floor crying. She begins to tell you of her brother's accident ...

Career counselling also may be a part of the role of clinical educators (Rassi & McElroy, 1992a) (see Case Study 2.6 and Chapter 7). In the role of career counsellor a clinical educator may discuss what it is like to be a practising health professional, be aware of job opportunities for students, provide professional contacts, discuss professional politics, and write letters of recommendation or references (Rassi & McElroy, 1992a).

Case Study 2.6

It is the third week of Harry's clinical placement. He comes to you one afternoon saying that he is disillusioned with his career choice and that he feels he needs to change professions.

In all of the above case studies, the clinical educator must use counselling skills to explore with the student, his or her response to the realities of practice.

2.4.7 RESEARCHER

Finally, it may be the role of clinical educators to conduct research into the clinical or clinical education process (American Speech-Language-Hearing Association, 1985; Stritter, Hain & Grimes, 1975). Clinical education is a relatively new field and much of the literature is anecdotal or descriptive. To facilitate the development of the field it is important that clinical educators conduct research into clinical education (see Chapter 8). Furthermore, students are excellent resources for conducting research into the clinical process. Graduate students in particular may find their setting for the clinical education programme to be ideal for gathering data for their research thesis. Collaboration between clinical educators and their students can be an excellent foundation for publishing clinically relevant research (for example, McLeod & Isaac, 1995).

Bloom (1995) described three models for incorporating research into the clinical education experience and socializing students to believe they are capable of conducting research. She advocated mutual fostering of research activity between students, clinical educators and university programmes through a highly structured format to ensure success. In each model faculty members work together with clinical educators and students to promote an integrative and applied approach to clinical research.

Although the role of researcher is valued across professional disciplines, it is not essential for clinical educators to be engaged in research. What is essential is the thought process of clinical inquiry and application of scientific method. Clinical educators need to model the process of actively thinking about the underlying assumptions which direct their clinical practice and continually ask if the proposed mechanisms of change are working. Clinical educators need to think like researchers and teach their students the process of clinical inquiry.

2.5 CONCLUSION

To be a clinical educator is both a demanding and complex task. Frequently clinical educators spend their time responding to the immediate demands of students, clients and other professionals. This chapter provides a framework for clinical educators to think about their philosophies of clinical education by examining models of clinical education and the roles and responsibilities of clinical educators. Clinical educators and students can benefit from clarifying which models they support. In this chapter, models of clinical education have been categorized five ways:

descriptive models, integration models, developmental models, interactive process models and collaborative models. The *Teacher-manager model* (Romanini & Higgs, 1991), which is a comprehensive model, has been presented in detail. Definition of the roles and responsibilities of clinical educators provide further insight into clinical education for both clinical educators and students. Seven roles have been presented: role model, colleague, teacher, evaluator, administrator-manager, counsellor and researcher.

REFERENCES

American Speech-Language-Hearing Association (1985). Clinical supervision in speech-language pathology and audiology (position statement). *Asha*, **27**, 57–60.

American Speech-Language-Hearing Association (1991). Supervision of student clinicians, *Asha*, **33**, 53.

Anderson, J. L. (1988). *The supervisory process in speech-language pathology and audiology*. Boston: College Hill Press.

Balsam, R. M. & Balsam, A. (1984). *Becoming a psychotherapist*. Chicago: University of Chicago Press.

Belenky, M. F., Clinchy, B. M., Goldberger, N. R. & Tarule, J. M. (1986). *Women's ways of knowing*. New York: Basic Books.

Benner, P. (1984). *From novice to expert*. Reading, MA: Addison-Wesley.

Bloom, J. S. (1995). Applied research during fieldwork: Interdisciplinary collaboration between universities and clinics. *American Journal of Occupational Therapy*, **49**, 207–13.

Borders, L. (1992). Learning to think like a supervisor. *The Clinical Supervisor*, **10**, 135–48.

Boud, D., Keogh R. & Walker, D. (1985). Promoting reflection in learning: A model. In D. Boud, R. Keogh & D. Walker (Eds). *Reflection: Turning experience into learning* (pp 18–40). London: Kogan Page.

Brasseur, J. (1989). The supervisory process: A continuum perspective. *Language, Speech, and Hearing Services in Schools*, **20**, 274–95.

Bruffee, K. A. (1987). The art of collaborative learning: Making the most of knowledgeable peers. *Change*, **19**, 671–4.

Christie, B. A., Joyce, P. C. & Moller, P. L. (1985). Fieldwork experience, Part 1: Impact on practice preference. *American Journal of Occupational Therapy*, **10**, 671–4.

Cogan, M. (1973). *Clinical supervision*. Boston: Houghton Mifflin.

Cohn, E. S. & Crist, P. (1995). Back to the future: New approaches to fieldwork education. *American Journal of Occupational Therapy*, **49**, 103–6.

Cohn, E. S. & Czycholl, C. M. (1991). Facilitating a foundation for clinical reasoning. In E. B. Crepeau & T. LaGarde (Eds). *Self-paced instruction for clinical education and supervision: An instructional guide* (pp 159–82). Rockville, MD: American Occupational Therapy Association.

Cohn, E. S. (1993). Fieldwork education: Professional socialization. In H. L. Hopkins & H. D. Smith (Eds). *Willard and Spackman's occupational therapy* (8th ed.)., (pp 12–19). Philadelphia: Lippincott.

Conohan, T. J., Rubeck, R. F. & Anderson, D. O. (1981). Rating the importance of clinical teacher attitudes. *The Arizona Medical Educator*, **11**, 1–3.

Crist, P. A. (1993, 13 January). Issues in fieldwork education. *Advance for Occupational Therapists*, 2.

Davies, I. K. (1971). *The management of learning*. London: McGraw-Hill.

DeClute, J. & Ladyshewsky, R. (1993). Enhancing clinical competence using a collaborative clinical education model. *Physical Therapy*, **73**, 683–97.

Dowling, S. (1979). The teaching clinic: A supervisory alternative. *Asha*, **21**, 646–9.

Dowling, S. (1992). *Implementing the supervisory process: Theory and practice*. Englewood Cliffs, NJ: Prentice Hall.

Emery, F. E. (1969). *Systems thinking*. Middlesex: Penguin Books.

Farmer, S. & Farmer, J. (1989). *Supervision in communication disorders*. Columbus: Merrill Publishing.

Goldhammer, R. (1969). *Clinical supervision: Special methods for the supervision of teachers*. New York: Holt, Reinhart & Winston.

Goldhammer, R., Anderson, R. & Krajewski, R. (1980). *Clinical supervision*. New York: Holt, Reinhart & Winston.

Hagler, P. & McFarlane, L. (1991). Achieving maximum student potential: The supervisor as coach. *Canadian Journal of Rehabilitation*, **5**, 5–16.

Hersey, P. & Blanchard, K. (1982). *Management of organizational behaviour: Utilizing human resources* (4th ed.). Englewood Cliffs, NJ: Prentice Hall.

Higgs, J. (1991). The role of the teacher and learner in fostering self-direction in independent learning programmemes. *Proceedings of the 11th International Congress of the World Confederation for Physical Therapy* (pp 177–9). London: WCPT.

Higgs, J. (1992). Managing clinical education: The educator-manager and the self-directed learner. *Physiotherapy*, **78**, 822–8.

Higgs, J. (1993). Managing clinical education: The programme. *Physiotherapy*, **79**, 239–46.

Higgs, J. & Jones, M. (1995). *Clinical reasoning in the health professions*. Oxford: Butterworth-Heinemann.

Higgs, J. & Mackey, M. (Eds) (1989). *Professional responsibilities, legal liabilities and insurance for clinical educators*. Sydney: Cumberland College of Health Sciences.

Horger, M. M. (1994). Cooperative learning and occupational therapy: A natural combination. *Education Special Interest Section Newsletter*, **17**, 1–2.

Irby, D. M. (1978). Clinical teacher effectiveness in medicine. *Journal of Medical Education*, **58**, 808–15.

Johnson, D. W. & Johnson, R. T. (1990). *Learning together and alone: Cooperative, competitive and individualistic learning*. Boston: Alyn & Bacon.

Kadushin, A. (1968). Games people play in supervision. *Social Work*, **18**, 23–32.

Kent, R. D. (1989–1990). The fragmentation of clinical service and clinical science in communicative disorders. *National Student Speech-Language-Hearing Association Journal*, **17**, 4–16.

Kolodner, E. L., Weiner, W. J. & Frum, D. C. (Eds) (1989). *Models for mental health fieldwork*. Rockville, MD: American Occupational Therapy Association.

Koontz, H., O'Donnell, C. & Weihrich, H. (1982). *Essentials of management* (3rd ed.). New York: McGraw-Hill.

Ladyshewsky, R. & Healey, E. (1990). *The 2:1 teaching model in clinical education: A manual for clinical instructors*. Toronto: University of Toronto, Department of Rehabilitation Medicine.

Ladyshewsky, R. (1993). Clinical teaching and the 2:1 student to clinical instructor ratio. *Journal of Physical Therapy Education, 7*, 31–5.

Lincoln, M. A. & McAllister, L. L. (1993). Peer learning in clinical education. *Medical Teacher, 15*, 17–25.

Lognabill, C., Hardy, E. & Delworth, U. (1982). Supervision: A conceptual model. *Counseling Psychologist, 10*, 1.

Maloney, D. & Sheard, C. (1992, February). *An interpersonal skills approach to the learning triad: Client, student and clinical educator.* Paper presented to Australian Association of Speech and Hearing Conference, Melbourne, Australia.

Mandy, S. (1989). Facilitating student learning in clinical education. *Australian Journal of Human Communication Disorders, 17*, 83–93.

Mattingly, C. & Fleming, M. H. (1993). *Clinical reasoning: Forms of inquiry in therapeutic practice.* Philadelphia: F. A. Davis Co.

Mawdsley, B. L. & Scudder, R. R. (1989). Integrative task maturity model. *Language, Speech, and Hearing Services in Schools, 20*, 305–19.

McLeod, S. (1989). Responsibility, authority and power: A perspective on the role of the student supervisor. *Australian Communication Quarterly, 10*, 10–12.

McLeod, S. & Isaac, K. (1995). Use of spectrographic analyses to evaluate the efficacy of phonological intervention, *Clinical Linguistics and Phonetics, 9*, 229–34.

McCrea, M. (1980). Supervisee ability to self-explore four facilitative dimensions of supervisor behaviour in individual conferences in speech-language pathology. (Doctoral dissertation, Indiana University, 1980). *Dissertation Abstracts International, 41*, 2134B.

Miller, P. H. (1993). *Theories of developmental psychology.* New York: W. H. Freeman & Co.

O'Neil, E. H. (1993). *Health professions education for the future: Schools in service to the nation.* San Francisco: The Pew Health Professions Commission.

Oratio, A. R. (1977). *Supervision in speech pathology: A handbook for supervisors and clinicians.* Baltimore: University Park Press.

Pickering, M. (1987). Supervision: A person-focused process. In M. Crago & M. Pickering (Eds). *Supervision in human communication disorders: Perspectives on a process* (pp 107–34). San Diego, CA: College-Hill Press.

Pickering, M., Rassi, J. A., Hagler, P. & McFarlane, L. (1992). Integrating classroom, laboratory, and clinical experiences. *Asha, 34*, 57–9.

Rassi, J. A. & McElroy, M. D. (1992a). Education in the clinic. In J. A. Rassi & M. D. McElroy (Eds). *The education of audiologists and speech-language pathologists* (pp 175–96). Timonium, MD: York Press.

Rassi, J. A. & McElroy, M. D. (1992b). Integration of person and process. In J. A. Rassi & M. D. McElroy (Eds). *The education of audiologists and speech-language pathologists* (pp 443–5). Timonium, MD: York Press.

Reed, K. L. (1984). *Models of practice in occupational therapy.* Baltimore: Williams & Wilkins.

Rogers, J. C. (1982). Sponsorship: Developing leaders for occupational therapy. *American Journal of Occupational Therapy, 36*, 309–13.

Romanini, J. (1995, June). *The teacher as manager in clinical education.* Paper presented to International Nursing Congress, Athens, Greece.

Romanini, J. & Higgs, J. (1991). The teacher as manager in continuing and professional education. *Studies in Continuing Education, 13*, 41–52.

Rosenthal, J. (1986). Novice and experienced student clinical teams in undergraduate clinical practice. *Australian Communication Quarterly, 2*, 12–15.

Rubin, I. (1980). Team development. In R. Schenke (Ed.). *The physician in manage-*

ment. Virginia: The American Academy of Medical Directors.

Sabari, J.S. (1985). Professional socialization: Implications for occupational therapy education. *American Journal of Occupational Therapy*, **39**, 96–102.

Schön, D. (1987). *Educating the reflective practitioner*. New York: Basic Books.

Shriberg, L., Filley, F., Hayes, D., Kwiatkowski, J., Schatz, J., Simmons, K. & Smith, M. (1975). The Wisconsin procedure for appraisal of clinical competence: Model and data. *Asha*, **17**, 158–65.

Sprinthall, N. A. & Thies-Sprinthall, L. (1983). The teacher as an adult learner: A cognitive-developmental view. In G. A. Griffin (Ed.). *Staff development* (pp 13–35). Chicago: National Society for the Study of Education.

Stern, K. (1994). Cooperative learning: Increasing achievement in the classroom. *Education Special Interest Section Newsletter*, **17**, 3–4.

Stritter, F. T., Baker, R. M. & Shahady, E. J. (1986). Clinical instruction. In W. C. McGaghie & J. J. Frey (Eds). *Handbook for the academic physician* (pp 99–124). New York: Springer Verlag.

Stritter, F. T., Hain, J. D. & Grimes, D. A. (1975). Clinical teaching re-examined. *Journal of Medical Education*, **50**, 876–81.

Tiberius, R. & Gaiptman, B. (1985). Supervisor-student ratio: 1:1 versus 1:2. *Canadian Journal of Occupational Therapy*, **52**, 179–83.

Tompkins, C. & McGraw, M. (1988). The negotiated learning contract. In D. J. Boud (Ed.). *Developing student autonomy in learning* (2nd ed.), (pp 17–39). London: Kogan Page.

Torbert, W. R. (1978). Educating toward shared purpose, self-direction and quality work: The theory and practice of liberating structure. *Journal of Higher Education*, **49**, 109–35.

Turney, C., Cairnes, L., Eltis, K., Hatton, N., Thew, D., Towler, J. & Wright, R. (1982). *Supervisor development programmemes: Role handbook*. Sydney: Sydney University Press.

Von Bertalanffy, L. (1969). The theory of open systems in physics and biology. In F. E. Emery (Ed.). *Systems thinking* (pp 70–85). Middlesex: Penguin Books.

Watts, N. T. (1990). *Handbook of clinical teaching*. Edinburgh: Churchill Livingstone.

Wellington, B. & Romanini, J. (1993, February). *The 'good' clinical supervisor: Perceptions of students in nursing*. Paper presented at the 5th National Practicum Conference, Sydney.

White, R. & Ewan, C. (Eds) (1991). *Clinical teaching in nursing*. London: Chapman & Hall.

Wittman, P. P. & Schwartz, K. B. (1991). Identifying the developmental needs of students. In E. B. Crepeau & T. LaGarde (Eds). *Self-paced instruction for clinical education and supervision: An instructional guide* (pp 125–36). Rockville, MD: American Occupational Therapy Association.

Professional development of students and clinical educators

3

Michelle Lincoln
School of Communication Disorders,
The University of Sydney, Australia

Diana Carmody
Department of Social Work,
New Children's Hospital, Sydney, Australia

Diana Maloney
School of Communication Disorders,
The University of Sydney, Australia

3.1 CHAPTER OVERVIEW

The issues discussed in this chapter will increase awareness of the complex process involved in educating students in clinical settings. This chapter considers aspects of motivation for both students and clinical educators. It includes information about students' professional development and ethical considerations for students and clinical educators. The role of feedback in clinical education is described and applied to a client-centred approach to clinical learning. The authors have developed the views expressed in this chapter as a result of critically reviewing literature in this area, continuing education and extensive experience in working in clinical settings. The seeds of the approaches to clinical education discussed in this chapter were planted by Rogers (1951) and nurtured to the present day by many in the fields of client-centred counselling, family therapy and communication management including Egan (1990), Anderson (1988), Nelson-Jones (1986) and Pickering (1987). The authors have used 'we' throughout the chapter when writing about their own views or experiences.

Postcard 3

Dear All

I love this place and the work here. It's so beautiful, if wet. The local people are lovely and so appreciative of what we are doing. The work is interesting in many ways. I'm learning so much about who I am as a person and what I value. The cultural differences are sometimes quite confronting. What we take to be norms of professional communication don't apply here. As you know, I'm pretty direct with people, and I find their indirectness or 'politeness' drives me nuts some days. I don't know where I stand and whether what I think we've agreed to, we really have. I'm also thinking a lot about what's 'professional'. I know the workers know a lot more about the ways things work in this community, the needs here and about CBR, but I worry about what looks to me like non-professional behaviour. Nothing is documented, there are no programme plans for the clients, and the workers talk about the families they have worked with during the day with their own families at night. I'm wondering whose role it is to raise these issues with them.

love Sally

This chapter provides essential information for clinicians in the field who are considering accepting students to their clinic, academics who have a clinical teaching component in their university contract, post-graduate students studying clinical education and undergraduate students involved in peer teaching in clinical settings.

This chapter moves from discussing the broad issues of motivation, anxiety, professional socialization and ethics to examining the interpersonal skills involved in communication and giving and receiving feedback. The chapter has been structured in this way in order to lead the reader from a consideration of how people come to be involved in clinical education, through to consideration of how they might be feeling about their involvement and what happens to them as they participate in clinical education, and finally to how clinical educators can grow themselves, and facilitate growth as students move through their clinical education experiences.

3.2. MOTIVATION FOR LEARNING IN CLINICAL PLACEMENTS

Clinical education is multifaceted and diverse. There are as many aspects to clinical education as there are students and clinical educators. Factors which motivate participation in courses may be common between clinical educators and students; for example, a common desire to achieve greater understanding of the theory underlying disorders and to increase skills in applying this knowledge successfully with clients in their chosen discipline.

We believe that examining the motivation of clinical educators and students is a good place to start when considering personal and professional development, because without motivation of some sort there would be no clinical educators or students. A person's reasons for engaging in clinical education are the starting point in professional development. Students' and clinical educators' motivation may change as a part of normal professional growth. Developmental models of clinical education (see Chapter 2) that discuss the progression of students through stages and how students make sense of their experiences may also be applicable to the developmental stages of clinical educators. For example the 'learner task maturity model' (Higgs, 1993) discussed in Chapter 2, could easily apply to the role development of clinical educators as well as students.

While we acknowledge that students and clinical educators may share some similar motivations, there are also differences which are unique to each group. An individual within each group may have many motivating factors which are probably related to personal and professional goals. For example, students who strive for high academic achievement may be motivated by a desire to achieve or to gain good employment (or any number of other factors).

3.2.1 STUDENT MOTIVATION

Students who have chosen to study in the health care field tend to be committed to curing, helping or empowering, and therefore enjoy feeling that they can do a good job. They are anxious to bring about change for the good of their clients. Other motivating factors for engaging in clinical education may include: passing the academic year, graduating, getting high marks and sometimes dealing with one's own pain or disability (for example, a divorcee going into marriage counselling).

Clinical practice provides an opportunity for students to test the relevance and usefulness of the theory they are taught. During students' first placements an understanding of the implications of a professional role and others' expectations of that role begins to develop. In the first placement some students will be motivated by the challenge of actually experiencing the chosen profession in reality. After at least one year (and sometimes more) of lectures, discussions, role playing and assignments in preparation for their chosen field, clinical placement provides the opportunity actually to try out some of this knowledge during interactions with colleagues and clients. Beginning social work students may glamorize their first placement because they have waited so long for it, the 'real world at last'! Medical students traditionally have not gone into hospitals until second or third year, but a current trend in medical education is to introduce an experiential strand of behavioural studies in first year. Wealthall (1994) recommends that medical students have early and ongoing contact with clients throughout their training.

Motivational factors are likely to change throughout students' clinical education experiences. Developing knowledge and understanding about their chosen profession and their own skills, attitudes and knowledge leads to a readjustment of personal and professional goals. It is likely that ongoing interactions with clients and clinical educators also have an impact on motivational influences. For example, a medical student who started out with financial goals may develop more altruistic motives as professional and personal growth occurs.

3.2.2 CLINICAL EDUCATOR MOTIVATION

People within their chosen profession have a variety of career paths they can follow. Clinicians who choose to be clinical educators increase their opportunities to meet new and challenging learning experiences with each group of students they manage. Factors influencing clinicians' decision-making about career pathways may include the impact of lecturers and clinical educators on their own learning as students and the vision they have for themselves in their chosen profession. Anderson (1988) suggests that before assuming a clinical education role, clinical educators should develop self-knowledge about their personal motivation for taking on this role.

The clinical education track can be one that provides many branches off the main path which ultimately lead back to continued learning and education for both the clinical educator and the students who learn with them. Clinical educators may want to supervize students to enhance their own professional development – another step up the ladder; access university seminars or post-graduate opportunities; update their theoretical knowledge; earn extra money or gain a title such as *student unit supervisor* or *clinical educator*. A career as a clinical educator can provide the opportunity to specialize in a specific area in the chosen professional field as well as learning about how to be an educator.

Some clinicians choose to be clinical educators because their experiences as advanced students, assisting beginning students, consolidated their own learning (Rosenthal, 1986). Others want to provide a more positive experience for students than the perception they have of their own clinical learning experience in some clinical settings. Certain professionals choose to be clinical educators because they feel the position provides the opportunity to combine continued 'hands on' skills with academic research. Some academic positions have a clinical education component (Urlich, 1992). Clinics and agencies may also require clinicians to take students or see students as human resources to help with surveys, studies, data collection and quality assurance. Other clinicians may feel professionally obligated to provide clinical opportunities, particularly if working in specialist areas and some professionals reluctantly undertake the clinical education role because placements are needed and they respond to pressure from the educational institution. With such diversity of factors motivating students and clinical educators as they come together in the clinical field, there may be several areas of normal anxiety for both.

3.3 NORMAL ANXIETY ABOUT LEARNING IN CLINICAL EDUCATION

3.3.1 STUDENT ANXIETY

The presence of anxiety in health-science students from various disciplines, whilst on clinical placements, has been reported in numerous publications (Anderson, 1988; Bogo, 1993; Chan, Carter & McAllister, 1994; Mitchell & Kampfe, 1990; Pagana, 1988; Pickering, 1989–1990; Turkoski, 1987). In general, mild levels of stress may enhance student performance, but excessive levels of anxiety may produce negative outcomes. Mitchell and Kampfe (1990) found that high levels of stress impacted on students' effectiveness, productivity, attitudes, professional behaviour and job satisfaction. Anderson (1988) purports that anxiety may 'distract from or inhibit learning' (p. 77). Social anxiety, which may be about students' feelings of adequacy in meeting their own standards or obtaining the approval of others (Nelson-Jones, 1986), can have a positive or negative impact on students' ability to learn in clinical placements.

Before a placement begins students can be expected to be anxious about:

- what will be expected of them (Pickering, 1989–1990)
- the clinical education setting itself and whether they will be upset by what they see (for example, aged people, palliative care, accident and emergency areas)
- their relationship with the clinical educator (will we like each other?)
- their ability to perform as well as other students have done or are doing
- whether the clinical educator will prefer other students, give low marks or expect too much
- whether the placement will live up to expectations and provide hoped for learning opportunities.

Such normal student anxieties can be handled in different ways, some more effectively than others, according to clinic and university resources.

(a) Reducing anxiety: Preparation for clinical placements

It is helpful if the university spends time in preparation for placements with students in a group, so that they realize these concerns are not unusual. The more aware students are of what is going to happen in a clinical placement, the more students will be able to handle these anxieties. Thus, when pre-placement interviews, clinic or agency visits are possible beforehand, students will feel more in control. With out-of-town and interstate placements, this could be difficult, but the clinic and clinical educator may be able to send information in advance, so that students can inform and prepare themselves. Background reading specific to the setting could also be provided (for example, a text on mental illness for students going into a psychiatric setting, or on palliative care and bereavement if going to a hospice). Most universities provide a *clinical education handbook* which should be made available to both students and clinical educators beforehand. When a clinic or agency provides regular ongoing placements one group of students could develop a handbook for future students. This handbook should contain specific information about clinic structures, policy and procedures, personnel, clinic mission statement, types of cases, pertinent references, and so on.

(b) Reducing anxiety: Student and clinical educator relationship

The anxieties specific to the student–clinical educator relationship will not be able to be addressed until early in the placement itself as the development of a competent working relationship takes time. This relationship can provide fertile ground for both students and clinical educators to examine the positive and negative effects of anxiety on the learning objectives for the clinical placement (Bogo, 1993). The opportunity for students or clinical educators to discuss such anxieties with peers is beneficial and could be built into the clinical education experience for both students (see Chapter 4 on peer learning) and clinical educators. For a clinic, or clinical educator with several students, there can be both formal and informal opportunities for peer discussion, but when a single student is in a clinic it is often necessary for the university to provide this forum. For example, social work students at the University of Sydney have 'placement seminars' during their block clinical placements where they can share their experiences away from the agency.

Chan, Carter and McAllister (1994), in a study about anxiety in speech therapy students, found that beginning students, in their first clinical placements, experienced anxiety which was a generalized response to the new situation. These students were aware of their lack of theory and were concerned about harming clients, despite knowing that clinical educators were responsible for total client management. This highlights the need to help students to achieve balance between the expectations they have for themselves and the expectations which are stated in course materials and assessments. For example, the use of Anderson's continuum of supervision (1988), discussed in Chapter 2, is one way to make explicit incongruencies in levels of expectation, of students and clinical educators, especially in relation to responsibility for client care. Both students and clinical educators can indicate where on Anderson's continuum they feel a student's current level of independence lies. They can then discuss the differences between their perceptions and expectations.

Chan *et al.* (1994) also reported that advanced students reported a high level of anxiety arising from factors not related to client care. It appears that concerns about client care had diminished with the acquisition of relevant theory and clinical experience. Advanced students' anxiety arose from factors that may be grouped as those that pose a threat to the student as an emerging professional. These factors included relationships with the clinical educators, the clarity of the clinical educators' expectations, the level of control in the clinic and issues about being assessed. Students in this group were close to graduation and the prospect of future employment was near. They had high expectations for themselves and probably were concerned about whether they were really 'good enough' to be entering the workplace. A mismatch between the style and level of supervision may contribute to students' anxiety. For example, a student able to function independently may have received a direct style of supervision (see Chapter 2). In our experience, students have felt disadvantaged and frustrated when they experience a mismatch in the style or level of supervision in their final placement (see Case Study 3.1).

Case Study 3.1 A mismatch in supervision level and style

Judy was a very conscientious, advanced level student, who had received excellent grades in all previous placements. Whilst on her final placement, Judy became so anxious about her ability to perform at the level and in a style acceptable to her clinical educator that she sought assistance from the director of her clinical education programme. The problem was identified as being a mismatch between Judy's sense of herself, as an emerging interdependent professional, and the clinical educator, who felt a need to keep tight control of client management. In discussions with the clinical educator, the clinical director found that the ethos of the clinic was hierarchical and staff members were not encouraged by the head of the department to make independent decisions. It was mutually decided by all stakeholders that the student would complete her commitments to the clinic but not be given a final assessment by the clinical educator.

Aspects of the assessment system (see Chapter 6) were also seen as factors contributing to the anxiety in advanced students. There was some conflict of values as students were expected to be self-directed, self-evaluating learners, but were still required to undergo mandatory external evaluation. This may possibly have resulted in students' questioning the reliability and validity of the external evaluation. The Chan *et al.* (1994) study demonstrated that anxiety related to clinical education is present throughout beginning, intermediate and advanced levels of experience. The source of this anxiety changes as students' levels of competence and personal growth change. Clinical educators therefore need to explore with each student the source of their anxiety and assess whether it is appropriate to the student's stage of development.

3.3.2 CLINICAL EDUCATORS' ANXIETY

Clinical educators may also experience normal anxiety before and during student placements. Balancing the needs of clients, to whom professionals have prime responsibility, against the learning needs of students is always challenging (Best & Franke, 1994). For example, occasionally it may be in the best interests of clients to discontinue contact with a student who is experiencing difficulties, despite the clinical educator's efforts to help the student. Consequently the subsequent feeling of failure which may be experienced by the clinical educator needs to be dealt with as constructively as possible via an established mechanism. This mechanism will usually contain elements of support by peers and senior staff so that ongoing learning will occur for the student and clinical educator.

Another source of anxiety may be when a student is unable or unwilling to fit in to an agency and to meet its norms in a professional manner (for example, by refusing to dress as required, or by inappropriately challenging the clinic's ethics). When this happens, it may cause embarrassment or even damage to the profession's image in the clinic. Consequently, clinical educators may be concerned that students' performance may be judged by clients and colleagues as a reflection of their own skills.

Clinical educators may also be anxious about the theoretical basis of their own practice (whether or not they are up-to-date with knowledge), and their ability to teach and model skills. Support from university educators, by way of provision of seminars, reading materials and support personnel with whom to discuss their task of clinical education, is helpful. As with students, group (or peer) learning and discussion amongst clinical educators is an invaluable tool for ensuring a high standard of practice and boosting the confidence of clinical educators. We have experienced one valuable model used in some hospital social work departments which is described as 'supervize the supervisor'. Here a staff supervisor, with close connections to the university, provides readings and discussion on a regular basis to all clinical educators in a group at the pace expected of the students. Thus clinical educators are able to share difficulties, make suggestions and plan strategies to cope with students' problems in a supportive educative atmosphere.

Specific anxieties may also arise in both students and clinical educators in relation to individual settings (for example, high stress areas such as Intensive Care Units), the type of patients or clients (people with mental or physical disabilities), personal experience and background (for example, a young mother working with seriously ill children), and biases or experiences (such as concern about supervising a member of the opposite sex, or an older student). Dealing with these anxieties requires open and honest dialogue between clinical educators and students, an ability to acknowledge the anxieties openly and to accept them as normal and real. Again, a forum for peer discussion, or access to a more experienced clinical educator in the clinic or university can facilitate this openness.

3.3.3 DEVELOPMENT OF SELF-AWARENESS

As the relationship between the clinical educator and the student develops and the student becomes more familiar with the clinical setting, changes will occur. These changes in attitudes, beliefs, views and skills may cause anxiety in either participant (Kadushin, 1968; Pickering, 1989–1990). This type of anxiety is normal and can be productive. Examination of the cause of the anxiety may lead to an increase in self-awareness. Egan (1990) states that, understanding clients is not enough. 'It is essential to understand your own assumptions, beliefs, values, standards, skills, strengths, weaknesses, idiosyncrasies, style of doing things ... and the ways in which these permeate your interactions with your clients' (pp 24–5). Egan goes on to say that he sees (clinical) education as an opportunity for professionals to 'grapple with personal issues, that will affect their ability to deliver services to clients. Effective training programmes (practicums) with high standards of quality are a better way of "licensing" helpers to practice than written exams' (p. 25).

Pickering (1989–1990) defines growth as 'Moving beyond stability, seeking change, and gradually becoming more comfortable with one's self and with one's place in the world' (p. 23). Pickering further states that the 'Supervisory process as an opportunity and reality for growth is undisputed' (p. 23).

Both students and clinical educators may have realistic concerns about their beliefs, prejudices, strengths and weaknesses as they work together in the supervisory relationship. It is essential for both to be open, honest and non-judgemental, and for the clinical educator to give appropriate feedback and invite self-disclosure when there appear to be difficulties for the student. We believe that increased self-awareness and personal growth will only occur in open non-judgemental relationships.

In summary, anxiety is a healthy basis for growth and self-awareness development in students during their clinical experience. Clinical educators would be perturbed if students had no concerns at all before beginning a placement or throughout a placement. When these anxieties are openly acknowledged and discussed, they become a springboard for further learning. If anxiety is denied and ignored, students are more likely to engage in surface learning (Brown, 1983), perform poorly in the placement, be less helpful to clients and perhaps less sure whether they have chosen the right profession (Mitchell & Kampfe, 1990). Dialogue and information-sharing between people from the clinic and university and between student and clinical educator hold the key to the satisfactory resolution of the anxiety. If anxiety is managed constructively then the student is able to move beyond it and begin to learn and develop a professional self.

3.4 DEVELOPING THE CLINICAL EDUCATOR ROLE

Beginning to supervize students on clinical placement is just as big a milestone for the clinician as handling one's first client alone, but this fact is often overlooked by both the university and the clinic! Just as a student needs to be self-aware when working with clients, so should the clinical educator accept his or her own anxieties and limitations and look for support in the new venture. We believe the university needs to provide detailed information about expectations of students and learning objectives for students at the different stages of clinical work and the theoretical material they have covered in their course to date. Methods of evaluating student progress in clinical settings should be supported by seminars, readings and contact with university educators. These mechanisms of support need to be more accessible for beginning clinical educators and those who have students exhibiting difficulties in a placement.

3.5 ESTABLISHING LEARNING CONTRACTS

A learning contract is one way of mapping the essential learning processes that must occur to achieve learning objectives (Ladyshewsky, 1995). Establishing a learning contract is one way of documenting the expectations, objectives, process and outcomes of professional development for students and clinical educators. We encourage clinical educators and students to negotiate the contents of the learning contract for each placement. If the formulation of the contract is not a negotiated process, the student may not take ownership of the learning objectives stated in the contract. The process of developing the contract provides excellent opportunities for clinical educators to provide information about the clinic, their expectations for the student and their clinical education philosophy. This process also provides the opportunity for students to give clinical educators information about their current academic status and their previous clinical experience.

The implementation of learning contracts as part of clinical education has many advantages for clinical educators. The following list of advantages were adapted from Pratt and Magill (1983). Learning contracts:

- instill personal responsibility for learning
- focus the clinical educator's energy towards specific students' learning needs
- define roles, responsibilities and expectations
- enhance communication and the quality of the relationship between students and clinical educators
- increase the quality of feedback since it focuses on what students want to learn.

Additionally, learning contracts can provide a structure for the working relationship between students and clinical educators. Thus, the contract is not only a useful way of exploring needs, establishing goals, dividing responsibilities and evaluating learning, but it can also be supportive and reassuring in spelling out the expectations each has of the other. It is beyond the scope of this chapter to discuss specific information about what to include in learning contracts and how to negotiate the contents and evaluate the outcomes of learning contracts. There are many texts and publications available which cover this topic in detail, for example Laycock and Stephenson (1994) and Boud (1992).

The discussion in this chapter, so far, has focused on the relationship between students and clinical educators as the primary facilitator of professional development. The next section discusses other influences on professional development. The process of personal and moral growth while moving from student to professional is explored in some detail.

3.6 PROFESSIONAL SOCIALIZATION

Professionalism refers to a set of values, attitudes, knowledge and skills which are displayed within the culture of a profession by practising professionals (White & Ewan, 1991). Students are expected to gain the knowledge and skills necessary to practise as well as become a professional during their training. The process of becoming a professional is referred to as 'professional socialization' (Ewan, 1988; White & Ewan, 1991).

Ewan (1988) suggests that professional socialization is part of a 'hidden curriculum' (p. 86). She suggests that students receive verbal and non-verbal messages from sources such as clinical educators, clients, other professionals and university educators about professionalism. We also feel that professional socialization is part of a 'hidden curriculum' because often little is taught in university courses about components of professional socialization such as ethics (Resnick, 1993). At the same time, in our opinion, professional socialization is rarely directly assessed. For example, students' skills in developing rapport with clients may be assessed but their ability to discuss the ethical issues involved in client management with clinical educators is not. Ewan (1988) suggests that clinical educators can assist students to develop professionalism by making the hidden curriculum explicit. This may involve discussing clinical educators' own definitions of professionalism with students.

Any discussion of professional socialization must include ideas about what the components of professionalism are. Students do not become professionals simply by learning theory or completing clinical experiences. A review of the literature relevant to the health sciences suggests that there are four components of professionalism. The component frequently identified is *technical competence* (Higgs, 1993; Purtillo & Cassel; 1989; Wealthall, 1994). A second component frequently identified is *professional interpersonal skills*. This encompasses the communication skills, values and attitudes of the professional (Andre, 1992; Corey, Corey & Callanan, 1993; Wealthall, 1994). The third component is *knowledge of professional standards of conduct* (Corey *et al.*, 1993; Ewan, 1988; White & Ewan, 1991). The fourth component of professionalism is *ethical competence* (Corey *et al.*, 1993; Davis, 1989; Purtillo & Cassel, 1989). Davis (1989) states that professionalism is essentially about moral obligation to those for whom professionals care. Simply put, professionals are obligated to make decisions in the best interest of their clients. The next section discusses how students become 'socialized' in each of these components.

(a) Technical competence

Technical competence is achieved through lectures, tutorials, practicals and supervized clinical experience. Typically, academic and clinical assessment focus predominantly on developing skills in this component (see Chapter 6). Shuval (1980) reports that technical competence rather than personal growth in a professional role is the objective of medical education. However, as Ewan (1988) asserts 'Technical competence does not ensure the ability to perform as a competent professional' (p. 87).

(b) Professional interpersonal skills

The second component is development of professional interpersonal skills. White and Ewan (1991) suggest that students bring their own personalities, dispositions and past experiences to the clinical setting and consequently give their own personal interpretation to the role of the professional. This component is about developing a clinical style which is comfortable for the individual, and facilitative and effective for clients. Throughout their clinical education students trial different styles in an attempt to find what suits them best. Some students may experiment with being authoritarian, exuberant, distant or vague. Careful feedback from the clinical educator or guided self-evaluation (see Chapter 4) about the impact of their interaction on their clients will help the student assess their style. Clinical educators often find this the most difficult area in which to give feedback (see section on feedback in this chapter). Students and professionals who do not develop a professional self-image may be at risk of professional dissatisfaction (Ellard, 1974; Schwartz, Swartzhurg, Lieb & Slaby, 1978). For this reason it is important that clinical educators provide thoughtful feedback about this area of personal and professional development (see Case Study 3.2).

Case Study 3.2 Encouraging students to develop a range of clinical styles

Susan is an intermediate level student. She describes herself as reserved and shy. Her clinical educator thinks that her interaction with a 4-year-old child is flat and unmotivating for the child. She discusses this with Susan who agrees to attempt to make her interaction with the child more exuberant and energetic. They compare videos of Susan's next treatment session with the previous week's session. They specifically collect data on the child's response rate and clinical progress. The child had progressed faster in the second session. Susan reported that she felt unnatural and 'fake' during the session and found it difficult to maintain this style of interaction even though she could see that it had benefited the child. Susan's clinical educator encouraged her to continue experimenting with her clinical style until she found one she was comfortable with and which was effective for the client.

(c) Professional standards of conduct

The third component, learning professional standards of conduct, generally occurs through awareness and knowledge of the professions' code of ethics. Teaching of ethical decision-making has received more emphasis in disciplines such as medicine, social work and occupational therapy than disciplines such as speech therapy and audiology (Pannbacker, Middleton & Lass, 1994; Resnick, 1993). Various authors have suggested that students need to be exposed to the theory of ethics and codes of ethics early and frequently during their professional education (Green, 1986; Reichert & Caruso, 1991).

Some standards contained in ethical codes do not require personal interpretation. For example, in the United States the code of ethics of the National Association of Social Workers (1990) states 'The social worker should provide clients with accurate and complete information regarding the extent and nature of services available to them' (p. 431). Other sections of this code however, do require personal interpretation; for example 'The social worker should afford clients reasonable access to any official social work records concerning them' (p. 432). The ethic pertaining to 'reasonable access' requires individual interpretation. When standards of conduct require interpretation the fourth component of professionalism becomes important.

(d) Ethical competence

Developing ethical competence (Purtillo & Cassel, 1989) involves developing a personal interpretation of the professional code of ethics where it is required. Students need to develop a good understanding and sense of the fundamental philosophical principles underlying most codes of ethics: autonomy, beneficence, justice, fidelity and non-maleficence (Beauchamp & Childress, 1989). Resnick (1993) suggests that the emphasis of ethics teaching should be directed towards avoidance of ethical problems rather than solving ethical problems. Stewart Gonzalez and Coleman (1994) report that students prefer to learn about ethics from student-led case studies of ethical situations rather than outside assignments and lectures. It is also helpful for students to observe clinical educators applying ethical principles in clinical settings and to have an opportunity to discuss ethical issues with clinical educators. Andre (1992) also suggests that students need 'time and scope for reflection' (p. 148), if they are to achieve moral growth.

Professional socialization may be conceived as a process in which students experiment with and test out their clinical skills, professional standards, ethical interpretations and professional personae. The notion of professional socialization may initially raise many concerns with students. They may interpret it as a *cloning process* in which clinical educators or groups of professionals seek to recreate themselves. We have found that discussion of the four components of professional socialization and emphasis on the development of individual interpretation of ethics, competencies and professional role may allay students' concerns about *cloning*.

3.6.1 INFLUENCES ON PROFESSIONAL SOCIALIZATION

Ewan (1988) suggests that professional socialization occurs through 'specialized social interactions in which students and the people with whom they come into contact develop expectations of themselves and others in the clinical context and respond to each other with those expectations in mind. Eventually, responses develop into behaviour patterns and ways of perceiving situations which accord with society's expectations of their role' (p. 85). Ewan is suggesting that professional socialization occurs through interaction with others. These interactions may be between student and client, student and university educator, student and clinical educator, student and student (Ewan, 1988) or between a student and another professional.

(a) Student–client interactions

What do clients expect when they visit a professional? Factors which may influence a client's expectations may include their cultural background, socio-economic status, educational level, the context in which the health care is delivered and the amount and type of previous contact with health professionals (Ewan, 1988). It is likely they expect a clean, tidy, neatly dressed person who interacts confidently with them at an appropriate level. They expect the person to know what they are talking about, to be organized, efficient, mature and thorough. They probably also expect the person to be warm, friendly and courteous. They may also expect the professional to have excellent communication skills. Ewan (1988) states that minimum expectations of patients of doctors include that they should be 'Competent, up to date, conscious of environmental and community influences, person centered, sympathetic, able to attend to some emotional needs, willing to foster long-term relationships, be family centered and willing to explain and share information' (p. 10).

What happens if the clinician or student does not meet the client's expectations? Perhaps the client will have little confidence in the clinician's abilities or perhaps he or she will feel that the person is unprofessional. Others may simply adjust their expectations of what a professional will be like.

The extract below is from a discussion paper we give to our beginning level speech therapy students to raise their awareness about professionalism (Lincoln, 1995). Our main aim is stimulate students thinking about the client's expectations of the student and about the students' previous experience of professional and unprofessional behaviour.

What do students expect of clients? This very much depends on the setting in which the students are placed and the caseload with which they are working. The individuals' values, beliefs, attitudes and biases will also influence their expectations. Corey *et al.* (1993) suggest that counselling professionals must be willing to focus on themselves as a person and as a professional, as well as on their clients. They suggest that professionals need a high level of self-awareness to ensure their own needs and biases do not obstruct the growth of the client. Similarly, professionals' expectations of clients may be influenced by the professionals' own needs and biases. In our experience, beginning level students tend to expect clients to be reliable, diligent and grateful. However, clients may not fulfill these expectations. We spend time in early clinical conferences exploring with students the place of the treatment in clients' lives, families and communities to help them gain perspectives other than their own on clients' attitudes and behaviours.

Extract from a discussion paper on professionalism (Lincoln, 1995)

'Generally clients will come to have a view of students as professionals if they are able to do the following things:

- Be punctual for client appointments.
- Develop rapport with clients but don't allow this to become a "friendship" type relationship [see Chapter 2].
- Make efficient and effective use of clinical time.
- Know your professional boundaries and be able to refer to other professions when appropriate.

- Have knowledge of other professions so referrals are appropriate.
- Be aware of appropriate self-disclosure.
- Demonstrate your professionalism by maintaining confidentiality, being aware of legal requirements, advocating the rights of clients and always showing concern and respect for clients.
- Be aware of your methods of communication and why you are using particular techniques.'

(b) Student–university educator interactions

University educators provide a role model as they lecture to students. Not only do they teach information and skills, they also communicate their own interpretation of what it means to be professional and the associated attitudes and values that go with their concept of professionalism. University educators also give models of ways of talking about topics and disorders. Students may draw on these models when they are required to talk to other professionals about clients and their disorders.

(c) Student–clinical educator interactions

Clinical educators interact with students in 'real' environments; hence, they may possibly be the greatest influence on the professional socialization of students. They provide a role model in the workplace; students are able to observe 'professionalism' in action (see Chapter 2). Green (1988) found that nursing students chose staff nurses or head nurses as preferred role models before clinical nursing instructors and university teachers. In a clinical setting, students observe the way clinical educators interact with other professionals, clients and peers. This includes the language, body language, level of formality, tone and emotional content of the interaction. Students can be encouraged to seek clarification from their clinical educators about specific interactions they observe and to ask 'how come' the clinical educator chose to interact in the way they did. Students may also observe how clinical educators introduce themselves and how they address clients. By observing several clinical educators throughout their professional education, students are able to compare clinical educators and formulate a 'professional persona' which they are comfortable with. Ewan (1988) suggests students need to experience, discuss and evaluate professional behaviour 'in order to extract personal meaning which can be incorporated into their own professional self image' (p. 87).

(d) Student interaction with other staff and agencies

Part of owning a professional role is feeling comfortable with it and therefore being confident, appropriately assertive, respectful and polite when interacting with those outside of the profession (this may be anybody from the cleaner to the medical director). Examples of professional behaviour include: polite requests to clerical staff for assistance, giving a cleaner a polite but clear message that it is necessary to clean the sink in your office each night, or communicating standards of practice to managers. Clinical educators should endeavour to observe these everyday interactions and look for signs of the development of professionalism in their students. Clinical educators should also provide opportunities for students to observe them in such interactions (for example, have students attend meetings and case conferences with the clinical educator, have students listen-in on phone calls to other agencies).

(e) Student–student interaction

As students may all have different clinical experiences throughout their education, discussion with other students will enable them to tap others' interpretations of the professional role (see Chapter 4 on peer learning). Wealthall (1994) suggests that 'peer exchange can give students feedback about the range of attitudes within a group and group pressure will give indications to students about what the standard, acceptable or desirable range of attitudes/behaviours in a particular situation is' (p. 32). Students can also demonstrate professionalism in the way they interact with each other. In a broad sense, this may include making sure clinic or interview rooms are left tidy and equipment is returned so other students are not inconvenienced. It may involve providing sensitive peer support and facilitating others learning through their interaction with them. It involves showing respect and acceptance of students from other cultures, as well as to those from their own (see Chapter 9).

3.6.2 PROFESSIONAL SOCIALIZATION: A CONTINUUM OF PERSONAL AND PROFESSIONAL GROWTH

Professional socialization undoubtedly occurs along a continuum of growth. As we have discussed, through exposure to clients, university educators, clinical educators, other professionals and fellow students, students learn what it means to be professional and begin to develop their own professional personae and personal interpretation of the relevant code of ethics. Concrete and specific feedback from clinical educators can assist students in their development. Feedback to beginning students may be about professional presentation, ways of talking to clients and other professionals, and issues around confidentiality. Feedback to more advanced students may seek to challenge their thinking on ethical issues or may seek to increase their awareness of their own expectations, attitudes and biases. Perry (1970) suggests that students' intellectual and ethical development progresses from seeing issues in polar terms (for example, right-wrong, good-bad) to seeing issues as contextualized and subtle. This suggests that students are better able to cope with diversity of opinion and diversity of contexts as they move along a continuum of growth. Developing self-awareness, confidence in their professional role and the development of personal ethics are all hallmarks of students' professional growth.

3.7 ETHICAL ISSUES IN CLINICAL EDUCATION

3.7.1 ISSUES FOR CLINICAL EDUCATORS

Clinical educators are ultimately responsible, both legally and ethically, for the actions of their students. They are responsible for protecting the welfare of the client, student, public and profession (Corey *et al.*, 1993; White, 1989). They are bound to behave ethically towards the clients and students they are supervizing. This can sometimes present some unique ethical dilemmas to which there are no clear-cut solutions. Identification and discussion of the dilemmas with colleagues may result in some clarification of what ethical behaviour to adopt. The list below includes some potential ethical dilemmas in clinical education.

Potential ethical dilemmas for clinical educators

- Communicating information about a student's past clinical performance and difficulties to a subsequent clinical educator
- Confidentiality in the client–student relationship – is there ever a case when a student should not pass confidential information on to their clinical educator in full?
- The question of how voluntary a client's 'consent' is to being seen by a student
- Handing a client that you have been seeing yourself over to a student
- Advising students on personal crises in their lives

Clinical educators are also faced with the challenge of teaching students about ethical behaviour. The list below is a summary of Best and Franke's (1994) suggestions for teaching students ethical behaviour in clinical settings. These suggestions are primarily about clinical educators providing excellent models of ethical behaviour (see also Case Study 3.3).

Suggestions for teaching ethical behaviour (Best & Franke, 1994)

- Respect student individuality, privacy and dignity.
- Provide a positive role model.
- Include ethical behaviour in student assessment.
- Continually reflect on your own teaching and clinical practice.
- Do not abuse the inherent power of the student–clinical educator relationship with romantic, intimate or business relations.

Case Study 3.3 Respecting individuality

A clinical educator was concerned about a student who presented on the first day of her clinical placement in a conservative neighbourhood wearing a nose ring and many earrings in each ear. The clinical educator was concerned about the student's professional presentation and the reaction of the parents and children she would be working with. It was evident during the student's first few clinical sessions that she had difficulty establishing rapport with parents and presented as lacking in confidence and assertiveness. The clinical educator decided to discuss her concerns about the student's lack of rapport with the client and parents. During the course of the discussion the clinical educator discussed with the student the potential impact her appearance may have on parents and children and whether this could be related to her difficulties in developing rapport. They also discussed strategies for developing rapport and developed a learning goal to specifically target this area. The student continued to wear her nose ring and earrings and her clinical educator accepted that it was her right to do so.

3.7.2 ISSUES FOR STUDENTS

Being a student can also present some unique ethical dilemmas. While all students are guided by the code of ethics of the profession they will be entering, issues specifically related to being a student may not be covered under the appropriate code. An example of this is a student being asked for professional advice by an acquaintance – is it unethical for the student to provide advice? Another example is if a client discloses information to a student which he or she requests is not passed on to the clinical educator – to whom is the student ethically responsible, the client or clinical educator? Appendix 3.1 contains extracts from the code of ethics of the Australian Association of Speech and Hearing (1986). Beneath each ethic listed in the appendix are behaviours which relate specifically to being a student clinician (Lincoln, 1995). These behaviours were developed in consultation with students from all years of the four-year bachelor programme at the School of Communication Disorders, University of Sydney. Davis (1989) also contains a 'Students Draft Ethics Policy' which was created by the students of the University of Miami School of Medicine. Awareness and reference to the version of the code of ethics presented in Appendix 3.1 in discussion with students has assisted us to make the code of ethics 'real' for students.

In order to help students develop professional skills, it is necessary for clinical educators to have competent communication skills. Similarly, in order for students to help clients they also need to develop effective communication skills. The following section discusses the communication skills needed in clinical education and the application of these skills when giving and receiving feedback.

3.8 COMMUNICATION SKILLS NEEDED IN CLINICAL EDUCATION

The communication skills required in clinical settings are different from those required in other settings, consequently students need to become aware of all aspects of their own and others' communication. Pickering (1987) suggests that 'supervision is a context for metacommunication, and the limitations on the richness of what is discussed come only from the participants themselves. The person-focused nature of the discourse, as well as of the process *per se*, suggests the importance of communicating about communication' (p. 126) (see Chapter 7). By engaging in *metacommunication* (talking about talking) students and clinical educators can increase their awareness about communication.

We believe that students' learning is extended when they are offered the opportunity to improve their communication and interaction skills through increased awareness, knowledge and practice with both clinical educators and clients. This view is also shared by many others who write about the value of using the student–clinical educator relationship as a forum for the development of interpersonal communication skills (Bamford, 1981; Blumberg, 1977; Bogo, 1993; Farmer & Farmer, 1989; Pickering, 1985, 1989–1990). It is important for students and clinical educators to have shared information about the communication skills that are required in the clinical setting. Discussion with students about these principles of communication listed below (based on Pickering, 1987), that are felt to be of particular relevance to clinical education, may facilitate the development of shared knowledge and further develop an effective working relationship between students and clinical educators.

Principles in communication (based on Pickering, 1987)

- Communication is complex.
- Communication is a 'process' not a 'thing'.
- Communication is circular not linear.
- Meaning, ideas, and information are conveyed through a variety of message systems, both verbal and non-verbal.
- Communication involves the total personality.
- Messages may have multiple levels of meaning.
- The message sent is not necessarily the message received.
- The self is created and maintained through interpersonal transactions.

The principles of communication listed above state that communication is a process. Whenever we are with another person we are communicating verbally and non-verbally. It is impossible not to communicate, even silence is a communication, although it may be difficult to know the meaning of silence. Clinical educators have the challenge of providing a climate that encourages, first, the exploration of communication, second, the recognition of assumptions and, third, the skills to seek clarification (to say 'I don't understand what you mean, would you please give me more specific information'). This specific information may relate to feelings, experiences or behaviours.

Clinical educators can use, and thereby model communication strategies which facilitate clarification of the views and issues being discussed. In our experience, based on feedback received from students, we believe that students 'flourish' in a learning environment where congruence exists between the content and the manner of discussion. Pickering (1989–1990) and Bogo (1993) believe that the communication skills needed for effective clinical education are the same as those used in effective client management. Consequently, the interpersonal communication skills which are developed through the clinical educator–student relationship will ultimately benefit clients.

Another important area for clinical educators and students to explore together is that of communication *difference*. The American Speech-Language and Hearing Association (ASHA) has taken initiatives to address the needs of persons from culturally diverse backgrounds in the revision of its accreditation and certification of student programmes (Campbell, 1994). Campbell states, 'There is a need for knowledge regarding cultural diversity as it pertains to all aspects of human communication and its disorders' (p. 41). The difference may be of culture, gender or age in either students or clinical educators or both. Differences can enrich our experience of working with students and clients, but unless the difference is recognized it may hinder communicative competence. For example, communication differences have been reported by students from Asian countries studying courses in the health sciences in Australia (McAllister, Chan, Rosenthal & Stewart, 1994). Some of the major problems reported were understanding Australian idiom, slang and humour, and problems with their speech being understood by clients and clinical educators. Clinical educators need to develop competent cross-cultural communication skills for working with clients and students (see Chapter 9 and Case Study 3.4).

Case Study 3.4

A social work student of Asian background complained of difficulties in looking directly at his clients. He discussed with his clinical educator that this is considered very ill-mannered and rude in his culture. However he is aware that Australian clients may perceive him as inattentive or disinterested.

3.8.1 A CLIENT-FOCUSED APPROACH TO CLINICAL EDUCATION

A central goal of clinical education is the integration of theory and practice. This includes the application of broad areas of knowledge to specific client problems. The fundamental responsibility of clinical educators is client care and as Hagler, Case and Des Rocher (1989) state 'the tertiary and ultimate indicator of supervisory effectiveness is probably client change' (p. 155). Students learning to develop options for client management in a clinical setting need to be *client-focused*. We believe students must aim to increase their skills in diagnosing client disorders and planning client management by observing the effect of themselves and others on clients' behaviours. Further, they must develop awareness of the feelings present in the clinician–client relationship. However, as beginning clinicians, they are often *self-focused*, and may be totally immersed in the plans and goals they have for a session, almost, at times to the exclusion of the client. It is important to remember that intermediate and advanced students may feel like and behave like beginning students when they are in a clinic placement or learning experience which is new or different. Fuller and Brown (1975) hypothesize that student teachers progress through three levels of awareness. Beginning students are at a 'survival' or self-orientated level, the second level is reached when an interest in teaching issues develops and the third level is when concern for pupils are the primary focus. A hallmark of the development of clinical competence in students appears to be when a shift from being self-focused to client-focused occurs.

(a) The benefits of a client-focused approach

We believe that a *client-focused* approach to clinical education provides a framework that is safe, empowers the learner, encourages independent and interdependent learning and results in the learner producing a range of options for problem-solving that is uniquely his or her own. A safe working relationship with their clinical educators allows students to apply theory to practice, as the focus is on the interaction between students and clients rather than on students' performance *per se*.

A client-focused approach encourages independent learning which is related to specific interactions. When clinical educators make observations and comments and raise questions about the client or student interaction, rather than providing instruction or prescriptions for change, independent learning is promoted. Students, focused on clients' needs, move back and forth between practical experiences with clients, feedback received from clinical educators and academic knowledge. This new awareness is then applied to the management of clients. This cycle of behaviour encourages 'the development of self-evaluation, and problem solving on the part of the individual being supervised' (American Speech-Language and Hearing Association, 1985, p. 57). This client-focused environment encourages students to be autonomous learners who take initiative for setting their own goals and diagnosing their learning needs (Knowles, 1990).

3.9 FEEDBACK

3.9.1 THE NATURE OF FEEDBACK IN CLINICAL EDUCATION

In recent times, universities have required their students to provide feedback on their courses at both the micro level of individual subjects such as clinical education, and at the macro level of the course as a whole. We believe that it is important for students to have a wide view of feedback and perceive it as a normal and routine part of their learning experience. Students benefit from a learning climate that states explicitly that feedback is reciprocal between students and educators (Bogo, 1993; Pickering,

1989–1990). If students only receive feedback from their clinical educators, with no opportunity to provide feedback to them about their clinical education experiences, they may perceive the experience as judgemental rather than educational. Bogo (1993) states 'That it is not unusual for students to feel wary about the power differential' (p. 30) between students and clinical educators. This power differential is emphasized if feedback is a one-way process.

The opportunity for students to experience a variety of feedback approaches from various sources will enhance their learning and encourage movement through the stages of the continuum of independence (Anderson, 1988) (see Chapter 2). The following are examples of some formal feedback procedures in which we have participated.

(a) Client feedback to the student and clinical educator

Appendix 3.2 contains examples from a client feedback form that was developed at the Communication Disorders Treatment and Research Clinic, The University of Sydney. Through this form, clients provide feedback to their student clinicians on the service they receive. Students increase their understanding of the value of giving and receiving feedback if they have the opportunity to respond to feedback from their clients whilst they are still treating them.

(b) Student feedback to university staff

The purpose of the procedure described in Appendix 3.3 is to provide students with an opportunity to reflect on the supervision they received during their placement, and then to provide feedback to the university staff member in charge of their clinical subjects. The feedback is collated, passed on and acted on as appropriate to ensure quality in clinical subjects.

(c) Student feedback to the clinical educator (see Appendix 3.4)

Student self-appraisal (McLeod, in press) provides a structured format for the giving and receiving of feedback between students and clinical educators. It is a procedure designed to facilitate mutual planning within a clinical education placement by eliciting collaborative feedback from students and clinical educators. The student self-appraisal procedure involves a structured discussion between students and clinical educators about their clinical placement. The aim of the discussion is for students to generate a list of goals for themselves, and suggestions for their clinical educator. A list of accomplishments during the clinical placement is also generated. McLeod (in press) surveyed clinical educators and found that this procedure is a valuable tool for feedback between students and clinical educators. Tiberius, Sackin, Slingerland, Jubas, Bell and Matlow (1989) discuss a comparison of different feedback procedures. They found that staff physicians improved their teaching performance and sustained it over successive student groups when they received feedback via a supervisory rating scale and by small group discussion. They found that feedback via the rating scale only was less effective in improving teaching performance.

We believe that learning about the concept of feedback, and its place in adult learning should occur prior to students' entry into clinical courses. Opportunity for discussion needs to be provided about the differences between providing anonymous feedback as a class member to a lecturer and providing feedback about an individual clinical educator with whom the student has a close working relationship. In many instances, clinical educators will have the dual responsibility of providing ongoing feedback to students about their clinical skills and also *assessing* students' performance. Therefore, it is essential that students have the opportunity to express concerns and fears they may have about the dual role of clinical educators. Students who have marked problems with issues related to power and authority can find giving and receiving feedback difficult (see Chapter 7).

(d) Student feedback

Students can be encouraged to give feedback on their own clinical practice as another way of taking responsibility for effective client management and for their own learning (see self-evaluation in Chapter 4). Alternative methods of feedback include peer evaluation (Lincoln & McAllister, 1993), self-evaluation (Knowles, 1990) and are also discussed in Chapter 4.

3.9.2 THE PURPOSE OF FEEDBACK

Students need to understand the purpose of feedback and to learn to give positive and negative feedback and to receive positive and negative feedback about their clinical practice. Deep learning (Brown, 1983) will occur as students reflect on their feelings about the feedback experience. Beginning students may benefit from participating in groups where they have the opportunity to hear advanced students giving feedback to their peers and clinical educators. With intermediate and advanced students it is important that students explore their experiences of giving and receiving feedback in previous placements with each new clinical educator. During orientation to the placement, students and clinical educators ascertain students' previous experience and knowledge of the feedback process. The type of the feedback individual students perceive they need to meet their learning goals is identified through discussion of what aided or did not aid their learning in previous placements. Some ideas about the purpose of feedback which may be useful in small group discussions are listed below. Clinical educators can also clarify with students their own personal position to giving and receiving feedback in the specific placement by discussing the list below.

Purpose of feedback

- To let students know how their interactions with clients and others are perceived by the clinical educator in the clinical setting
- To increase the awareness of the effect of one person's behaviour, verbal and non-verbal, on another person
- To provide observation on effective and ineffective modes of interpersonal communicative behaviours
- To increase awareness of effective modes of behaviour (for example, teaching strategies, behaviour modification strategies and communication skills)
- To provide factual information and access to resources for beginning clinicians or advanced clinicians assessing/treating a new client group
- To assist students to evaluate their progress in relation to their stated clinical learning goals in a specific placement
- To provide written or verbal comments on the content and process of clinical interactions
- To provide specific information on a specific technique and its effectiveness with a target population
- To give feedback on adherence to scientific principles in work practices

---

Feedback and evaluation from the clinical educator to the student has been the primary method used to facilitate students' growth and learning (Anderson, 1988) and will be discussed as a way of facilitating understanding and learning between the *triad* of client, student and clinical educator. We contend that it is the very individuality of each client that beginning student clinicians find threatening. They often want to make the client fit the treatment. In contrast, advanced students find the individuality of clients to be challenging and this extends their learning. Feedback provides an opportunity to address the uniqueness of the client and student pair, and can promote students' feelings of responsibility for client management whilst ensuring the client receives excellent care. All participants increase their skills and options for understanding identified problems. Feedback to beginning students may be concrete, specific and factual, based on observation of behaviours, whilst feedback to advanced students may be in the form of philosophical questions about individual styles of relating to clients.

3.9.3 BOUNDARIES WITHIN THE FEEDBACK PROCESS

Boundaries may relate to both the physical and territorial aspects of the placement, as well as to the dynamics of the relationship between students and clinical educators. It is important for clinical educators to introduce the concept of boundaries in the early stages of establishing an effective working relationship with students. During orientation to the clinic placement, clinical educators provide information about the 'rules' related to the administrative procedures for the clinic as a whole and those specifically relating to students attending the clinic. Some of this information will relate to physical boundaries; for example, the specific room allocated to students and those rooms not available for student use. Other boundaries will relate to availability and emotional space for both students and clinical educators.

Clinical educators may choose to provide reading material for students on boundaries if it is part of the nature of their work and if this is a possible issue in client–student interactions (for example, Stone & Olswang, 1989; Zebrowski & Schum, 1993). Clinical educators may make clear to students that discussion about interactions between them may provide opportunities for extending the students' understanding of their interpersonal style and skills. The opportunity for this type of learning experience needs to be negotiated, and is dependent on the stage of students' clinical experience.

(a) Negotiation of boundaries

To create a *safe* learning environment, boundaries need to be negotiated between each individual student and clinical educator and they need to be flexible over the life of the placement. In discussing boundaries in relation to counselling, Stone and Olswang (1989) state 'in order for relationships to be satisfying and successful, participants must share an understanding of what material, events and experiences will or will not be part of the interaction' (p. 27). Discussion about boundaries should continue throughout placements and participants can alert each other when they feel someone may have overstepped the boundary, be this student, client or clinical educator.

Clinical educators can build into the feedback process mechanisms that provide boundaries in the clinical educator–student–client relationship, thus giving a structure which allows risk taking by all participants. The clinical educator states clearly to the student that principles relating to the ethical management of clients will be adhered to at all times and are considered to be within the boundaries of the working relationship. That is, all material, events and the student's experiences relating to client management are considered to be within the boundaries of the feedback process and will be discussed.

(b) Provision of boundaries within client-focused feedback

A client-focused approach draws a boundary around the content and process of the student–client interaction. Client-focused feedback provides opportunities for clinical educators to give feedback on actual behaviours related to intention (Pickering, 1989–1990) and to address assumptions made by the student within the context of the student–client interaction. This approach may reduce the potentially personal nature of feedback, as it is reframed in relation to client needs rather than student behaviours.

3.9.4 CONSTRUCTIVE OR DESTRUCTIVE FEEDBACK

Feedback can be either constructive or destructive, depending on whether it stems from the needs of the person giving the feedback or the person receiving the feedback. *Good* feedback is given with the honest intention of providing assistance and increased understanding for the receiver. The aim is for the receiver to find the feedback useful in developing clinical skills and interpersonal effectiveness. The person giving the feedback should be clear about his or her reasons for providing the feedback and have established acceptable boundaries with the receiver.

Bad feedback stems from the needs of the person giving the feedback rather than the needs of the receiver. It can be punishing and judgemental. On occasions, the person receiving the feedback may have a sense of being attacked personally because it goes outside the established boundaries. This feedback is not helpful and does not provide the receiver with further useable knowledge about their clinical or interpersonal skills. This type of feedback is likely to cause distance between the student and clinical educator and does not aid student learning. The subject of feedback is discussed further in Chapter 7.

3.10 CONCLUSION

Students and clinical educators approach the clinical education task with similarities and differences in their basic motivations. We contend that students and clinical educators' motivations will influence the course of their professional development. Throughout professional development experiences, students are socialized into their chosen profession. Part of this socialization process is the development of ethical competence and professional communication skills. Clinical educators in clinical settings are influential in helping students develop competence in these areas.

We believe that an ideal learning environment is one that nurtures a student's abilities to take risks and learn from their 'mistakes'. It is also an environment that values students' ability to be self-directed learners who develop and carry-out their own learning contracts. In our experience, the negotiation of boundaries within a specific placement, and client-focused feedback play an essential part in the successful clinical education of all students.

APPENDIX 3.1: EXCERPTS FROM SPEECH PATHOLOGY STUDENT CODE OF ETHICS (LINCOLN, 1995)

Note the sections in italics are from the Australian Association of Speech and Hearing code of ethics (1986).

1 *Members shall use every resource available, including referral to other professionals, to provide the best possible service.*
   - It is the students' responsibility to provide their clinical educator with all client information so joint decisions can be made about this information.
   - Students should maintain close contact with their clinical educator at all times regarding client welfare and management.
   - Students should not assume that their clinical educator has observed all of every interaction and therefore should pass on new and important information which may arise in each session.
   - Students shall accept responsibility for and strive to achieve the best possible clinical result for each client. This includes being well prepared and clear about rationales behind management decisions and techniques.
2 *Members shall not reveal to unauthorised persons any professional or personal information from the client served professionally, unless required by law or unless necessary to protect the welfare of the client or the community.*
   - Students shall be vigilant about maintaining confidentiality. For example, video and audio tapes of sessions should not be played to people other than those directly involved in client care.
   - Client reports, especially those that are word processed should not be accessible to others. For example, do not leave client reports on the hard disk of a shared computer.
   - Do not use clients' full names when discussing them with peers.
   - Do not remove any identifying information about clients from the clinic area (for example, files).
3 *Members shall maintain adequate records of professional services rendered.*
   - All reports should be completed promptly.
   - All progress notes and file entries should be complete and up-to-date.

APPENDIX 3.2: CLIENT FEEDBACK FORM

All clients and students attending the Communication Disorders Treatment and Research Clinic at The University of Sydney are asked to independently rate the areas listed below on a five-point scale. The students compare their ratings with the client's and following discussion with the clinical educator they may address any identified problem areas with the client.

The following are some of the areas rated on the feedback form:

- the client or caregiver's understanding of the communciation disorder (for example, I understand the nature of my/my child's communication disorder)
- the amount of the improvement that has occurred over a specified time period (for example, I think my/my child's communication disorder has improved over the last ... months)
- the active listening skills of the student (for example, The student clinician listened to me when I talked about my/my child's communication disorder)
- effective use of clinic time (for example, I think the student clinician made effective use of therapy time).

The provision of a formal feedback system for clients is seen as a way of encouraging them to provide feedback to students and clinical educators throughout the semester.

APPENDIX 3.3: CLINICAL EDUCATOR FEEDBACK FORM

All students in the School of Communication Disorders at The University of Sydney provide feedback about their clinical educators to the Director of Clinical Education at the end of each clinical placement. The feedback is provided anonomously and students can elect to have the feedback passed on to the clinical educator or not. Most students are willing to allow clinical educators access to their feedback. The Director of Clinical Education uses the student feedback to identify areas of continuing education for clinical educators and the suitablity of clinical placements. The feedback form requires the students to rate their clinical educators on a variety of aspects of their clinical education as well as to answer open-ended questions. The following is a summary of some of those aspects:

- encouragement of self-evaluation (for example, Did your clinical educator encourage self-evaluation? Were your contributions in discussion and feedback times expected and valued?)
- negotiation of the supervisory relationship (for example, Was the supervisory process discussed and negotiated with you?)
- provision of feedback (for example, Did your clinical educator

positively acknowledge your skills and abilities? What type of feedback did you receive from your clinical educator? Was this feedback appropriate to your needs and skills?)
- encouragement of independent learning (for example, Did your clinical educator encourage your growing clinical independence?)
- identification and resolution of problems in the supervisory relationship (for example, Did you have any problems in your interactions with your clinical educator? (a) If yes, describe. (b) How were they addressed? Did you feel that you could discuss negative aspects of your placement with your clinical educator?)
- knowledge of the field (for example, Did your clinical educator ensure optimal treatment for the client?).

APPENDIX 3.4: STUDENT SELF-APPRAISAL (McLEOD, IN PRESS)

A structured discussion occurs between students and clinical educators. The aim of the procedure is to produce a list of student and clinical educator goals and accomplishments. The following questions are discussed:

- What have been the most satisfying aspects of your placement over this review period? What have been the high points?
- What do you consider are the most important activities you have performed over this review period?
- What do you think of the quantity and variety of your caseload?
- What are the activities you would like to be doing that you are presently unable to do? What other tasks or roles would you like to try?
- What are the particular difficulties/frustrations you have encountered in this placement? What have you done to improve them? What else can be done?
- What further ways could you see your clinical educator facilitating your clinical work and satisfaction?
- Comment on the opportunities provided for your ongoing education and self-development.
- Are there any other issues you wish to discuss?

REFERENCES

American Speech-Language Hearing Association (1985). Clinical supervision in speech-language pathology and audiology (position statement). *Asha*, **27**, 57–60.

Anderson, J.L. (1988). *The supervisory process in speech-language pathology and audiology*. Boston: College Hill Press.

Andre, J. (1992). Learning to see: Moral growth during medical training. *Journal of Medical Ethics*, **18**, 148–52.

Australian Association of Speech and Hearing (1986). Code of ethics of the Australian Association of Speech and Hearing. Melbourne: Australian Association of Speech and Hearing.

Bamford, P. (1981). Communication in teaching practice supervision. In P.W. Marland (Ed.). *Aspects of supervision in teaching practice* (pp 115–32). Townsville: James Cook University of North Queensland.

Beauchamp, T. & Childress, J. (1989). *Principles of biomedical ethics* (3rd ed.). New York: Oxford University Press.

Best, D.L. & Franke, M.L. (1994). *Quality supervision: Theory and practice for clinical supervisors*. Melbourne: Faculty of Health Sciences, La Trobe University.

Blumberg, A. (1977). Supervision. An interpersonal intervention. *Journal of Classroom Interaction*, **13**, 23–32.

Bogo, M. (1993). The student/field instructor relationship: The critical factor in field education. *The Clinical Supervisor*, **11**, 23–36.

Brown, G. (1983). Studies of student learning, implications for medical teaching. *Medical Teacher*, **5**, 52–6.

Boud, D. (1992). The use of self-assessment schedules in negotiated learning. *Studies in Higher Education*, **17**, 185–200.

Boydell, D. (1986). Issues in teaching practice supervision research: A review of the literature. *Teaching and Teacher Education*, **2**, 115–25

Campbell, L.R. (1994). Learning about culturally diverse populations. *Asha*, **36**, 40–1.

Chan, J., Carter, S. & McAllister, L. (1994). Sources of anxiety related to clinical education in undergraduate speech-language pathology students. *Australian Journal of Human Communication Disorders*, **22**, 57–73.

Corey, G., Corey, M. S. & Callanan, P. (1993). *Issues and ethics in the helping professions* (4th ed.). Pacific Grove, CA: Brooks/Cole.

Crago, M. & Pickering, M. (1987). Supervision in human communication disorder. Cambridge, Massachusetts: College Hill Press.

Davis, C. (1989). *Patient practitioner interaction. An experiential manual for developing the art of health care*. New Jersey: Slack Incorporated.

Egan, G. (1990). *The skilled helper. A systematic approach to effective helping* (4th ed.). Pacific Grove, CA: Brooks/Cole Publishing Company.

Ellard, J. (1974). The disease of being a doctor. *Medical Journal of Australia*, **21**, 318–22.

Ewan, C. E. (1988). The social context of medical education. In K. Cox & C. E. Ewan (Eds). *The Medical Teacher* (2nd ed.) (pp 85–9). Edinburgh: Churchill Livingstone.

Farmer, S. & Farmer, J.L. (1989). *Supervision in communication disorders*. Columbus: Merrill Publishing Company.

Fuller F. F. & Brown O. H. (1975). Becoming a teacher. In K. Ryan (Ed.). *Teacher education the 74th NSSE yearbook* (pp 9–14). Chicago: University of Chicago Press.

Green, W. W. (1986). Professional standards and ethics. In R. M. McLauchlin (Ed.). *Speech-language pathology and audiology: Issues and management* (pp 135–60). New York: Grune & Stratton.

Green, G. (1988). Relationships between role models and role perceptions of new graduate nurses. *Nursing Research*, **37**, 245–7.

Hagler, P., Case, P. & Des Rocher, C. (1989). Effects of feedback on facilitative conditions offered by supervisors during conferencing. In D. Shapiro (Ed.). *Proceedings of the Supervision: Innovations. A National Conference* (pp 155–8). Sonoma County, CA: The Council of Supervisors in Speech Language-Pathology and Audiology.

Higgs, J. (1993). Physiotherapy, professionalism and self-directed learning. *Journal of the Singapore Physiotherapy Association*, **14**, 8–10.

Kadushin, A. (1968). Games people play in supervision, *Social Work*, **13**, 23–32.

Knowles, M. (1990). *The adult learner: A neglected species*. Houston, Texas: Gulf Publishing Company.

Ladyshewsky, R. (1995). *Clinical teaching*. Canberra, Australia: HERDSA Gold Series.

Laycock, M. & Stephenson, J. (1994). *Using learning contracts in higher education*. London: Kogan Page.

Lincoln, M. (1995). Professionalism. In L. McAllister & D. Maloney (Eds). *Clinic Handbook*. Sydney: School of Communication Disorders, University of Sydney.

Lincoln, M. & McAllister, L. (1993). Facilitating peer learning in clinical education. *Medical Teacher*, **15**, 17–25.

McAllister, L., Chan, J., Rosenthal, J. & Stewart, M. (1994). *An investigation of perceptions and experiences of clinical education in NESB/international students*. Melbourne: Foundation for Quality Supervision Conference.

McLeod, S. (in press). Student self-appraisal: Facilitating mutual planning in clinical education. *The Clinical Supervisor*.

Mitchell, M. M. & Kampfe, C. M. (1990). Coping strategies used by occupational therapy students during field work: An exploratory study. *American Journal of Occupational Therapy*, **44**, 543–50.

National Association of Social Workers (1990). Code of ethics (Rev. ed.). Silver Springs, MD: Author. In G. Corey, M. Corey & P. Callanan (1993). *Issues and ethics in the helping professions* (4th ed.). Pacific Grove, CA: Brooks/Cole.

Nelson-Jones, R. (1986). *Human relationship skills: Training and self-help*. Sydney, Australia: Holt-Saunders.

Oratio, A.R. (1977). *Supervision in speech pathology: A handbook for supervisors and clinicians*. Baltimore: University Park Press.

Pagana, K.D. (1988). Stresses and threats reported by baccalaureate students in relation to an initial clinical experience. *Journal of Nurse Education*, **27**, 418–24.

Pannbacker, M., Middleton, G. & Lass, N. (1994). Ethics education for speech-language pathologists and audiologists. *Asha*, **September**, 40–2.

Perry, W.G. (1970). *Forms of intellectual and ethical development in the college years: A scheme*. New York: Holt, Rinehart & Winston.

Pickering, M. (1985). Interpersonal communication constructs and principles: Applications in clinical work. In C.S. Simon (Ed.). *Communication skills and classroom success: Therapy methodologies for language learning disabled students* (pp 95–110). San Diego, CA: College Hill Press.

Pickering, M. (1987). Supervision: A person-focused process. In M. Crago & M. Pickering (Eds). *Supervision in human communication disorders: Perspectives on a process* (pp 107–34). San Diego, CA: College Hill Press.

Pickering, M. (1989–1990). The supervisory process: An experience of interpersonal relationships and personal growth. *National Student Speech Language Hearing Association Journal*, **17**, 17–28.

Pratt, D. & Magill, M.K. (1983). Educational contracts: A basis for effective clinical teaching. *Journal of Medical Education*, **58**, 4462–7.

Purtillo, R.B. & Cassel, C.K. (1989). *Ethical dimensions in the health professions*. Philadelphia: W.B. Saunders Company.

Reichert, A. & Caruso, A. (1991). Ethical standards in the university clinic: A student perspective. *National Student Speech-Language Hearing Association Journal*,

18, 137–41.

Resnick, D.M. (1993). *Professional ethics for audiologists and speech-language pathologists*. San Diego, CA: Singular Press.

Rogers, C. (1951). *Client-centred therapy*. Boston: Houghton Mifflin Company.

Rosenthal, J. (1986). Novice and experienced student clinical teams in undergraduate clinical practice. *Australian Communication Quarterly*, **2**, 12–15.

Schwartz, A., Swartzhurg, M., Lieb, J. & Slaby, A. (1978). Medical school and the process of disillusionment. *Medical Education*, **12**, 182–5.

Shuval, J. (1980). *Entering medicine: The dynamics of transition*. Oxford: Pergamon Press.

Stewart Gonzalez, L. & Coleman, R. (1994). Ethics education: Students prefer case study approach. *Asha*, **August**, 47–8.

Stone, J.R. & Olswang, L.B. (1989). The hidden challenge of counseling. *Asha*, **31**, 27–31.

Tiberius, R.G., Sackin, H.D., Slingerland, J.M., Jubas, K., Bell, M. & Matlow, A. (1989). The influence of student evaluative feedback on the improvement of clinical teaching. *Journal of Higher Education*, **60**, 665–81.

Turkoski, B. (1987). Reducing stress in nursing students' clinical learning experience. *Journal of Nursing Education*, **26**, 335–7.

Urlich, S.R. (1992). Supervision: Issues for academia. *Asha*, **August**, 51–2.

Wealthall, S. (1994). Socialisation or educational institution: Auckland School of Medicine's attempt to increase humanistic attributes in students. *Australasian and New Zealand Association for Medical Education Bulletin*, **21**, 26–37.

White, K. (1989). Ethical responsibilities of clinical educators. In J. Higgs & M. Mackey (Eds). *Professional responsibilities, legal responsibilities and insurance for clinical educators* (pp 5–7). Sydney: Cumberland College of Health Sciences.

White, R. & Ewan, C. (1991). *Clinical teaching in nursing*. London: Chapman & Hall.

Zebrowski, P.M. & Schum, R.L. (1993). Counseling parents of children who stutter. *Asha*, **May**, 65–73.

Learning processes in clinical education

4

Michelle Lincoln
School of Communication Disorders,
Faculty of Health Sciences,
The University of Sydney, Australia

Lynette Stockhausen
Faculty of Health and Behavioural Sciences,
Griffith University, Australia

Diana Maloney
School of Communication Disorders,
Faculty of Health Sciences,
The University of Sydney, Australia

4.1 CHAPTER OVERVIEW

This chapter discusses learning processes which clinical educators and students can use to aid clinical learning. Reflection, self-evaluation, journalling and peer learning are learning processes which can be facilitated by clinical educators and utilized by students to promote independent learning. Explanation, awareness and practice of these processes places an array of self-supervision tools in the hands of the beginning clinician. Some of the content of this chapter comes from reflection on our experiences as clinical educators and some draws on the work of other researchers and writers in the field. Statements beginning with 'we' have been used throughout the chapter to indicate when the authors are writing about their experiences and thoughts. The chapter is essentially about facilitating growth along the continuum of supervision towards the self-supervisory stage.

Postcard 4

Dear All

I wish we had some more students here. Not only is there so much to do, but I miss having someone to 'debrief' with at the end of the day! You get so used to having other students around in the clinic there, to grab for a quick question or a long whinge, that you don't appreciate how much your peers help your learning, not to mention staying sane. Under my mosquito net at night, I spend a lot of time thinking about what I'm doing, and I do talk to one of the English nurses working at the hospital about our 'cross-cultural disasters of the day'! You'll laugh to know that I'm keeping my learning journal going, even here. I'm amazed at how writing about what's going around (and around) in my head and how I'm feeling really does help me clarify what's happening and what I could do next. Besides which, I don't want to forget one second of this time here, if I can help it. It's all so special. There's a fax here at the hospital.

love Sal.

Fax reply to Postcard 4

Dear Sally,

I can really see and feel your current environment from your cards and I enjoy the feelings you talk about as you reflect on your experiences. You always had such a capacity to reflect in discussions. I'm glad journalling has proved useful.

Perhaps, like us, you'll write a book!

Best wishes

Di

4.2 REFLECTION

Educators throughout time have espoused the idea that students learn from experience. If, however, we believe, as does Dewey (1933), that there can be no true growth in learning by mere experience alone, but only by reflecting on experience, then reflective practice must be taken seriously by those facilitating students' clinical education. Schön (1983) asserts that through reflective practice students develop a critical understanding of 'the repetitive experiences of a specialized practice' (p. 61), and can make new sense of situations of uncertainty or uniqueness which they experience. Whilst reflection has come to have multiple meanings (for example, intuitive thought, metacognition and thoughtful action), there remains a dimension to reflection that is personal, developmental and embedded in experience (Boud, 1988).

As graduates enter the professional field of their practice, they are required to be independent, critical thinkers who are able to perform in their profession. Universities are now challenged to make creative use of field or clinical experiences (see Chapter 9). Reflective practice helps students make sense of their experiences and become competent practitioners. It is the responsibility of educators, therefore, to provide students with strategies to facilitate reflective practice. The model of reflection described below has proved helpful for clinical educators and students in many health science disciplines.

4.2.1 A MODEL OF REFLECTION

The following is a description of a three-stage model of reflection developed by Boud, Keogh and Walker (1985) and applied to clinical education by Mandy (1989).

(a) Stage 1: Returning to experience

This stage involves recalling the events and emotions associated with an experience. In effect, it is a chronological 'replaying' of the experience. This may be done by writing a description of the experience (see journalling section 4.4), replaying the experience in the student's mind (see self-evaluation section 4.3) or describing the experience to another (see peer learning section 4.5). Boud *et al.* (1985) suggest that the student's descriptions should pay close attention to detail and should not contain judgments. Any emotions the student felt during the experience may also be noted. This process allows re-examination of the actual events that occurred rather than what the student wished had happened.

(b) Stage 2: Attending to feelings

Boud *et al.* (1985) suggest that 'utilizing positive feelings is important because they give us the impetus to persist in challenging situations, help us see events more sharply and provide the basis for new affective learning' (p. 29). It may help the student believe in his or her own skills and capabilities and receive satisfaction from the task being undertaken.

Negative emotions may cause barriers to learning. It may be uncomfortable or distressing for a student to return to an experience which resulted in negative emotions. They may simply repress the experience. Other students who experienced negative emotions, such as anger or embarrassment, may find it difficult to recollect events clearly or to see other perspectives or interpretations of the experience. Boud *et al.* (1985) suggest that when this occurs the feelings need to be discharged or transformed in some way so the learning process can proceed.

(c) Stage 3: Re-evaluating the experience

Boud *et al.* (1985) state that there are four aspects of re-evaluating the experience: association, integration, validation and appropriation. Association is the combining of thoughts and feelings during the experience and during reflection. Integration refers to the synthesis of these thoughts and feelings into a whole, new perspective, idea or attitude. Validation occurs as the student 'tests out' the new understanding they have to see if it is consistent with other information, other opinions or other experiences. Finally, appropriation occurs if the new knowledge becomes a part of the student him/herself. For example, the student may have developed a new attitude or value as a result of the reflective learning process.

4.2.2 PURPOSES OF REFLECTION

Most students spontaneously reflect on experiences in an unconscious manner. The purpose of encouraging planned and conscious reflection is to ensure that students make decisions out of awareness. Through conscious reflection they can evaluate their ideas and thinking, and make active decisions (Boud *et al.*, 1985). Unconscious reflection may have resulted in the same decision, but the student would have been unaware of how they arrived at that decision and would have missed out on the learning that occurred as a result of the generation and consideration of other possibilities during the decision-making process.

Students may use reflection for specific purposes. For example, a medical student may reflect to evaluate how well he or she performed a technical skill. The student recalls in detail every aspect of his/her administration of a technical procedure and identifies that several times during the administration he/she felt uncertain about what to do next. The student attends to these feelings and recognizes that this occurred because the client was not responding to the procedure in the same way as previous clients. The student then thinks through possible reasons for this and decides on the most likely scenario. This is then added to his or her knowledge about clients' responses during the procedure. By returning to the experience in detail, attending to feelings and re-evaluating the experience this student has integrated new knowledge with existing knowledge.

Students may also reflect to find personal or professional meaning in experiences. For example, beginning occupational therapy students may be required to observe experienced practitioners. After the observation students are asked to reflect on what they learned about the roles of an occupational therapist. This task requires students to integrate new with existing knowledge about the role of occupational therapists and to begin to predict towards a career for themselves in occupational therapy. As some students test out the reality of this new and integrated knowledge, they may realize that they are unsuited or unmotivated to pursue such a career. Others may begin internalizing the professional and personal qualities they observed.

Students may also reflect to evaluate critically their knowledge base. They may return to the experience to check that what occurred was consistent with their theoretical knowledge. This may result in discarding a theory, the adoption of another theoretical stance or the development of a new theory. While the purposes of reflection are many and varied, conscious reflection is planned and deliberate. The intention of the student who engages in reflection is to learn!

4.2.3 THE DEVELOPMENT OF REFLECTION

Boud *et al.* (1985) suggest that the ability to reflect is developed to different levels in different students. They postulate that this is why some students learn more effectively from experiences that others. Bingham (1993) argues that reflection is a learned process. He suggests that before reflective processes can be effective the student must have good observation skills and be able to store key information in memory. Further to this, he suggests that at a beginning level students' observation skills are limited by their contextual and theoretical knowledge. Advanced students are able to reduce their information load because they know what is relevant, while beginning students use most of their processing capacity sorting information and deciding what is important when observing and reflecting. Consequently the content and outcome of reflection will be different depending on the stage of the student. He suggests that supervisory conferences with beginning level students should continually focus on the important elements of the event. Advanced level students could be encouraged to identify their thinking processes and evaluate the soundness of these. He concludes that 'the teaching of thinking, such as reflection, does not require huge changes in what we teach but it may require a change in emphasis and some change in how we directly teach thinking skills' (Bingham, 1993, p. 13).

4.2.4 TYPES OF REFLECTION

Schön (1987) describes two types of reflection: reflection-in-action and reflection-on-action. As the descriptors suggest, reflection-in-action occurs during the event or experience. Students recognize problems or puzzling circumstances during an experience and make changes on-line. Reflection-on-action occurs after the event or experience and involves *post hoc* exploration and interpretation of the event. Health professionals need to be able to reflect in- and on-actions. We suggest that students find it easier to reflect on-action than in-action. The ability to reflect in-action, and as a result make on-line changes, is a hallmark of students moving from an intermediate to advanced level of clinical skills.

Clinical educators can assist students to become reflective clinicians. Boud *et al.* (1985) suggest that learners can be assisted by 'providing a context and space to learn, giving support and encouragement, listening to the learner and providing devices which may be of use' (p. 38). They go on to propose that 'Perhaps the most important role (of the educator) is to alert people to the nature of reflection in the learning process' (p. 38). The remainder of this chapter discusses ways of alerting learners to the value of reflection and 'devices' which may be helpful.

The following sections discuss three learning processes which have reflection as their core process. Ways of facilitating reflection using these processes are discussed. Students' choices concerning which of these learning processes they will use are influenced by many variables. For example, the students' preferred learning style may determine which process they use (see Chapter 1). Some students prefer to learn in groups where learning occurs through interactions with peers, while others prefer to reflect alone through writing and yet others may prefer to reflect and discuss with their clinical educator. Other variables such as time constraints, the nature of the placement and facilities it provides, and clinical educators' preferred reflection mode will also influence students' choices.

4.3 SELF-EVALUATION

The terms *self-evaluation* and *self-assessment* are often used synonomously in the clinical education literature (Boud & Brew, 1995). We contend that the two terms reflect the same learning process. However, self-evaluation refers to learning activities where the goal of the activity is *to learn*, and self-assessment refers to learning activities where the goal of the activity is *to assess* performance (generate grades, scores, etc.), and in doing so, possibly learn. Boud and Brew (1995) take a different perspective on the use of these terms. They suggest that the defining characteristic of self-assessment is 'students identifying standards or criteria to apply to their work and making judgments about the extent to which they have met these criteria or standards' (p. 130). Further they suggest that there are connections between self-assessment and reflection. However, self-assessment has as its outcome specific judgments about performance, whereas reflection can be more exploratory and may not lead to a definitive outcome. In other words 'all self-assessment involves reflection, but not all reflection leads to self-assessment' (p. 131). In this chapter we have chosen to use the term *self-evaluation* because we are discussing a learning process in which individual students set goals for their clinical work and evaluate their progress towards these goals, but are not responsible for ultimately producing grades or marks about their performance. This chapter will discuss self-evaluation as a learning tool; Chapter 6 discusses self-assessment as an assessment and learning tool.

Mercaitis (1989) defines self-evaluation as the ability to evaluate competently the adequacy of one's clinical behaviours. The authors of this chapter suggest that in the clinical context, self-evaluation is essentially reflection about the adequacy of one's clinical skills and professional conduct. Self-evaluation can involve reflection in and on events and experiences. Boud (1989) asserts that 'The need to monitor one's own performance is one of the defining characteristics of professional work' (p. 21). These definitions suggest that self-evaluation is part of the daily work of practising clinicians and that self-evaluation is an integral part of being a professional. Boud (1992) also suggests that the ability to self-evaluate requires attention and practice just as other intellectual skills do. If life-long learning is one of the goals of clinical education, then self-evaluation provides a tool for students to evaluate their performance, monitor their progress and set meaningful learning goals.

The facilitation of self-evaluation is congruent with adult learning theory. It allows the adult to determine what they need to learn and how they are going to go about it. It also allows adults to draw on past experience when evaluating and problem-solving about their clients. Self-evaluation elicits evidence of achievements and provides an opportunity for students to make judgments about how successful or otherwise they have been in meeting their predetermined goals. Consequently students can 'diagnose' their own learning needs and gain increasing clinical independence.

Much research effort has been devoted to determining the validity and accuracy of student self-assessment (see Chapter 6); however, no research exists about self-evaluation as a learning tool. For example, it is unknown whether self-evaluation skills are developmental or whether they can be taught and practised. It is unknown whether self-evaluation results in higher order learning when compared with other methods of receiving feedback about performance and it is also unknown if any particular ways of self-evaluating are more effective than others. Despite this lack of empirical evidence it can be theoretically argued that self-evaluation is an important skill.

4.3.1 CONDITIONS CONDUCIVE TO SELF-EVALUATION

Many of the conditions which are needed for the effective giving and receiving of feedback which were discussed in Chapter 3 are needed for effective self-evaluation. Additionally when reading or listening to students' self-evaluations, clinical educators or peers respond, not to the accuracy of the recount of events, but rather to the level of insight and awareness students demonstrate about their own and others' behaviours during the experience. For students to self-evaluate honestly they must know that they will not be assessed negatively if they evaluate their own performance negatively. Rather, in this context the clinical educator rewards the student for being aware that he or she performed negatively and encourages him/her to explore the event or experience and make sense of what occurred. The goal of this interaction for the clinical educator would be to assist the student to develop strategies for managing similar experiences or events in the future and goals for managing future contacts with the client. The goal for the student is to evaluate his or her performance accurately and reflect about what could have been done differently or what needs to be done in the future.

4.3.2 WAYS OF SELF-EVALUATING

Clinical educators cannot assume that their students are able to self-evaluate independently. As Bingham (1993) and Boud (1992) contend (see section 4.2.3), self-evaluation skills need to be facilitated. The supportive environment of the student–clinical educator relationship is the ideal place for these skills to be encouraged and developed. Each student will need to experiment with different ways of self-evaluating so he or she can find the most comfortable and effective method. The following are options for clinical educators and students to explore when discussing how self-evaluation will occur.

(a) Supervisory conferences

Clinical educators can encourage students to self-evaluate during supervisory conferences. Kenny and McAllister (1995) suggest that it is best if the purpose and goals of self-evaluation are discussed with the student before the conference and that the student comes to the conference knowing that self-evaluation will occur. Additionally they suggest that clinical educators should attempt to be non-directive and facilitative during the conference.

(b) Videos

It is often helpful for students to self-evaluate their performance by watching videos of themselves conducting client sessions (for example, treatment sessions, educational sessions, procedures, client counselling). Students who are experiencing difficulty self-evaluating may benefit from guidance in what to pay attention to. McGovern and Wirz (1980) present an analysis scheme for students to use to evaluate their interaction skills and the pacing of their treatment sessions. The type of evaluation clinical educators expect students to undertake will vary depending on their place on the supervisory continuum (see Chapter 2). For example, a beginning level student may be directed to observe how many times he or she said 'OK' during a session (Mawdsley, 1987), an intermediate level student may be asked to observe the effect of his or her own behaviours on the client's behaviour and an advanced level student may be asked to consider other facilitative responses he or she could have used during a counselling session.

(c) Written self-evaluations

Journals provide an excellent means of encouraging self-evaluation. We encourage students to write after a session, while reflecting on the pre-session plan which was submitted. The student is encouraged to write about why things did or did not go to plan. Again, beginning level students may need a structured questionnaire to help them begin self-evaluating. Some of the questions we use as prompts for students to assist them to self-evaluate are shown below.

Prompts to assist students in self-evaluation

- What was your overall impression of the session?
- What things went well during the session, and what did you learn from this?
- What things went wrong during the session, and what did you learn from this?
- What emotions can you remember feeling during the session?
- Did you observe or think about any client behaviours during the session?
- Did you observe or think about any of your own behaviours during the session?
- Did the session follow your plan? Why or why not?
- What theoretical knowledge did you use, or could you have used, during the session?
- What past experiences did you use, or could you have used, during the session?
- What do you need to learn or find out about before the next session?
- Do you need to meet with your clinical educator?
- Do you want your clinical educator to observe the next session?

4.3.3 DIFFICULTIES WHEN SELF-EVALUATING

From our experience it seems some students are 'natural' self-evaluators. That is they self-evaluate spontaneously and regularly. Other students have more difficulty. This may be the result of students being at different stages in the development of self-evaluation skills (see section 4.2.3). The kinds of difficulties we have typically observed in students are described below.

(a) Inability to move beyond the dominant feeling or perception

If the dominant feeling or perception is negative, some students are unable or unwilling to return to an event and reflect on it (see section 4.1). Similarly if the dominant feeling or perception is positive some students do not feel a need to reflect on the experience. However, valuable learning can occur about why the experience was positive, for example what was done well or correctly, so this can be repeated in the future.

(b) Inability to evaluate self positively or negatively

Some students find it difficult to evaluate their own performance positively; they continually identify weaknesses or errors. Typically, these students will complete an essentially positive experience and will focus all self-evaluation on one error or difficulty without acknowledging the positive things they achieved. Our experience has shown us that these students quickly 'burn out' in clinical practice because they are unable to maintain their self-esteem and achieve work satisfaction. Of relevance here is the study by Carney and Mitchell (1994). They found that 71 per cent of first- and third-year medical students evaluated their overall competence level below that of faculty assessors, despite efforts within their academic and clinical work to encourage self-evaluation. Students who only evaluate experiences positively also need assistance with self-evaluation. There is an element of risk taking when students self-evaluate negatively with a clinical educator. Students may need assistance from the clinical educator to identify what is preventing them from taking risks. It may also help to offer them other options for self-evaluating, such as those discussed in section 4.3.2.

(c) Inability to solve problems

Some students are unable to complete self-evaluation because they are unable to solve problems independently. Beginning level students may not have developed professional problem-solving skills. The clinical educator may need to allow students to self-evaluate up to the problem-solving stage and then assist them to complete the evaluation. Students may also be unable to solve problems because they do not have enough information. Consequently, through self-evaluation they may identify what information they need and how to get it with or without a clinical educator's assistance. Again this may be the case with a beginning clinician who does not know the necessary theory to work effectively with a client or it may also be the case with advanced students who are undertaking a new experience.

This section has discussed the process of self-evaluation as a potential reflective device for learners to utilize. Clinical educators can create an environment which is conducive to self-evaluation through awareness and negotiation. Students can choose from an array of procedures to assist their self-evaluation. We believe that the successful use of self-evaluation is dependent upon a commitment from both the student and educator to maintain the 'self' in self-evaluation. In other words, the focus must stay on the students' recollections, perceptions and thoughts. Without this focus, student growth will not occur.

Self-evaluation is essentially a solitary learning process and while it is a necessary skill to develop, self-evaluation may not always be students' first choice of learning process to employ. Journalling may be a more effective way of reflecting for some students. The next section offers insight into the educational benefits of journal writing and strategies to utilize journals effectively in clinical education.

4.4 JOURNAL WRITING

Journal writing is a learning process that also facilitates reflection. Journal writing, learning logs or diaries are perhaps the most extensively used, and in some cases abused, reflective devices. In our day-to-day lives we write to remember, to organize our lives and our thoughts, to communicate and clarify our ideas and emotions. Educators have realized the potential of journals as a means of exploring students' insights into their thoughts and feelings as they engage in clinical experiences (Cothern, 1991; Hahnemann, 1986; Holly, 1987). The possible educational benefits of journal writing (Heinrich, 1992; Holly, 1987; Smith, 1987) makes it essential for us to examine this as a tool that fosters reflective practice.

We believe that journalling is a form of writing to learn, a way of learning that promotes critical thinking. It is not just a re-write of a textbook or previous classroom content, 'but reflective questioning and exploration of those concepts applied to the realities of the clinical environment' (Stockhausen & Creedy, 1994, p. 77). Encouraging students to write journal entries 'enhances their ability to move progressively to higher levels of abstraction and conceptualization' (Stockhausen & Creedy, 1994, p. 77).

In addition 'writing-to-learn' as a reflective process becomes speculative; that is, it 'is not used primarily to communicate with others, but rather it orders and represents one's own learning and thinking' (Stockhausen & Creedy, 1994, p. 77). It can be a dialogue with oneself that allows a defining of oneself and one's beliefs. It is essentially reflection-on-action (Schön, 1987).

Writing can be used to help students make sense of practical experiences or events, the people involved and situations which arise during their clinical placements. Gore (1987, p. 37) acknowledges that in this sense students may come to value their 'practical knowledge' instead of viewing it as inferior to the scientific knowledge produced by researchers. Deliberation and critique help students test their experiences against the ideas of others involved in the profession: their clinical educators, peers, clients and other health care professionals (Macrorie, 1987). Knowledge cannot be given (Blais, 1988), it must be constructed, and understanding is an internal process of creating knowledge through the ways one thinks about the world. 'When students write in terms of their own experiences, reactions and responses, they are learning that their ideas are as potentially powerful as any others' (Stockhausen & Creedy, 1994, p. 78).

We are aware that journal writing is also used by many clinical educators to reflect on their own experiences as an educator. Journal writing provides educators with an avenue to reflect on teaching and learning strategies, and structuring and managing clinical experience possibilities. When the clinical educator acts as a positive role model and values the importance of reflection and journal writing, students observe and identify with this behaviour as a professional activity.

4.4.1 WHEN TO WRITE

Holly (1987) suggests that journal entries can be made close to the time of the experience or to reflect back over a day or number of days. Holly (1987) also discusses the significance of writing immediately after (or as close as possible to) the initial event, in order to capture the original experience before it becomes coloured or shaped by events that may obscure or change the reflection. Students and clinical educators may use journals prior to an experience to document plans and to consider the expectations of the context and people involved in the clinical experience. However, anytime may be the appropriate time to write. If the clinical educator or the students feel the need to write, then it is probably the most appropriate time to do so.

Writing close to or soon after the event can sharpen significant experiences or focus on significant personal questions arising from a clinical experience. We suggest an allocation of time, say 10 minutes, may be set aside before or after the clinical experience, tutorial or debriefing session. This allows the students and clinical educator the opportunity to pose

questions, or focus on a particular theme raised by the students or significant events that have occurred through a clinical day (Stockhausen &
Creedy, 1994).

Students and clinical educators may find it more effective to write at
home. This may promote a deeper reflection as the participants are
removed from the pressure of writing with others or within time constraints (Stockhausen & Creedy, 1994). Writing away from the context of
the experience may also generate different ideas or responses to events.

Using different settings may stimulate the writing process. Examples of
this are going outside and sitting under a tree, writing alone, writing with
a peer or while conversing with a client or another health care worker.
This strategy can facilitate the student to enter into a meaningful dialogue
with the person by discussing what has been written. Often music can create a mood, a range of feelings or memories that can be linked in a meaningful way to current experiences.

4.4.2 HELPING STUDENTS TO WRITE

Students often struggle with what to include in their journals or how to get
started. Huse-Inman (1980) and Holly (1987) offer suggestions such as
motivators and starters. Some of their suggestions to guide student's reflective journalling are shown below. In an effort to focus, direct or redirect students in their thinking in parts of their journals during clinical practice
these key questions or prompts may be used. Often, a suggested topic or
title can be used to entice students to write. Significant key questions may
also be posed to relate theory already presented to students in lectures or
act as a stimulus to theory yet to be presented. The advantage of this is that
students can see an equal emphasis on both theory and practice.

Motivators and starters for writing journals (adapted from Huse-Inman
[1980] and Holly [1987])

- I was amazed when ...
- I was frightened when ...
- What caught my attention today?
- The most exciting experience today!
- The importance of self-discipline/motivation
- I responded to the situation as I did because ...
- What puzzled me?
- What did I enjoy, dislike, accomplish during clinical today?
- What did I learn from the discussion?
- How was my performance during clinical practice?
- How did I feel doing an interview/physical assessment/injection/wound care?
- What happened when ...?
- What was my role during the event?
- What was the flow of events?

- What were the important elements of the event?
- How will I probably react next time?
- What feelings and senses surrounded the event?
- What did I do and how did I feel about what I did?
- What might I be aware of if this event occurs again?

- How did the other participants in the event react?
- What am I most/least confident about?
- What do I need to do to prepare for tomorrow?
- What things have you learned that you think are most important and tell how you perceive you learned them?

Smith (1987) has suggested the use of structured diaries (journals) as a method of helping students extract learning from experiences. He suggests that by incorporating observational and analytical prompts, systematic and comprehensive learning from experience is encouraged. The prompts suggested by Smith to support structured journalling are shown below.

Prompts to assist students write structured journals (Smith, 1987)

1 *Brief description of the practice encounter* The people, the sequence of events, the situation, what you did.
2 *Important observations of the practice encounter* What you observed about the experience, your own behaviour, what others observed about the event or your role or behaviour.
3 *What you learnt from the practice encounter* What you believe you learned should be stated as confirmations or deviations from your expectations.
4 *How this learning relates to theories or concepts you have read, heard*

about, or constructed yourself Decide whether your theories, actions, hypotheses or behaviours are supported, overturned or deviate as a consequence of your experience, readings, involvement or collaboration with others.
5 *What you would like to change* Be specific, stating exactly what it is you hope to change: behaviour, standards, policies or procedures and under what conditions.
6 *How you will change these* Set review procedures and dates, identify how you will assess your changes.

The structured journal has the advantages of being easy to follow, developing skill in learning how to learn, and empowering students to be more involved and have more control over their learning. The structured journal can be used as an adjunct to other reflective strategies, such as debriefing (Smith, 1987). Smith's structured journal approach could also incorporate an avenue for students to vent frustrations and their sense of feelings experienced during the events.

The authors of this chapter have also used transcripts of actual dialogue between students and clients as the starting point for journalling. We have asked students to transcribe a recorded dialogue between themselves and a client and then journal about the dialogue. Some common student comments we read in their journals are 'I can't believe I didn't respond when she said ...', 'I was waffling and they knew it!', 'I thought I was listening to the client, but I wasn't' and 'It didn't really sound like me'. Reflecting on a specific interaction and then journalling may be an easier starting point than reflecting on an entire interaction.

4.4.3 PROMOTING REFLECTIVE JOURNAL WRITING

Besides encouraging students to write with the aid of prompts, it is also necessary for students and clinical educators to have a clear idea or purpose as to *why* they are writing. This is of particular importance if the journal or entries from the journal are to be assessed. Journalling must be seen as a tool to explore and develop reflection and be valued by all. Deciding as a group on a set of principles for journal writing is an appropriate beginning point. It is necessary that these principles support individual differences and diversity of abilities and interests. Fostering a climate of trust and mutual respect for one's writing is imperative. If journal writing is to allow students to develop reflective thinking and effective skills for life-long learning, then opportunities to have a meaningful choice over how they demonstrate their learning is important. This choice empowers students to write honestly and with more intent.

(a) Dealing with issues of confidentiality

Establishing the process of journal writing can be facilitated by clinical educators negotiating with students on a number of issues. These issues can include confidentiality, policies and procedures for sharing the content with peers or clinical educators, how often entries will be recorded, and how often and perhaps what type of feedback may be sought. Heinrich (1992) suggests that it should be explicitly stated that no reader can share journal material without the writer's expressed permission. A suggestion for providing feedback may be to have students leave space on every page for peer or clinical educator feedback or comments.

Students cannot be forced to write. If the journal entries do not form a component of the assessment, then students' decisions not to write should be respected. If students insist that the clinical educator does not read their journal, then privacy should be respected. If students wish the clinical educator or peers not to read a section of their journal, the students may fold in half the pages they do not want read. Similarly, students could place journal entries in a loose-leaf folder and simply remove any pages they do not wish others to see.

Similarly client confidentiality must also be protected when using journalling. Students should be instructed not to include any identifying information about clients in their journals. For example the clients' surnames and addresses and specific information about their workplace should not be included.

(b) Making the effort worthwhile

For those students just beginning to journal, a clinical educator's comments can help expand the students' writing and exploration of practice and make the journals more useful as a learning tool. Also, some students believe that if a journal is not read by the clinical educator as an essential component of the experience, then journalling has no worth. Students may also feel that journals must count for something, as must every requirement in a university setting. If clinical educators do not view or offer critique of the journals, students sometimes do not understand how they could be of value.

Extending journal writing into supervisory conferences further enhances the reflective process and allows the students to reflect on their writing and experience and share these with others. Rather than have students write only in the vacuum of their own thoughts, sharing of their experiences, thoughts and perceptions can augment students' personal views to incorporate the views of others sharing similar experiences. This can motivate students to write thoroughly, honestly and with meaning (Stockhausen, 1994). 'In this sense journal writing, as a reflective tool, fosters self-critical disclosure and allows for open collegial relationships to develop with peers and clinical educators sharing the same experience' (Stockhausen & Creedy, 1994, p. 81).

We have found that a common complaint by students and clinical educators when they undertake journal writing activities is that journalling takes time. Not only does it take time to reflect and write, but it also takes time to read and respond to these writings. It is important to remember if journal writing is to be valued by students that time needs to be set aside for students to write. The rewards for this time investment are a more individualistic, personal understanding by clinical educators of students' efforts to come to terms with professional issues and practices.

(c) Creativity in journalling

Providing students with the scope to be creative in their journals can also increase motivation and opportunities. Students can be given the freedom to explore other avenues besides writing in their journals which still demonstrate reflection. Students may be encouraged to design images that reflect their perception of their journals, use different coloured pens or colour code entries to reflect moods. Photographs, comic strips, jokes, sketches, diagrams, poems and doodles may also be included in journals (Heinrich, 1992).

4.4.4 ASSESSMENT

Perhaps the greatest controversy in using journals is associated with assessment (Stockhausen & Creedy, 1994). Those educators using journals face a moral dilemma: Should journals, as personal writings, be assessed? There are a number of creative ways that journals can be integrated into assessment and these shall be discussed shortly. However, if journal writing is to be used as an assessment item several issues need to be addressed.

Clear guidelines as to the purpose, type of assignment and appropriate assessment criteria are imperative. If journals are to be assessed then assessment criteria may be negotiated and agreed upon with students. Again this allows for individual differences to be taken into consideration and empowers students to have an active voice in their education.

Self-critique of journal entries empowers students to identify issues of importance to them. Assessment of journals should be used as a learning device that extends students' learning experiences beyond the initial observation, activity or reflection. Encouraging students to examine their journals for recurring themes allows students to develop their own voice.

One way of assessing journals is to ask students to report a significant or critical incident that has occurred during their clinical practice and examine the important elements of the event. They may write about the significance of the people involved in the event, their roles, relationships and responses. Russell (1989) and Holly and Smyth (1989) offer some insights into how the journals can be analyzed to reveal hidden meanings of the writer.

Writing assignments offer a more structured approach to assessment but can still incorporate students' personal experiences and writing. The following are suggestions for journal writing assignments that can be used for grading purposes.

(a) Writing self-evaluations of journals

Ask students to write entries in which they evaluate their own journals. Pose questions such as: Which entries make the greatest impact on you now?; Which seem least worth doing?; What patterns do you find from entry to entry? For some students, this writing may be the clarifying activity of the semester.

(b) Setting time to write as part of the clinical placement

Students may be requested to write for a required length of time (for example, 15 minutes) on a topic suggested by the clinical educator, which may have arisen as a consequence of the clinical experience or be set purposefully to integrate classroom learning. After giving five such journal assignments, ask each student to select their best piece of writing, rewrite it and pass it in for a mark. Students can be encouraged to relate personal experiences, theoretical knowledge and research to the topic. This type of journal assignment is consistent with adult learning theory because it asks students to integrate theory and personal practice which creates greater motivation.

(c) Journalling by contract

Another option requires students to write at least once a week. Here students are given a list of writing topics and sign contracts to write on a given number of topics that have personal experiential significance. The topics are broad in scope and encourage students to explore themselves, their values, and their environment. Writing in their journals about provocative issues helps students to see their positions more clearly and even to discover new ideas. Ethical and moral dilemmas of practice usually provide an initial starting point for this type of journal assessment item. Debriefings or tutorials on controversial issues are likely to foster healthier and informed debate, as well as be more dynamic if students have first written about these issues in their journals. Marks may be awarded for preparation and involvement in debriefings or tutorials. After the first week of journal writing, the students may suggest topics for use in the following week. This option not only encourages individual writing, but since students are all writing on the same topic, they will be interested in others' view points.

(d) Journalling to provide material for class discussion

Negotiate with students to keep a journal record of their responses to a current issue. On a given day these responses can form the basis for a more formal class discussion. Writing in a journal requires students to go one step beyond thinking vaguely about their responses, but it stops short of the formal written assignment which may cause unproductive anxiety over form, or question interpretation. However, even in the most specialized fields some free, imaginative speculation helps and when that speculation is recorded in the journal, students have a record to look at later that documents where they've been and may suggest where to go next.

(e) 'Free writing'

Students and clinical educator can 'free write' on what is important to them in the context they are in. Free writes involve asking students to take about three minutes to respond to a particular question or topic. Both clinical educators and students write at the same time. It is important to do something active and deliberate with what the students have written. An example of this is to share the free write with a fellow student (Heinrich, 1992).

(f) Looking for patterns in the journals

The journal may also provide evidence of one's own values and beliefs which have surfaced as a result of writing. These can be detected by examining the journal entries for recurring themes, metaphors or words.

4.4.5 PROVIDING FEEDBACK TO STUDENTS ABOUT THEIR JOURNALS

The art of responding sensitively to journal entries involves permitting students to risk trial and error approaches and not censoring entries (Stockhausen & Creedy, 1994). Clinical educators can write a few comments in the margins or a brief note at the end of journals. These responses should always be positive and very specific, such as praise for insight or analysis. If entries appear too brief, challenge the student with probing questions, make a positive suggestion for next week's journal. Aim to extend the student.

Fostering further curiosity through constructive feedback on student entries has the potential to increase students' self-esteem and motivation as well as to broaden their perspectives on their observations, involvement in activities and reflections. Posing probing questions extends descriptions to analysis. Positive comments in the margin may foster feelings of achievement. The following three case studies are examples of feedback on journal entries by students undertaking an undergraduate nursing degree.

Case Study 4.1

Excerpt from journal
6th September, dressed an ulcer on Mr W's ankle with ...
11th September, dressed Mr W's ankle, I feel more confident in doing dressings now.

Clinical educator's response
Alison, its encouraging to see you are becoming more confident in carrying out wound care and aseptic technique. There were five days between you initially attending to Mr W's ankle ulcer. What changes in the wound did you notice between these times? Was the dressing regime changed during this period? If so, why? What was the function of the ...?

Case Study 4.2

Excerpt from journal
I monitored the patient's strict fluid balance.

Clinical educator's response
Monitoring is an important nursing function. Have you considered what the significance of the strict fluid balance was? How did this relate to the patient's condition?

Case Study 4.3

Excerpt from journal
During the procedure I just sat there and held the patient's hand. When everything was finished I remained at his bedside listening to him talk about his family. As I left the room he thanked me for just 'being there' for him and he said he felt I would make a caring nurse. This made me feel great and created a sense in me that I had provided him with more than just physical care.

Clinical educator's response
Rhonda, this incident has given you insight into several aspects of caring. Your empathy and insight into the patient's anxiety regarding the procedure is demonstrated by the patient's appreciation. You may like to examine why you held the patient's hand and what made you stay.

Developing an ongoing dialogue between students and clinical educator helps students progress to a deeper analysis of issues and themes. It is not so much the writing that is assessed, but how the students demonstrate their reflection on practice, that leads them to a deeper abstraction of the practice.

4.4.6. THE VALUE OF JOURNAL WRITING FOR CLINICAL EDUCATORS

Encouraging students to write in a journal also has many advantages for clinical educators. Reading students' journals may give clinical educators insight into their students' understanding and learning. This provides the clinical educators with feedback about the clinical experiences they are providing and the effectiveness of their teaching. Reading and commenting on students' journals also reinforces the reflective process and demonstrates to the students that reflection is expected and valued. Finally, reading a student's journal individualizes the student for the clinical educator. This may be particularly helpful for clinical educators who are assigned large numbers of students.

4.4.7 CONCLUSION ON JOURNAL WRITING

Journal writing as a reflective process does reveal new possibilities for clinical educators to understand what is occurring in practical experiences. Reflection through journal writing has the potential to allow clinical educators to penetrate and explore students' cognitive and 'tacit knowledge' and intuitive thought, as well as their own knowledge and thoughts. Journalling offers new insights into what students really think and feel about the numerous situations they are faced with in their clinical environment. Journal writing becomes a process in which students are encouraged to use their own practice and interpretations as a legitimate source of knowledge and personal learning. Journal writing provides an avenue to promote reflectivity and develop writing as a life-long skill. As students think about problems, they integrate personal and academic knowledge across the curriculum and disciplines. The personal writing process and sharing of ideas exposes misconceptions which can be challenged, modified and understood; making knowledge of the self and the world more meaningful (Stockhausen & Creedy, 1994).

While the educational benefits of journal writing to aid the reflective process have been embraced, there has been some criticism that little empirical evidence exists to support this stance (Bean & Zulich, 1989). However, the abundance of educational literature attesting to the value of journal writing and case studies involving journal extracts provides an impetus to examine further the use of journal writing as a means to determine, promote and extend students' reflections and build their clinical knowledge. Wibel (1991, p. 45) perhaps best describes the contribution that journal writing can make to reflection: 'No other medium provides this growth and empowerment. Writing in reflection bridges the void, creates the opportunity, secures the risk, and ensures a response'.

Both self-evaluation and journal writing are to some extent solitary reflective practices. After solitary reflection using either of these processes, the student may share their reflections with their clinical educator or a peer or they may prefer to have peers facilitate their reflection. The next section discusses peer learning as a reflective process. Peer learning may appeal to some students because it is a more social and interactive learning process. Once again peer learning encourages reflection-on-action.

4.5 PEER LEARNING

In the context of clinical education, 'peer learning' refers to learning which occurs through interactions with fellow students in clinical settings. Other terms which include the term 'peer' such as peer tutoring, peer teaching, peer review and peer evaluation refer to procedures designed to facilitate the process of peer learning (Lincoln & McAllister, 1993). These are analogous with other learning procedures such as seminars, lectures and demonstrations. This section discusses the peer learning process and then some formal and informal procedures for facilitating peer learning.

4.5.1 ADULT LEARNING AND PEER LEARNING

The application of the peer learning process is consistent with how adults learn. The characteristics of adult students described by Knowles (1990) (see Chapter 1) appear to be compatible with the peer learning process. For example, sharing and reflecting upon experiences with a peer may facilitate the knowledge of why something has to be learned and its relevance to real-life situations. Peer interactions allow adults to maintain their independence and control their learning. The peer learning process may also affirm the adult's self-esteem, self-concept and perceptions of usefulness which may increase internal motivation.

4.5.2 APPROACH TO LEARNING

It is known that students utilize both surface and deep approaches to learning (Kolb, 1988; Marton, 1983) and that reflection is an important part of clinical learning (Mandy, 1989) (see Chapter 1). Peer learning procedures may facilitate deep learning and reflection by encouraging application, reorganization and questioning of knowledge which may have been previously learned at a surface level only. Components of the peer learning process such as mutual problem-solving, brainstorming, joint analysis, observation of peers, and self- and peer evaluation may facilitate deep learning (Lincoln & McAllister, 1993).

The expression and analysis of negative emotions through reflection with peers may enhance learning. We believe that interaction with peers in similar learning situations is more likely to facilitate the expression of negative and positive emotions than interactions with educators. It is possible that emotions may be more freely expressed with peers because there may be more empathy and less risk of judgment. The safe and supportive environment of a peer group may facilitate analysis of these emotions.

4.5.3 GOALS OF CLINICAL EDUCATION

Clinical education aims to produce independent clinicians who are capable of evaluating their own skills and performance and participating in life-long learning. One of the most common ways practising health workers facilitate their own learning is through peer interactions at formal and informal levels. Therefore, professional education programmes would benefit from encouraging and valuing this skill in students.

There are few reports in the literature of applications of the peer learning process with adults. However, it is possible to hypothesize why the peer learning process may be beneficial to students. Consequently this section is divided into hypothesized and reported benefits of the peer learning process.

4.5.4 HYPOTHESIZED BENEFITS

(a) Broadening perspectives

Adults bring a wealth of past experience to interactions which have the potential to facilitate learning by peers. Students develop a wider view or a different perspective of a client, disorder, placement site or interaction as a result of hearing about another student's past experience. This may facilitate reorganization and re-analysis of thoughts.

(b) Developing professional interaction skills

Participation in peer learning may facilitate the development of professional interaction skills which are necessary in the workplace. For example, students may have the opportunity to practise conflict resolution, negotiation and appropriate assertiveness with peers. The peer learning process may promote collegial relationships between peers. It is worthwhile to encourage co-operation between peers because it is an essential skill for health and education professionals in their work environment.

(c) Promoting professional socialization

Peer learning may assist students to develop their professional identity and sense of belonging to their chosen profession. In future years, this may result in the establishment of a united professional group which values members' expertise and whose members actively consult each other (Lincoln & McAllister, 1993).

4.5.5 REPORTED BENEFITS OF PEER LEARNING

Many of the reports describing the benefits of peer learning approaches when used with adults contain anecdotal evidence only.

(a) Promoting independent learning skills

In the academic learning environment a goal of teaching is the production of autonomous students who can apply, analyze and synthesize information (Collier, 1983). Collier discusses a technique called 'syndication', which is used in higher education to achieve the above goals, through peer learning. Students form 'syndicates' and members are responsible for researching and teaching allocated topics to the other members. He considers that the benefits to the syndicate members include heightened motivation, increased involvement in academic work, development of higher order intellectual skills (for example, critical thinking, problem-solving), a deep learning approach to content and the facilitation of self-directed and independent learning skills. The benefits of peer group learning and teaching were reported by a group of nurses working in a clinical environment (Hart, 1990). These are listed below.

Reported benefits of peer learning (Hart, 1990)

- Recognizing group members as untapped resources and acknowledging professional expertise
- Allowing feedback on individual contributions
- Creating a feeling of equality
- Creating group power
- Improving small group skills
- Taking pressure off individuals
- Encouraging information sharing
- Making it OK to admit problems

- Providing reassurance
- Providing different perspectives
- Giving direction for actions
- Increasing self-esteem and confidence
- Spreading enthusiasm
- Developing listening and facilitation skills
- Encouraging a professional approach to problems
- Helping to organize information
- Alleviating/diffusing conflict

(b) Dealing with emotions in learning

Hart (1990) also reports that a group of nurses involved in teleconferences with peers experienced reduced feelings of professional isolation, were able to gain different perspectives on professional issues and were provided with reassurance.

(c) Broadening knowledge and perspectives

Dowling (1979) reported that peers increase their clinical knowledge beyond the scope of their own cases and that self-supervisory skills increased through observation, analysis and problem-solving during a peer-teaching session (the 'teaching clinic'). Dowling's teaching clinic is discussed in more detail in section 4.5.6 and Chapter 2. A further article by Dowling (1983) evaluated the interaction between supervisors, peers and clinicians during a 'teaching clinic'. It confirmed that this method of supervision fostered self-supervisory behaviours and increased conference participation, problem-solving and strategy development.

4.5.6 PROMOTION OF PEER LEARNING

(a) Unstructured approaches

'An unstructured approach to facilitating peer learning refers to the creation of an environment which is conducive to peer learning' (Lincoln & McAllister, 1993, p. 21).

Multiple student placements

A clinical programme in which individual students are placed in individual clinics would not be conducive to peer learning. In contrast, a programme which places several students in the same or different years in a single setting would be more conducive to peer learning (Lincoln & McAllister, 1993). Several authors, including Callan, O'Neill and McAllister (1993), McFarlane and Hagler (1993) and Harris and Ludington (1993), have written about the benefits of multiple student placements. Rosenthal (1986) reported on a programme which utilized peer learning in speech therapy clinical education. Beginning students in their first clinical placement were teamed with advanced students who were in their final clinical placement (see Chapter 2 for further details). This approach would best be described as a peer tutoring procedure (Lincoln & McAllister, 1993).

Case Study 4.4

'I don't know if the student I was watching was doing the right treatment, but it was good to see that she was as nervous as I usually am!'

Beginning level student

Observation facilities

The provision of observation facilities, such as one-way viewing windows encourages students to watch their peers working with clients. The provision of a meeting room for students to meet and discuss clinical issues and concerns without fear of judgment by clinical educators is also conducive to learning. With careful planning it is possible to create an environment which encourages peer learning even in a small clinic with only two students; for example, by making sure students have a time and a place for discussion with each other.

Clinical educator modelling

Clinical educators also facilitate peer learning in an unstructured manner. They can model the process by consulting with colleagues in the presence of students. They may suggest that students observe peers, manage cases jointly, use a peer to get an objective opinion, give another student feedback on a session with a client, consult more advanced students or students with a similar client, caseload or problem (Lincoln & McAllister, 1993). An awareness of the benefits of peer learning could maximize clinical educators' uses of natural educational resources in the clinic.

Peer facilitation

Rather than focusing on the clinical educator facilitating peer learning, students could be taught how to facilitate each other's learning. The inclusion of a course in learning theory which has a unit on peer learning, early in the students' education, might facilitate this process. Role playing could be used to teach students how to ask questions of their peers that facilitate problem-solving and deep learning in the clinical education context. Farmer and Farmer (1989) suggest that broad or open-ended questions, divergent questions and evaluative questions are the most facilitative of students' learning. By providing students with this information about facilitative questioning, educators are empowering students to maximize their own, as well as their peers' learning experiences.

(b) Structured approaches

'Structured approaches to facilitating peer learning refer to organized, formalized activities. These are procedures which are instituted to take advantage of the known benefits of the peer learning process' (Lincoln & McAllister, 1993). Examples of structured approaches are discussed below.

Teaching clinic

Dowling (1979) used a procedure called a 'teaching clinic', based on the concept of peer-group supervision, to facilitate peer learning in speech therapy clinical education. This technique is discussed in detail in Chapter 2.

Peer tutoring

Strober Escovitz (1990) reported on the use of advanced medical students to give feedback to beginning students about their client interviewing skills. The advanced students watched vidoes of the beginning students' interviews and provided them with written and verbal feedback. The advanced students were paid for attending training, watching the videos and providing feedback. The author reports that the use of peers for feedback was a positive learning experience for both the advanced and beginning level students.

Supervisory conferences

The use of 'conferencing' in clinical education is advocated by many experts in the field (Anderson, 1988; Farmer & Farmer, 1989). Group supervisory conferences are an excellent venue for facilitating the peer learning process. By assuming a non-dominant, facilitatory role during a conference, the clinical educator may promote the peer learning process through case presentation, mutual problem-solving, idea sharing, role playing, discussion and goal setting. Conference group members may offer each other support, recognize each other's contributions, promote confidence and self-esteem of members and form a group identity. Further research is needed to identify which clinical educator behaviours are facilitative of peer learning in this context and what structures may be needed for successful interaction (for example, rule setting and group size).

Structured observation

Structured peer learning may also be facilitated by formalizing the observational process. By requiring students to observe their peers interacting with clients, their exposure to different clients and disorders is increased. Learning from the observation is assured by further requiring students to discuss their observation with the students they observe, collect specific data on the interaction or write feedback to the clinician.

Supervision in absentia

Farmer and Farmer (1989) describe a technique called 'supervision in absentia'. This type of supervision is recommended for advanced students. Farmer and Farmer report students meet as a group to discuss an agenda which may have been set by the students, clinical educators or both. Clinical educators are not present during conferences. However, conferences are videotaped and any unresolved issues or questions are directed to the camera to solicit input from the clinical educator at a later time. The clinical educator meets with the students at a negotiated time and discusses the unresolved issues and the self-supervision process. We suggest this structured technique would be highly facilitative of peer learning (Farmer & Farmer, 1989). However, Farmer and Farmer stress that this technique is only suitable for use with advanced students, as less experienced students require more support and direct input from the clinical educator.

Case Study 4.5

Our experience when using supervision in absentia with advanced level students has been very positive. The students report that they develop more confidence in their clinical skills and feel less apprehensive about commencing clinical practice.

Case Study 4.6

'When I knew I could solve problems with my peers help and didn't need my clinical educator I felt I was ready to graduate.'

Advanced level student

4.5.7 USING PEER LEARNING ALONG THE CONTINUUM OF SUPERVISION (ANDERSON, 1988)

Different strategies for facilitating peer learning may be appropriate at different stages of the continuum from dependence to independence in clinical work. Beginning clinicians may be resistant to learning from anyone other than an authority figure. Hence, strategies used at this stage need to be subtle; for example, unstructured observation, modelling, multiple student placements or supervisory conferencing. However, students who are close to graduating should be encouraged to maximize learning via this strategy. In this case 'supervision in absentia' would be a more appropriate strategy to employ.

4.5.8 CAUTIONS WHEN FACILITATING PEER LEARNING

Clinical educators need to be aware that peer learning is not an appropriate strategy to use in all instances. The level of dependency of the student needs to be considered before encouraging peer learning. For example, if one student in the peer interaction is dependent on the other to a greater degree, then the relationship will lack equality and learning will not be maximized. The dependent student may or may not develop independence and self-direction during the relationship. However, the non-dependent student may feel frustrated and constrained by their peer's dependency.

The application of the peer learning process may result in decreased competition between students, as they may focus on group goals and achievements. On the other hand, it may highlight differences between students and contribute to competition. The outcome with regard to competition largely depends on the personalities of the students and their understanding and experience of the peer learning process. In our experience non-competitive clinical interactions between peers is a hallmark of professional and personal growth.

The peer learning process also may not be facilitative of learning when the students involved have either very strong or very weak clinical skills. In both these cases, learning is not likely to be maximized because the interaction may not be at an appropriate level (too high or too low) to allow integration, reorganization and synthesis of learning. Peer learning between students who have a 'personality clash' may also have potentially negative learning consequences. In the worst-case scenario, no learning would result. If the problem can be identified early in the relationship by the students or clinical educator, then this situation also has the potential to be a valuable learning experience. From this experience students can learn negotiation, teamwork and coping skills. This situation may mirror some issues which need to be dealt with in client–clinician relationships or collegial relationships when the student is working in his or her chosen field. Clinical educators need to handle this situation sensitively and provide support and guidance to the peers involved if a successful result is to be achieved. Again, the student's ability to deal with the situation is a hallmark of professional and personal growth.

This section has discussed the benefits and application of the peer learning process to clinical education. Increasing students' awareness and skills in using this process will provide them with a self-supervision tool which they will use throughout their professional career.

4.6 CONCLUSION

The three learning processes (self-evaluation, journalling and peer learning) discussed in this chapter have many commonalties. We suggest that they all foster the reflective learning process and that the ability to reflect on clinical practice is an essential skill for health practitioners. We also contend that these learning processes facilitate deep learning of academic material and that this results in informed and flexible practice. Self-evaluation, journalling and peer learning are all learning processes which are congruent with adult learning theory and the goals of clinical education. Finally, these three processes are self-supervision tools which clinicians can use to facilitate life-long learning.

REFERENCES

Anderson, J. (1988). *The supervisory process in speech-language pathology and audiology*. Boston: College Hill.

Bean, T.W. & Zulich, J. (1989). Using dialogue journals to foster reflective practice with preservice content-area teachers. *Teacher Education Quarterly*, Winter, 33–40.

Bingham, B. (1993). *Teaching for professional thinking: Issues and understandings in promoting reflection*. Brisbane, Queensland: Australian Catholic University, Queensland Division, McAuley Campus.

Blais, D. M. (1988). Constructivism: a theoretical revolution in teaching. *Journal of Developmental Education*, **11**, 2–7.

Boud, D. (1988). How to help students learn from experience. In K. Cox & C. Ewan (Eds). *The medical teacher* (2nd ed.) (pp 68–73). Edinburgh: Churchill Livingstone.

Boud, D. (1989). The role of self-assessment in student grading. *Assessment and Evaluation in Higher Education*, **14**, 20–31.

Boud, D. (1992). The use of self-assessment schedules in negotiated learning. *Studies in Higher Education*, **17**, 185–200.

Boud, D., Keogh R. & Walker, D. (1985). Promoting reflection in learning: A model. In D. Boud, R. Keogh & D. Walker (Eds). *Reflection: Turning experience into learning* (pp 18–40). London: Kogan Page.

Boud, D. & Brew, A. (1995). Developing a typology for learner self-assessment practices. *Research and Development in Higher Education*, **18**, 130–5.

Callan, C., O'Neill, D. & McAllister, L. (1993). Adventures in two to one supervision: Two students can be better than one. *SUPERvision*, **18**, 15.

Carney, S. L. & Mitchell, K.R. (1994). The development of self-evaluation skills during an undergraduate medical programme. *Australasian and New Zealand Association for Medical Education Bulletin*, **21**, 36–41.

Collier, G. (1983). *The management of peer group learning: Syndicate methods in higher education*. Windsor: Society for Research into Higher Education, NFER Nelson.

Cothern, N. (1991). *Seizing the power of personal journal writing*. Indiana University, Fort Wayne. ERIC document, ED 340044

Dewey, J. (1933). *How we think*. Boston: D. C. Heath.

Dowling, S. (1979). The teaching clinic: A supervisory alternative. *Asha*, **21**, 646–9.

Dowling, S. (1983). Teaching clinic conference participant interaction. *Journal of Communication Disorders*, **16**, 385–97.

Farmer, S. & Farmer J. (1989). *Supervision in communication disorders*. Colombus, Ohio: Merrill Publishing Company.

Gore, R. (1987). Reflecting on reflective teaching. *Journal of Teacher Education*, **37**, 33–9.

Hahnemann, B. (1986). Expert clinical teaching. In National League of Nursing (Ed.) *Curriculum revolution: Reconceptualising nurse education*. New York: National League of Nursing.

Harris, H. & Ludington, J. (1993). Adventures in two to one supervision: Two students can be better than one. *SUPERvision*, **18**, 16.

Hart, G. (1990). Peer consultation and review. *The Australian Journal of Advanced Nursing*, **7**, 40–6.

Heinrich, K. (1992). The intimate dialogue: Journal writing by students. *Nurse Educator*, **17**, 17–21.

Holly, M. L. (1987). *Keeping a personal–professional journal*. Geelong, Victoria: Deakin University Press.

Holly, M. L. & Smyth, J. (1989). The journal as a way of theorising teaching. *The Australian Administrator*, **10**, 3–4.

Huse-Inman, K. (1980). *Reflections*. South Dakota: South Dakota Dept. of Education and Cultural Affairs.

Kenny, B. & McAllister, L. (1996). *Self-evaluation: A vital skill for life-long learners*. Conference of the New Zealand Speech-Language Therapists Association and The Australian Association of Speech and Hearing. Auckland, New Zealand.

Knowles, M. (1990). *The adult learner: A neglected species*. Houston, Texas: Gulf Publishing Company.

Kolb D.A. (1988). *Experiential learning: Experience as the source of learning and development*. Eversley Cliffs: Prentice Hall.

Lincoln, M. & McAllister, L. (1993). Facilitating peer learning in clinical education. *Medical Teacher*, **15**, 17–25.

Macrorie, K. (1987). Forward. In T. Fulwiler (1987). *The Journal Book*. New Hampshire: Boyton-Cook.

Mandy, S. (1989). Facilitating student learning in clinical education. *Australian Journal of Human Communication Disorders*, **17**, 83–9.

Marton, F. (1983). How students learn. In N.J. Entwistle & D. Hounsell (Eds). *How students learn* (pp 125–38). Lancaster: University of Lancaster.

Mawdsley, B. (1987). Kansas inventory of self-supervision. In J. Anderson (1988). *The supervisory process in speech-language pathology and audiology* (pp 373–80). Boston: College Hill Publication.

McFarlane, L. & Hagler, P. (1993). Collaborative treatment and learning teams in a university clinic. *SUPERvision*, **18**, 13–14.

McGovern, M.A & Wirz, S.L. (1980). The use of video tape in the training of speech therapy students – The development of an observational schedule. *British Journal of Disorders of Communication*, **15**, 65–74.

Mercaitis, P. A. (1989). Strategies for helping supervisees to participate actively in the supervisory process. *Proceedings, Supervision: Innovations, A National Conference on Supervision*. Sonoma County, CA: Council of Supervisors in Speech-Language Pathology and Audiology.

Rosenthal, J. (1986). Novice and experienced student clinical teams in undergraduate clinical practice. *Australian Communication Quarterly*, **2**, 12–15.

Russell, T. (1989). Documenting reflection-in-action in the classroom: Searching for appropriate methods. *Qualitative Studies in Education*, **2**, 275–84.

Schön, D. (1983). *The reflective practitioner*. London: Temple Smith.

Schön, D. (1987). *Educating the reflective practitioner*. California: Jossey-Bass.

Smith, B. (1987). Structured diaries. *Training and Management Development Methods*, **1**, 3.13–3.16.

Stockhausen, L. (1994). The clinical learning spiral: A model to develop reflective practitioners. *Nurse Education Today*, **14**, 363–71.

Stockhausen, L. & Creedy, D. (1994). Journal writing: Untapped potential for reflection and consolidation. In S. Chen, R. Cowdroy, A. Kingsland & M. Ostwald (Eds). *Reflections on problem based learning* (pp 73–85). Sydney: Australian Problem Based Learning Network.

Strober Escovitz, E. (1990). Using senior students as clinical skills teaching assistants. *Academic Medicine*, **65**, 733–4.

Wibel, W. H. (1991). Reflection through writing. *Educational Leadership*, March, 45.

Learning to make clinical decisions

5

Joy Higgs
School of Physiotherapy,
Faculty of Health Sciences,
The University of Sydney, Australia

Postcard 5

Dear All

Had a lovely weekend. Walked to the next town with some staff from the hospital to have a look at a festival that was going on there. The temples were all done up and there were thousands of people in their best clothes. I find the religious differences fascinating. I wish I understood more of what was going on! Another interesting week. I've got the team writing program plans and notes of contacts with the clients and families. The plans are pretty sketchy at this stage but they are getting the idea. What's amazing is that they all look much the same, irrespective of the client needs. It's like they are operating with some formula; in fact, they are – I asked to have a look at their CBR training manuals from when they did their course in [the capital] and got the interpreter to explain some of the model plans. They are treating every child as if they were deaf, even if they aren't. Not sure how to tackle this – thought I'd try mind-mapping them through steps in matching program plans to client needs.

Any ideas?

love Sally

Fax response to Postcard 5

Dear Sally

Great to hear from you! Just an idea about how to get the CBR workers to match their programs to client needs. Do you remember when you were in year 2 and you wanted the clients to fit the program rather than the other way around? Your clinical educator moved you on from this stage by getting you to think about the client as a 'whole' rather than only a communication disorder and then to problem solve about how programs could be adapted to suit the client's unique needs. After this the clinical decisions you made were much more in tune with your client's needs. We know you have the skills to deal with this 'hurdle'. Let us know how you get on.

Best wishes

Lindy, Michelle, Sharynne and Di

5.1 CHAPTER OVERVIEW

To be a health professional requires making decisions and using these decisions to implement autonomous actions for which the professional is responsible. Therefore, the skill of decision-making or clinical reasoning is central to effective clinical practice. This chapter will examine the nature of clinical reasoning and the roles of educators and students in facilitating the development of clinical reasoning skills, particularly in the clinical setting.

5.2 UNDERSTANDING THE CONCEPT OF CLINICAL REASONING

Understanding the full depth and potential of clinical reasoning and gaining expertise in this complex ability is an ongoing discovery which occurs throughout the clinician's career. For the educator attempting to initiate or develop student skills in clinical reasoning, it is essential to gain a good understanding of clinical reasoning prior to commencing teaching in this area.

The term clinical reasoning refers to the thinking and decision-making processes associated with clinical practice. The three core elements of clinical reasoning are knowledge, cognition or thinking and the process of metacognition (which refers to the awareness and monitoring of cognition). Metacognitive skills can also be thought of as higher order cognitive skills that are necessary for the management of knowledge and the management of other cognitive skills.

5.2.1 RESEARCH INTO CLINICAL REASONING

Clinical reasoning has traditionally been described as being a process of hypothesis generation and testing, or *hypothetico-deductive reasoning*. A second major interpretation is the notion of *pattern recognition*. Recently, emphasis in understanding clinical reasoning has centred upon *knowledge-reasoning integration*. These three interpretations will be discussed below.

(a) Hypothetico-deductive reasoning

Early medical research into clinical reasoning (Barrows, Feightner, Neufield & Norman, 1978; Elstein, Shulman & Sprafka, 1978; Feltovich, Johnson, Moller & Swanson, 1984; Gale, 1982) focused on hypothetico-deductive reasoning as a model of clinical reasoning. This process involves collecting and analyzing information, generating hypotheses concerning the cause or nature of the client's condition, investigating or testing these hypotheses (through further inquiry) and determining the optimal diagnostic and treatment decisions based on the data obtained. Hypothetico-deductive reasoning involves both inductive reasoning (moving from a set of specific observations to a generalization, i.e. the generation of hypotheses on the basis of probability) and deductive reasoning (moving from a generalization to a conclusion in relation to a specific case) (Ridderikhoff, 1989). Deductive reasoning is widely used in the health sciences in the presentation of arguments to defend our decisions and actions. As the next section will indicate, inductive reasoning is frequently used by experienced clinicians who utilize experience-based learning as the foundation for applying clinical judgements to the case in question.

The hypothetico-deductive reasoning model is supported across many health professions. It has been seen as the dominant model of clinical reasoning in medicine for some time (Elstein *et al.*, 1978; Feltovich & Barrows, 1984), as a commonly used approach in physiotherapy (Jones, 1992), as one of the modes of reasoning in occupational therapy (where it is linked to the concept of 'procedural reasoning') (Fleming, 1991), and as an approach used by nurses as part of diagnostic reasoning (Padrick, Tanner, Putzier & Westfall, 1987).

In a number of the health professions other models and modes of reasoning are gaining prominence. In occupational therapy, clinical reasoning is currently viewed as involving multiple strategies, such as procedural, interactive, conditional and ethical reasoning (Chapparo & Ranka, 1995; Fleming, 1991). In nursing there is growing evidence that much of nurses' reasoning does not focus on either diagnosis or hypothesis generation (Fonteyn, 1991). In physiotherapy clinical reasoning models are emphasizing decision-making in relation to many aspects of clinical practice beyond diagnosis (Jones, 1992) and the role of metacognition in clinical reasoning (Higgs, 1992).

Hypothetico-deductive reasoning is a useful model for beginning students, particularly in professional situations which rely on the medical model. For example, students in undergraduate medical and physiotherapy programmes can examine the nature of reasoning and learn the skills of formulating and testing diagnoses using hypothetico-deductive reasoning strategies.

(b) Pattern recognition

Pattern recognition or inductive reasoning (i.e. moving from a set of specific observations to a generalization) is another interpretation of the clinical reasoning process (in particular, diagnostic reasoning). This model has been supported by a number of researchers (for example, Gorry, 1970; Hamilton, 1966). Groen and Patel (1985) and Johnson (1988) concluded that experts' reasoning in non-problematic situations resembled pattern recognition or direct retrieval from an extensive, well-structured knowledge base. Elstein *et al.* (1990), by comparison, argue that experts 'clearly do consider and evaluate alternatives when confronted with problematic situations' (p. 10) (as opposed to direct automatic retrieval of learned diagnostic/management hypotheses, etc.).

Pattern recognition has both strengths and weaknesses. While it lacks certainty, this reasoning strategy allows conclusions to be reached in situations characterized by imprecise data and limited premises. For instance, a clinician faced with contradictory signs and symptoms and wishing to avoid the use of potentially harmful invasive diagnostic tests, may derive a functional diagnosis (for example, low back pain of musculoskeletal origin) as the basis for initial management planning. Albert, Munson and Resnick (1988) argue that while we would prefer certainty to probability, we are often faced in medical situations with a lack in the level of information needed for correct, acceptable deductions and so we need to depend upon inductive inferences. Such clinical judgements need to be defensible and credible. They may well depend heavily on professional craft knowledge in particularly imprecise or complex human situations when logical, rational reasoning relying on propositional (scientific or theoretical) knowledge is inadequate. Pattern recognition is characterized by speed and efficiency (Arocha, Patel & Patel, 1993; Ridderikhoff, 1989). By comparison, hypothetico-deductive reasoning, particularly the phase of backward/deductive reasoning, is generally regarded as being a slower, more demanding and more detailed process than inductive reasoning (Arocha *et al.*, 1993; Patel & Groen, 1986; Patel & Groen, 1991; Ridderikhoff, 1989).

Pattern recognition may be used successfully by beginning students in situations where the case is simple and the student has had some experience in matching his or her textbook knowledge with real-life experience. By comparison, expert clinicians have a considerable depth of experience of both 'textbook' conditions and the variability within and between medical conditions, and can demonstrate a greater expertise in using pattern recognition when dealing with the complexity of cases where clients are simultaneously suffering from multiple conditions.

(c) Knowledge-reasoning integration

Recent research in the health sciences (for example, Schmidt, Norman & Boshuizen, 1990) has demonstrated that clinical reasoning is not a separate skill that can be developed independently of relevant professional knowledge and other clinical skills, such as investigative skills. There is increasing evidence to support the importance of domain-specific knowledge and an organized knowledge base in clinical problem-solving expertise (Bordage & Zacks, 1984; Elstein *et al.*, 1990; Grant & Marsden, 1987; Norman, Brooks & Allen, 1989; Patel, Evans & Kaufman, 1990; Patel & Groen, 1986; Schmidt *et al.*, 1990). However, it is the interaction between such knowledge and reasoning skills (cognitive and metacognitive) which is essential for effective thinking and problem-solving (Alexander & Judy, 1988; Barrows & Pickell, 1991).

5.2.2 A MODEL FOR CLINICAL REASONING

Clinical reasoning can be characterized as a process of reflective inquiry, in collaboration with the client (if possible), which seeks to promote a deep and contextually relevant understanding of the clinical problem, in order to provide a sound basis for clinical intervention. The essential elements of effective clinical reasoning are cognition (reflective inquiry), a strong underpinning of discipline-specific knowledge and metacognition (which provides the integrative element between cognition and knowledge). Figure 5.1 illustrates the essential interaction of these three core elements in the process of clinical reasoning.

This model or analogy of clinical reasoning was developed (Higgs & Jones, 1995a) to transcend disciplinary boundaries and contexts in order to present both the essence and elements of clinical reasoning. In this analogy, clinical reasoning is represented by an upward and outward spiral. This image is intended to demonstrate clinical reasoning as both a cyclical and a developing process. Each loop of the spiral incorporates data input, data interpretation/re-interpretation and problem formulation/re-formulation to achieve a progressively broader and deeper understanding of the clinical problem. Based on this deepening understanding, decisions are made concerning intervention, and actions are taken. The clinician may, for instance, decide not to intervene, to collect further data, to conduct a treatment or to provide care. Throughout the reasoning process, the core elements of knowledge, cognition and metacognition interact.

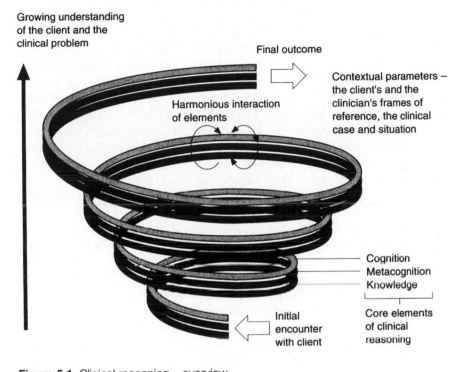

Figure 5.1 Clinical reasoning – overview
Reproduced with permission from J. Higgs & M. Jones, *Clinical Reasoning in the Health Professions*; published by Butterworth-Heinemann, 1995.

This model seeks to draw together the major dimensions of the current dominant clinical reasoning models in the literature. These include: the hypothetico-deductive reasoning, pattern recognition, problem-solving (Payton, 1985), the phenomenological model adopted in occupational therapy (Mattingly, 1991), models of backward reasoning and forward reasoning (Patel & Groen, 1991; Ridderikhoff, 1989), models as in nursing which emphasize intuition (Benner & Tanner, 1987; Rew & Barrow, 1987) or a combined model as presented by Higgs and Jones (1995a). In this interpretation of clinical reasoning the roles of various forms of knowledge in the reasoning process are numerous and are closely linked to the context (of the client, profession, situation) in which the knowledge is being utilized.

5.2.3 EXPERTISE IN CLINICAL PRACTICE AND CLINICAL REASONING

Benner (1984) describes the transition from novice to expert as a movement from reliance on abstract principles to the use of knowledge gained from experience as paradigms, and as a change in perception from a compilation of equally relevant pieces of data to an appreciation of the whole clinical picture with selectively relevant parts. In relation to cognitive skills, Benner and Tanner (1987) argue that other aspects of judgement apart from feature-detection or template-matching are needed to enhance pattern recognition in the process of decision-making, including similarity/dissimilarity recognition, deliberate rationality and a sense of salience. These skills appear to be innate human abilities, but their effectiveness is largely dependent upon an adequately structured knowledge base derived from experience. Expert clinicians utilize these skills in sub-consciously accessing their clinical experience (Benner & Tanner, 1987). In addition, the effective use of metacognitive skills in monitoring the cognitive process enhances problem-solving and decision-making (Biggs & Telfer, 1987).

Boshuizen, Schmidt and colleagues (Boshuizen & Schmidt, 1992; Schmidt *et al.*, 1992) have developed a stage theory of the development of expertise which emphasizes the parallel development of knowledge acquisition and clinical reasoning expertise. This model is based upon the notion and observation that developing knowledge and resultant reasoning expertise is largely the result of changes in knowledge structure. This process begins with students' reasoning which relies heavily on biomedical knowledge and the generation and testing of multiple hypotheses. With experience, knowledge is restructured, encapsulated and is structured around 'illness scripts' (i.e. abstract categories of illness features), and the associated reasoning, utilizing the illness scripts is a much more streamlined operation. Ongoing clinical experience results in the accumulation of 'instantiated scripts' (i.e. actual detailed cases/specific instances) in the clinician's knowledge base which provide the basis for prompt and automatic reasoning with similar cases in the future. Conscious reasoning and recourse to less clinically-structured and more basic knowledge occurs in complex situations. Patel and Kaufman (1995) regard the above interpretation as 'idealized'. They argue that the key role played by knowledge gained from the basic and applied sciences underlying clinical practice may be in facilitating explanation and coherent communication, rather than in facilitating clinical reasoning itself. Further research is needed to clarify the role of both biomedical knowledge and all knowledge types in professional practice.

Simon (1980) has suggested that it takes at least ten years' experience to obtain proficiency in any profession. However, experience alone does not result in expertise. Harris (1993) contends that for experience to lead to expertise, people must be able to learn from experience and they must be able to distinguish order and regularities in practice. Boud (1988) contends that expertise requires an ability to undertake a reflective process that includes associating experiences and integrating them in terms of patterns.

Clinical expertise (including clinical reasoning) can be viewed as a continuum along multiple dimensions. These dimensions include clinical outcomes, personal attributes such as intuition, clinical skills (for example, manual and technical ability, communication and interpersonal skills), personality characteristics (for example, empathy), and knowledge, cognitive and metacognitive proficiency (for example, logical, creative and reflective reasoning) (Higgs & Jones, 1995a).

In relation to the clinical reasoning component of clinical expertise, there are a number of dimensions of expertise which can be examined. Glaser and Chi (1988, pp xvii–xx), for example, provide seven knowledge and cognitive dimensions of expertise:

- 'Experts excel mainly in their own domains.'
- 'Experts perceive large meaningful patterns in their domain.'
- 'Experts are fast: They are faster than novices at performing the skills of their domain, and they quickly solve problems with little error.'
- 'Experts have superior short-term and long-term memory.'
- 'Experts see and represent a problem in their domain at a deeper (more principled) level than novices; novices to tend to represent a problem at a superficial level.'
- 'Experts spend a great deal of time analyzing a problem qualitatively.'
- 'Experts have strong self-monitoring skills.'

Higgs and Jones (1995a) add another dimension; to recognize and value the place of the client in the decision-making process (if possible) or at least giving consideration to the client's needs as a person, i.e. 'Experts have a deep understanding of the clinical problem including the client's perspective.' This factor is especially important in clinical settings where the professional paradigm expects clinical care to involve a partnership approach between clinician and client. In occupational therapy, for instance, considerable emphasis is placed on the utilization of a client-centred approach in which the focus is on people's rights to develop the skills and habits required for a balanced, wholesome life (Shannon, 1977).

The eight characteristics of experts as listed above emphasize the different levels of knowledge and cognitive/metacognitive skills which comprise clinical reasoning expertise. Less expert clinicians may only possess general knowledge of their profession while experts possess specialized knowledge. While this may account for superior outcomes with regard to diagnostic accuracy, other non-domain-specific knowledge and personal attributes will play a large role in determining how clinicians are perceived and judged by health care recipients. Similarly, while domain-specific knowledge and associated cognitive skills, such as pattern recognition, are characteristic of experts, cognitive strategies such as hypothetico-deductive reasoning, which are less dependent upon domain-specific knowledge and skills, are crucial when clinical patterns are not easily recognized. Acquisition of expertise must be approached with consideration of all aspects influencing clinical outcomes as viewed from both the clinician's and the client's perspectives.

5.3 ADULT LEARNING: A FRAMEWORK FOR TEACHING CLINICAL REASONING

The ideal choice of educational philosophy and framework for clinical reasoning programmes is adult learning. This is because both clinical reasoning and adult learning involve an essential link between the knowledge base and the cognitive strategies of the individual. Both processes involve an ability to seek information and knowledge as required (to learn or to make clinical decisions), a capacity to engage in self-monitoring, evaluation and development and responsibility, for decisions taken.

According to Finger (1990), adult learning provides a means of achieving transformation of the student and their situation by helping the student find a solution to a problem situation. Therefore, using adult learning approaches to teach clinical reasoning enables students to learn through their experience of solving their learning problems and at the same time learn about clinical reasoning or the transformation of clinical problems into solutions. Ramsden regards the notion of 'changing students' conceptions of aspects of the world around them' as 'the core of education' (Ramsden, 1988a, p. vii). Education can be enhanced, argues Ramsden (1988b), by understanding how students are thinking and learning, by helping students learn to understand how subject experts see relevant phenomena and by enabling students to change their conceptions of these phenomena. The principles and practice of adult learning come closest to this goal. Students in adult learning programmes need to take an active part in the learning process. In addition, clinical educators and students are engaged in interdependent learning and learning is directed towards growth of students.

The educational arguments presented above underpin the clinical reasoning teaching programmes developed by the author (Higgs, 1990). In particular, our programmes in the classroom and in clinical education have endeavoured to create adult learning conditions (such as motivation, acceptance of the student as a person, autonomy, emphasis on experience) and promote effective adult learning behaviours including: problem-solving, active participation in learning, interdependence, critical reflection, active seeking of meaning, experiential learning. (Refer to Terry & Higgs,

1993, for a discussion of learning environments which foster the development of reasoning skills.)

5.4 DEVELOPING CLINICAL REASONING SKILLS: TEACHING IN CONTEXT

Clinical reasoning is inextricably linked to the unique knowledge base of the professional discipline (and indeed to the individual clinician), therefore clinical reasoning needs to be taught in context. Thus, the educator's choice of clinical reasoning model for a given programme of study needs to take into consideration such factors as the conceptual framework of the health science discipline in question (for example, nursing), the specific learning environment or curricular context and the stage of development of the students. For instance, practice in the use of the hypothetico-deductive reasoning model may be highly desirable for undergraduate medical students who are learning how to collect and process a multitude of clinical data and make diagnostic and intervention decisions. By comparison, exploration of the phenomenological model may be best suited to occupational therapy students learning within a 'wellness' framework rather than a traditional medical model. And, for a group of postgraduate students with a wealth of clinical expertise, examination of clinical reasoning using a pattern recognition model may enable them to critique their prior learning, deepen their knowledge bases and gain a greater understanding of, and expertise in the use of clinical reasoning strategies.

In the absence of a commonly accepted model of clinical reasoning, it is desirable for students to develop their own understanding of the clinical reasoning process and of how they reason, as the first step in facilitating improved clinical reasoning. This can be accomplished through exploration of how others describe or have investigated clinical reasoning, examination of the differences between reasoning in novices and experts, reflection on their own reasoning and discussions with other students. In developing an understanding and awareness of their own learning students can learn to value cognition and knowledge as valuable tools to facilitate effective clinical practice and to develop expertise in the use of higher level cognitive skills (including metacognition or critical reflection-in-action). Through these means students can learn how to manage their reasoning rather than acquiring expertise (or perhaps erroneous thinking practices and knowledge) via trial and error or chance.

Clinical reasoning may be taught in a separate subject within a curriculum or as an integral aspect of all areas/subjects within the curriculum. The first strategy has the advantage of drawing attention to this skill rather than diffusing it among the various other learning goals of the curriculum. More time can be spent in refining individual students' clinical reasoning skills, or in identifying and addressing deficiencies in their knowledge and reasoning abilities. The more general approach has the potential advantages of reinforcing reasoning and the integration of knowledge in all areas of learning, and promoting transfer of learning from classroom to clinical settings. In either case, the goal of promoting deep (i.e. meaningful) learning of the nature and strategies of clinical reasoning should ideally be the learning goal.

Exploration of clinical reasoning can occur either in the classroom, or in the clinic. In the classroom students can learn from mistakes, explore alternative treatment decisions, change their minds and examine many detailed aspects of knowledge use and evaluation in the absence of both time constraints and the potential negative effects for clients of changing, uncertain or incorrect clinical decisions which can occur in the clinical context. The classroom setting also allows for discussion of students' thinking and the potential outcomes and relative merits of their decisions, and encourages feedback from both peers and university educators. However, attention must be also devoted to transfer of these skills from the classroom to the clinical context.

On-campus teaching in structured learning activities within health science curricula can be designed to promote the development of clinical reasoning skills and the integration of knowledge that students have gained both from life experiences and classroom and fieldwork studies. These structured learning activities can include small-group learning tutorials, peer teaching, cognitive mapping, role play, verbalizing interpretation of client data in simulated clinical settings, and experts discussing their interpretation of a problem.

As well as developing reasoning skills and knowledge in the classroom, students need to test the application of this knowledge in appropriate contexts. Clinical education provides this opportunity. During clinical placements much of the daily activity of health science students relates to clinical problem-solving since students are continually seeking, absorbing, interpreting, evaluating and summarizing clinical information and making clinical decisions on the basis of this information (Whelan, 1988). Experiences during clinical education promote an understanding of clients' conditions and needs, as well as the students' own abilities in meeting these needs. Students also learn valuable skills in information use and management, including how much information is necessary and desirable to collect to enable both effective and efficient clinical decision-making.

The reality of the clinical setting has many advantages even though it provides constraints to the exploration of clinical reasoning in action, such as time pressures and potential dangers to the client. Holmes (1975) has proposed that clinical education is vital for students to gain confidence in handling clients, develop their clinical/technical skills and acquire skills in decision-making. The clinical setting also provides the complex context and conditions (for example, consequences of their actions, variability and personalities of clients) which students will face in practice. Studies have shown that a number of groups of health personnel have been found to reason better in real treatment situations than in simulated situations (Gale & Marsden, 1982). Practice broadens experience, and therefore enhances performance. It has also been found (Norman, 1990) that the context in which learning occurs has a profound effect on the student's ability to recall learning, with recall occurring best in situations similar to that in which it was learned. Finally, the role of clients in teaching and providing feedback is a particular advantage of clinical settings (see Chapter 3 on client feedback). It is necessary, therefore, that health science curricula actively utilize both classroom and clinical settings to develop their clinical reasoning competence.

5.5 PREPARING STUDENTS FOR CLINICAL EDUCATION

Numerous strategies for teaching clinical reasoning skills in the classroom and the clinic have been suggested (Higgs & Jones, 1995b). The following section briefly outlines two such strategies.

5.5.1 EXPERIENTIAL COURSE IN CLINICAL REASONING

An experiential learning course in clinical reasoning has been conducted in Sydney for several years for postgraduate manipulative physiotherapy students (Higgs, 1990). In this programme, classes involve three to four students exploring a hypothetical/simulated case in front of an audience of their peers. The students are questioned about their clinical reasoning and knowledge by an 'expert' panel comprising physiotherapy educators/ clinicians and applied science educators who challenge the students' knowledge and their clinical reasoning strategies. The experts engage students in exploration of the relative advantages of different inquiry methods, investigation techniques and intervention strategies. Of particular concern is helping students evaluate the validity of their own knowledge and critically review their clinical evaluation strategies. Other students role play the client and provide information about the client.

5.5.2 COGNITIVE MAPPING

Another strategy for developing clinical reasoning skills and knowledge is by engaging students in drawing cognitive maps which visually represent aspects of their unique knowledge base. Cognitive maps can be formulated in many ways such as flow charts, annotated diagrams, images or maps illustrating interconnected ideas (Novak & Gowin, 1984). This exercise helps students assess and revise their knowledge bases in terms of accuracy, comprehensiveness and organization, and learn how to organize and access their knowledge more effectively. They can also gain feedback from peers and educators on knowledge content and the links being made between concepts and explore different forms of knowledge.

5.6 DESIGNING CLINICAL EDUCATION TO FACILITATE THE DEVELOPMENT OF CLINICAL REASONING SKILLS

The first step in designing clinical education programmes is to establish the contribution of clinical education as part of the overall curricular goals. Common goals in health science education include the development of technical and clinical reasoning competence, interpersonal skills, knowledge and self-directed learning skills. Self-directed learning skills and the ability to perform as adult students are particularly important attributes of health professionals in this age of rapid technological advancements. These skills provide students with the ability to generate knowledge and clinical skills in order to deal both proactively and responsively with their own learning needs and with changes in society's health care needs (see Chapter 9).

Clinical reasoning skills learned in the classroom can be transferred into the clinical setting. To achieve this transfer effectively, clinical educators need to develop a clear understanding of their students' learning needs by exploring the students' reasoning and use of knowledge and providing feedback on students' performance in these areas. In addition, since clinical reasoning competence lies at the centre of professional autonomy, it is desirable for clinical educators to create adult learning environments, facilitate adult and self-directed learning and promote students' evaluation and enhancement of their own reasoning skills. Thus, the ideal clinical education environment to foster clinical reasoning skills development combines both guidance and freedom to learn in a meaningful (deep learning) manner. Rogers (1983) refers to this type of environment as one of 'responsible freedom'. It may also be described as a 'liberating programme system' (Higgs, 1993) (see discussion in Chapter 1).

5.7 DEVELOPING CLINICAL REASONING IN THE CLINICAL SETTING

5.7.1 THE CONTEXT OF THE CLINIC

In clinical practice reasoning occurs within the immediate and personal context of the individual client, the unique multi-dimensional context of the client's clinical problem, the actual clinical setting in question, the personal and professional framework of the clinician, the broad context of health care delivery and the complex context of professional decision-making. Therefore, clinicians are faced with a mass of information to deal with and they need to develop strategies to reason effectively within these circumstances.

Clinicians need to develop the ability to make sense of the problems that individual clients present with, which can be 'confusing and contradictory, characterized by imperfect, inconsistent, or even inaccurate information' (Kassirer & Kopelman, 1991, p. vii). Also, they need to acquire a broad understanding of the environment in which they work, including knowledge of the factors influencing health (for example, the environment, socio-economic conditions, cultural beliefs and human behaviour). Furthermore, they need to be able to incorporate into clinical decisions the personal needs and preferences of their clients, health care professionals and to be able to deal effectively with an increasing body of scientific, technical and professional knowledge. The use of information technology support systems may be a useful aid to data management in some circumstances.

Thus clinicians need to be able to perform competently in situations which are often unclear or indeterminate (Kennedy, 1987; Schön, 1987). To achieve this outcome, Schön (1987) contends that clinicians need to be 'reflective practitioners' and thereby shape and reshape actions as required by the context. Clinical reasoning learning programmes should therefore foster the development of metacognitive skills including reflection and self-evaluation. (See Case Study 5.1 for an example of this process in action.)

5.7.2 LEARNING THROUGH EXPERIENCE

The processing of experience through reflection is particularly important for the development of clinical reasoning expertise (Rivett & Higgs, 1995). This is because reasoning is not an observable or directly demonstrable behaviour (such as a psychomotor skill) where performance can be assessed and feedback provided more readily. Instead, reasoning is a highly complex cognitive ability which is unobservable to others and often difficult to comprehend and communicate by the reasoner him/herself. These difficulties arise because clinical reasoning utilizes complex cognitive and metacognitive skills, including critical evaluation of data, the use of maximizing principles that facilitate optimal processing, and the evaluation and use of knowledge. Errors in reasoning may not be apparent in ensuing actions and sound reasoning strategies may appear to be adopted without adequate knowledge or accurate interpretation of clinical data. Reflection on reasoning and communication of knowledge and reasoning, therefore, are valuable mechanisms for enabling both the student and the teacher to examine the student's knowledge and reasoning strategies.

Case Study 5.1 Example of a clinical educator encouraging reflection and self-evaluation

Scene Debriefing session after student's treatment of a client

Clinical educator: I noticed that you tried several lines of inquiry to obtain information from the client while you were taking his history. How did you think the client was feeling?

Student: He appeared be very anxious at first and I was uncertain about what was making him anxious – perhaps his worries about his own condition or because you were assessing me and he knew I was rather anxious. He seemed OK beforehand.

Clinical educator: Could you explain your strategy for dealing with his anxiety.

Student: Well partly, I guess I was just trying at first to keep things going by trying to repeat the questions more clearly and aiming to reassure him. Then, when he seemed to relax a bit more I was able to ask him some simple questions which gave me time to listen carefully to his answers and start making some sense out of what he was saying. After that it was easier to get back into a more normal pattern of questions.

Clinical educator: Tell me a bit more about 'making sense out of what he was saying'.

Student: I mean that I was trying to put the pieces together and to identify what was key information.

Clinical educator: So, this helped to start to develop ideas about his diagnosis – or perhaps it helped with the next areas you needed to question him about ...?

Student: Yes, that's it! I had started to think of several hypotheses, particularly related to previous cases ...

Notes: The clinical educator first sought to help the student relax by asking exploratory questions focused on the client. Then she explored some of the student's responses in order to prompt reflection on the student's reasoning strategies and to challenge the student to consider new possibilities.

Related to active reflection as a means of enhancing learning are the skills of self-evaluation and metacognition (or reflective self-awareness). These skills are essential for processing information to make sound clinical decisions. In developing a greater awareness of their cognition individuals are better able to perform these mental processes. This argument supports the use of learning activities which prompt students to use, articulate, critique and review their clinical reasoning. In doing this, students are able to raise their awareness of their thinking and develop an enhanced capacity for responsible self-direction and decision-making.

In addition to facilitating the development of their cognitive and meta-cognitive reasoning skills, the clinical setting provides an important opportunity for students to generate and test their knowledge and to develop a knowledge base which is sound and well-organized. This can be done by students seeking to discover their own meaning through self-directed learning, and by endeavouring to make sense of their clinical learning experiences. Achieving these goals entails students questioning what they are learning or have learned, reflecting on their thoughts and actions, exploring the validity and effects of different ways of achieving their clinical goals, experimenting with new ideas and discussing thoughts and experiences with others.

5.7.3 CLINICAL REASONING DEVELOPMENT: WORKING WITH THE CLIENT

The clinical reasoning behind clinical performance encompasses not only diagnostic and management-oriented problem-solving, but also deals with clients' unique personal experience of their problems (i.e. the specific meaning and influences of their clinical problems). As such, clinical performance and the associated clinical reasoning cannot be judged solely on the basis of clinical results, such as whether the surgery or therapeutic intervention worked. The recipient of health care may have regained his or her health or function yet still feel the clinician's performance was inadequate. Thus, clinical reasoning cannot be fully understood or evaluated when only the clinician's perspective is considered. Shared decision-making between client and clinician is important if 'success' is to be realized from the client's perspective.

Clients' choices, rights and responsibilities in relation to their own health are changing. Payton, Nelson and Ozer (1990) advocate client involvement in decision-making which pertains to the management of their health and well-being. They argue that this process of client participation is based on the 'recognition of the values of self-determination and the worth of the individual' (p. ix). Using their understanding of their clients' rights and responsibilities, students and graduate clinicians need to develop their own guidelines for when and how much involvement the client should have in reasoning and decision-making. Mutual decision-making and two-way communication require skills in negotiation as well as explaining (see Chapter 3 on communication skills). The clinical setting is a highly appropriate context in which to refine these skills under the guidance of clinical educators. (Refer to Case Study 5.2.)

5.7.4 DEALING WITH RULES AND PROTOCOLS

Health professionals often use routines during data collection, for example, client questionnaires or standardized assessment protocols. Although this

---

Case Study 5.2 Example of involving the client in clinical decision-making

Student (To client): Since you'll be going home tomorrow, we need to organize a home programme of exercises that you could follow. I recommend that you go for an hour's walk each day. OK?
Client: I'll try.
Clinical educator (To student): Perhaps you could discuss several options of exercise with Mrs S and you could both consider the advantages of each and determine which option Mrs S would prefer? What about swimming, for instance?
Client: Swimming? Well, maybe – the local pool is quite close – but I don't go there often. On the other hand, it'll be rather dark for a long walk by the time I'll get home from work.
Student: OK. Then let's think about the alternatives and see what's best for you ...

Notes: The clinical educator is prompting the student to proceed beyond a preliminary step of 'consultation' to involve the client in decision-making.

---

may imply rigidness in procedures and lack of variation in response to individuals or to situations, data collection routines may also be regarded as useful scanning activities (as described by Barrows & Tamblyn, 1980) which aim to identify cues requiring further investigation. Such routines or protocols can assist in ensuring that adequate data is collected, thereby avoiding premature closure of hypothesis generation during clinical reasoning.

On the other hand, strict and unthinking use of data collection routines can be inefficient and can result in collection of excessive, confusing and perhaps irrelevant data causing difficulty in data analysis, particularly for students. The skilled clinician may choose to use data collection routines strategically. Therefore, it is useful to encourage students to explore the value of using planned strategies or routines as a basis for comprehensive and efficient data collection and to help them learn how to use such routines strategically when or if desirable.

5.7.5 COMMUNICATING REASONING

It is important for health professionals to be able to communicate their clinical reasoning to their clients and other people for several reasons, including facilitation of communication and mutual decision-making and demonstration of accountability. In addition to behaving in a competent, ethical and professional manner, clinicians need to be able to explain, clearly and credibly, the scientific and therapeutic basis for their actions and the expected outcomes, within the context of the individual client's needs, wishes and situation. Students can learn to communicate and justify their decisions effectively through clinical reasoning learning activities, such as verbalizing their interpretation of client data, and justifying their choice of intervention.

Through interactive learning activities (such as group discussions or role plays where students verbalize their reasoning) students can learn the valuable skill of communicating and testing their knowledge and reasoning. By communicating thoughts, arguments and rationales students are required to understand and organize what they know and how they use knowledge. Experience in such teaching (Higgs, 1990, 1992) has shown that when students are attempting to communicate their thoughts they learn a great deal about the nature, breadth, and scope of their own knowledge, the way they organize and link their knowledge, the way they access, accept and/or test knowledge and collected data, and the value and validity of their knowledge. They also develop a critical appreciation of how they reason, the errors in reasoning they or others make, strategies to reason effectively and efficiently and the process of metacognition. (See Case Study 5.3.)

5.7.6 ASSESSING STUDENTS' CLINICAL REASONING

Assessing clinical reasoning performance is not a simple task. Firstly, reasoning is not readily observable since it is an internal process. Secondly, it is difficult to measure since there is neither one perfect reasoning process nor is there only one way of interpreting any given case/situation. Thirdly, much of reasoning and knowledge is not only part of the developing and imprecise clinical sciences, but is also ideally part of a human interaction process where choice, human preferences and the art of clinical practice are essential elements.

Kennedy (1987), for instance, argues that professional judgement within the ambiguous or uncertain situations of health care is an inexact science and that judging clinical decisions by a priori standards of rationality is inappropriate. Thus the importance of individual perspectives rather than a priori criteria (Jungermann, 1986) and the defensibility of these perspectives could be more valuable evaluation criteria in the case of professional clinical judgements/decisions. Skills of professional judgement and critical self-evaluation are also needed to cope with information processing constraints or 'bounded rationality' (as per Newell & Simon, 1972) which result in limitations on the individual's ability to access knowledge and solve problems (Bransford, Sherwood, Vye & Reiser, 1986; Feltovich, 1983).

What is evaluated when assessing students' clinical reasoning? The individual's level of clinical reasoning expertise includes the ability to use

Case Study 5.3 Example of a student verbalizing her clinical reasoning

Scene Clinical tutorial – discussion of the management of a particular client assigned to a student. The student has just outlined her client's condition to the group

Clinical educator: At this point – before we discuss management – could you go through your clinical findings and explain your process of reasoning to us, in terms of the working hypotheses you developed and tested in reaching your diagnosis.

Student: From the beginning when the client walked into the room I started to think about low back pain and a right hip problem. Then as I collected more information I added a local muscle problem to the list. The main information I used to generate these hypotheses was the gait pattern, posture and the location and behaviour of the pain reported by the client. As I proceeded further through the history taking and physical examination, it became clearer that there were two clinical problems: a lumbar spine disorder and an unrelated knee problem.

Clinical educator: Could you describe your process of testing your various hypotheses. Did you set out to eliminate certain hypotheses or confirm others for instance?

Student: I guess right from the start I assumed it was a spinal problem and everything seemed to confirm that.

Clinical educator: (Leads students into further discussion on strategies for reasoning and scanning/searching techniques and on errors in reasoning such as premature closure of hypothesis generation.)

Notes: The student is encouraged to explain her reasoning approach/pattern in her own words and is then (with the group) prompted to explore and critique this reasoning aloud.

an organized, accessible knowledge base, to access this knowledge in relation to clinical problems, to generate and test working hypotheses related to various areas (such as diagnosis and intervention, skills in evaluating and using clinical data during reasoning), to use metacognition to monitor and influence one's own reasoning and to engage in self-evaluation of clinical reasoning (through reflection and review). In addition assessment of effective clinical reasoning would include assessing students' ability to communicate their reasoning process and the reasons behind the clinical decisions made, to generate knowledge (for example, by reflecting on clinical experiences), and to develop their knowledge bases (by critiquing and as needed revising the content, accessibility and organization of existing knowledge).

Since no single method of assessment can adequately evaluate clinical reasoning a variety of methods are therefore desirable. In the clinical education context these could include oral assessment, direct observation of performance with explanations, in real or simulated situations, self-assessment and peer assessment. In general, assessment of the process of reasoning is best examined in situations where the student's thoughts are made explicit and can be explored during reasoning.

In formative assessment situations, where feedback and learning rather than grading are important, desirable assessment methods are those which involve the exploration and application of thoughts with time during or after the exercise for discussion. For instance, during a debriefing session after a student treats a client, the clinical educator could ask the student to explain the rationale for the intervention implemented. Students' explanation could be prompted at times with questions to probe more deeply into the rationale provided and to encourage students to expand on 'shorthand' or 'glib' reasons/comments. In addition, students could be asked to reconsider the validity of their knowledge base and the reliability of the knowledge and clinical data they have used as the basis of their reasoning.

Alternatively, students could be encouraged to take the initiative during their clinical placements to discuss real or hypothetical clinical cases with clinical educators. Clinical educators, acting as 'sounding boards', can engage in reflective interactions seeking both to provide feedback (reinforcement as well as correction) to students and also to foster students' critical self-assessment.

In designing and conducting assessment procedures to facilitate the development of clinical reasoning skills, the nature of the assessment process and how it is presented to and perceived by the students is very important. The method of assessment also needs to be appropriate for the phenomenon (for example, knowledge, the ability to reason) being evaluated and to be a sound procedure (for instance in terms of reliability, validity and feasibility of use) (see Chapter 6).

5.8 CONCLUSION

In this chapter many aspects of the nature and teaching of clinical reasoning have been examined. Clinical reasoning has been presented as a complex phenomenon, but one which is vital to developing expertise in clinical practice. The clinical education context provides a valuable environment for students to develop, understand and explore their clinical reasoning abilities. A number of factors and strategies which will enable these goals to be achieved have been examined.

REFERENCES

Albert, A. D., Munson, R. & Resnik, M. D. (Eds) (1988). *Reasoning in medicine: An introduction to clinical inference.* Baltimore: The John Hopkins University Press.

Alexander, P. A. & Judy, J. E. (1988). The interaction of domain-specific and strategic knowledge in academic performance. *Review of Educational Research*, **58**, 375–404.

Arocha, J. F., Patel, V. L. & Patel, Y. C. (1993). Hypothesis generation and the coordination of theory and evidence in novice diagnostic reasoning. *Journal of Medical Decision Making*, **13**, 198–211.

Barrows, H. S., Feightner, J. W., Neufield, V. R. & Norman, G. R. (1978). An analysis of the clinical methods of medical students and physicians. *Report to the Province of Ontario Department of Health*, McMaster University, Hamilton, Ontario.

Barrows, H. S. & Pickell, G. C. (1991). *Developing clinical problem-solving skills: A guide to more effective diagnosis and treatment.* New York: Norton & Co.

Barrows, H. S. & Tamblyn, R. M. (1980). *Problem-based learning: An approach to medical education.* New York: Springer.

Benner P. (1984). *From novice to expert: Excellence and power in clinical nursing practice.* London: Addison-Wesley.

Benner P,. & Tanner, C. (1987). Clinical judgment: How expert nurses use intuition. *American Journal of Nursing*, **87**, 23–31.

Biggs, J. B. & Telfer, R. (1987). *The process of learning* (2nd ed.). Sydney: Prentice Hall.

Bordage, G. & Zacks, R. (1984). The structure of medical knowledge in memories of medical students and practitioners: Categories and prototypes. *Medical Education*, **18**, 406–16.

Boshuizen, H. P. A. & Schmidt, H. G. (1992). On the role of biomedical knowledge in clinical reasoning by experts, intermediates and novices. *Cognitive Science*, **16**, 153–84.

Boud, D. (1988). How to help students learn from experience. In K. Cox & C. Ewan (Eds). *The medical teacher* (2nd ed.), (pp 68–73). Edinburgh: Churchill Livingstone.

Bransford, J., Sherwood, R., Vye, N. & Rieser, J. (1986). Teaching thinking and problem solving: Research foundations. *American Psychologist*, **41**, 1078–89.

Chapparo, C. & Ranka, J. (1995). Clinical reasoning in occupational therapy. In J. Higgs & M. Jones (Eds). *Clinical reasoning in the health professions* (pp 88–102). Oxford: Butterworth-Heinemann.

Elstein A. S., Shulman L. S. & Sprafka S. S. (1978). *Medical problem solving: An analysis of clinical reasoning.* Cambridge, MA: Harvard University Press.

Elstein, A. S., Shulman, L. S. & Sprafka, S. A. (1990). Medical problem solving: a ten year retrospective. *Evaluation and the Health Professions*, **13**, 5–36.

Feltovich, P. J. (1983). Expertise: Reorganizing and refining knowledge for use. *Professions Education Researcher Notes*, **4**, 5–9.

Feltovich, P. J. & Barrows, H. S. (1984). Issues of generality in medical problem solving. In H. G. Schmidt & M. L. De Volder (Eds). *Tutorials in problem-based learning; A new direction in teaching the health professions.* Assen: Van Gorcum.

Feltovich, P. J., Johnson, P. E., Moller, J. H. & Swanson, D. B. (1984). LCS: The role and development of medical knowledge in diagnostic expertise. In W. J. Clancey & E. H. Shortliffe (Eds). *Readings in medical artificial intelligence: The first decade* (pp 275–319). Reading: Addison-Wesley.

Finger, M. (1990). Does adult education need a philosophy? Reflections about the function of adult learning in today's society. *Studies in Higher Education*, **12**, 81–98.

Fleming, M. H. (1991). The therapist with the three track mind. *American Journal of Occupational Therapy*, **45**, 1007–14.

Fonteyn, M. (1991). *A descriptive analysis of expert critical care nurses' clinical reasoning*. Doctoral Dissertation, University of Texas, Austin, Texas.

Gale, J. (1982). Some cognitive components of the diagnostic thinking process. *British Journal of Educational Psychology*, **52**, 64–76.

Gale, J. & Marsden, P. (1982). Clinical problem solving: the beginning of the process. *Medical Education*, **16**, 22–6.

Glaser, R. & Chi, M.T.H. (1988). Overview. In M. T. H. Chi, R. Glaser & M .J. Farr (Eds). *The nature of expertise* (pp xvi–xxviii). Hillsdale, NJ: Lawrence Erlbaum Associates.

Gorry, G. A. (1970). Modelling the diagnostic process. *Journal of Medical Education*, **45**, 293–302.

Grant, J. & Marsden, P. (1987). The structure of memorized knowledge in students and clinicians: An explanation for diagnostic expertise. *Medical Education*, **21**, 92–8.

Groen, G. J. & Patel, V. L. (1985). Medical problem-solving: Some questionable assumptions. *Medical Education*, **19**, 95–100.

Hamilton, M. (1966). *Clinicians and decisions*. Leeds: Leeds University Press.

Harris, I. B. (1993). New expectations for professional competence. In L. Cuddy & J. Wergin (Eds). *Educating professionals* (pp 17–52). San Francisco: Jossey-Bass.

Higgs, J. & Jones, M. (1995a). Clinical reasoning. In J. Higgs & M. Jones (Eds). *Clinical reasoning in the health professions* (pp 3–23). Oxford: Butterworth-Heinemann.

Higgs, J. & Jones, M. (Eds) (1995b). *Clinical reasoning in the health professions*. Oxford: Butterworth-Heinemann.

Higgs, J. (1990). Fostering the acquisition of clinical reasoning skills. *New Zealand Journal of Physiotherapy*, **18**, 13–17.

Higgs, J. (1992). Developing knowledge: a process of construction, mapping and review. *New Zealand Journal of Physiotherapy*, **20**, 23–30.

Higgs, J. (1993). The teacher in self-directed learning: manager or co-manager? In N. J. Graves (Ed.). *Student managed learning* (pp 122–31). Leeds: World Education Fellowship.

Holmes, B. (1975). The compleat physiotherapist. *Physiotherapy Canada*, **27**, 90–1.

Johnson, E. (1988). Expertise and decision making under uncertainty: performance and process. In M. Chi, R. Glaser & M. Farr (Eds). *The nature of expertise* (pp 209–28). New Jersey: Lawrence Erlbaum.

Jones, M. A. (1992). Clinical reasoning in manual therapy. *Physical Therapy*, **72**, 875–84.

Jungermann, H. (1986). The two camps on rationality. In H. R. Arkes & K. R. Hammond (Eds). *Judgment and decision making: An interdisciplinary reader* (pp 627–41). New York: Cambridge University Press.

Kassirer, J. P. & Kopelman, R. I. (1991). *Learning clinical reasoning*. Baltimore: Williams & Wilkins.

Kennedy, M. (1987). Inexact sciences: Professional education and the development of expertise. *Review of Research in Education*, **14**, 133–68, American Education Research Association, Washington, DC.

Mattingly, C. (1991). The narrative nature of clinical reasoning. *American Journal of*

Occupational Therapy, **45**, 998–1005.

Newell, A. & Simon, H. A. (1972). *Human problem solving*. Englewood Cliffs, NJ: Prentice-Hall.

Norman, G., Brooks, L. R. & Allen, S. W. (1989). Recall by expert medical practitioners and novices as a record of processing attention. *Journal of Experimental Psychology: Learning, Memory, and Cognition*, **15**, 1116–74.

Norman, G. R. (1990). Editorial: problem-solving skills and problem-based learning. *Physiotherapy Theory and Practice*, **6**, 53–4.

Novak J. D. & Gowin D. B. (1984). *Learning how to learn*. Cambridge: Cambridge University Press.

Padrick, K., Tanner, C., Putzier, D. & Westfall, U. (1987). Hypothesis evaluation: A component of diagnostic reasoning. In A. McClane (Ed.). *Classification of nursing diagnosis: Proceedings of the seventh conference* (pp 299–305). Toronto, Canada: C.V. Mosby.

Patel, V. L. & Kaufman, D. R. (1995). Clinical reasoning and biomedical knowledge: Implications for teaching. In J. Higgs & M. Jones (Eds). *Clinical reasoning in the health professions* (pp 117–28). Oxford: Butterworth-Heinemann.

Patel, V. L. & Groen, G. J. (1986). Knowledge-based solution strategies in medical reasoning. *Cognitive Science*, **10**, 91–116.

Patel, V. L. & Groen, G. J. (1991). The general and specific nature of medical expertise: A critical look. In A. Ericsson & J. Smith (Eds). *Toward a general theory of expertise: Prospects and limits* (pp 93–125). New York: Cambridge University Press.

Patel, V. L., Evans, D. A. & Kaufman, D. R. (1990). Reasoning strategies and use of biomedical knowledge by students. *Medical Education*, **24**, 129–36.

Payton, O. D. (1985). Clinical reasoning process in physical therapy. *Physical Therapy*, **65**, 924–8.

Payton, O. D., Nelson, C. E. & Ozer, M. N. (1990). *Patient participation in programme planning: A manual for therapists*. Philadelphia: F.A. Davis.

Ramsden, P. (1988a). Preface. In P. Ramsden (Ed.). *Improving learning: New perspectives* (pp vii–ix). London: Kogan Page.

Ramsden, P. (1988b). Studying learning: Improving teaching. In P. Ramsden (Ed.). *Improving learning: New perspectives* (pp 13–31). London: Kogan Page.

Rew, L. & Barrow, E. M. (1987). Intuition: A neglected hallmark of nursing knowledge. *Advances in Nursing Science*, **10**, 49–62.

Ridderikhoff, J. (1989). *Methods in medicine: A descriptive study of physicians' behaviour*. Dordrecht: Kluwer Academic Publishers.

Rivett, D. & Higgs, J. (1995). Experience and expertise in clinical reasoning. *New Zealand Journal of Physiotherapy*, **23**, 16–21.

Rogers, C. R. (1983). *Freedom to learn for the 80's*. Ohio: Charles E. Merrill.

Schmidt, H. G., Boshuizen, H. P. A. & Norman, G. R. (1992). Reflections on the nature of expertise in medicine. In E. Keravnou (Ed.). *Deep models for medical knowledge engineering* (pp 231–48). Amsterdam: Elsevier.

Schmidt, H. G., Norman, G. R. & Boshuizen, H. P. A. (1990). A cognitive perspective on medical expertise: theory and implications. *Academic Medicine*, **65**, 611–21.

Schön, D. A. (1987). *Educating the reflective practitioner*. San Francisco: Jossey-Bass.

Shannon, P. (1977). The derailment of occupational therapy. *American Journal of Occupational Therapy*, **31**, 229–34.

Simon, H. A. (1980). Problem solving and education. In D. T. Tuma & F. Reif (Eds).

Problem solving and education: Issues in teaching and research (pp 81–96). Hillsdale, NJ: Lawrence Erlbaum Associates.

Terry, W. & Higgs, J. (1993). Educational programmemes to develop clinical reasoning skills. *Australian Journal of Physiotherapy*, **39**, 47–51.

Whelan, G. (1988). Improving medical students' clinical-problem-solving. In P. Ramsden (Ed.). *Improving learning: New perspectives* (pp 199–214). London: Kogan Page.

Using assessment to promote student learning

6

Sandra Robertson
Department of Psychology and Speech Pathology,
Manchester Metropolitan University, United Kingdom

Joan Rosenthal
School of Communication Disorders,
The University of Sydney, Australia

Vickie Dawson
Department of Speech and Hearing,
The University of Queensland, Australia

Postcard 6

Dear All

Well I'm half way through my visit here, I can't believe how quickly the time has gone. This is the time during a normal placement that I would be assessed by my clinical educator. It's great not to have that stress around! I have decided though, to take some time this week and evaluate my own performance so far and set some personal goals for the remainder of my stay. I already know that I need to do some more work on the content and manner in which I'm giving feedback to the CBR workers. I've also decided to ask the CBR workers for feedback about how they think I'm going and also the paediatrician on the team. I'll let you know what they say.

Love Sally

6.1 CHAPTER OVERVIEW

This chapter discusses some of the issues surrounding the complex area of student assessment within the clinical setting. Specific methods of clinical assessment such as viva voce and case studies are not discussed. Rather, concepts and processes which underlie assessment are analyzed. Assessment within the context of adult learning is examined and some fundamental questions are addressed with regard to the why? and how? of the assessment process. Some insights into students' views of clinical assessment are considered, together with thoughts on peer assessment. Finally, some examples will illustrate the wide variety of assessment methods. Some of these are well-tried and proven, while others describe innovative pilot studies in progress.

6.2 ASSESSMENT: WHAT DOES IT MEAN?

The *Concise Oxford Dictionary of Word Origins* (1989) informs us that the term 'assessment' is derived from the verb 'to assess' whose original meaning was linked with the settling of amounts of taxation and has come to mean also the determining of the value of something. The Old French and Latin origins also carry the idea of 'to sit by' and hence the 'doer', the 'assessor' is someone who 'sits as assistant or adviser ... with a judge or magistrate to give advice on technical matters'. The dictionary also highlights the relation to the adjective 'assiduous', meaning 'attend or apply oneself; persevering, diligent'.

For all those involved in the process of assessing students in the clinical setting, there is a fascinating link in the definitions above. There is, firstly, the idea of determining value, but it is for the reader to decide whether this refers to the student or the 'outcome' or the 'product' of the education process. This issue will be considered later in the chapter.

Secondly, in relation to our definition, the 'doer', the person who 'assesses', may be considered as an assistant or adviser. There is no apparent hierarchy in the definition of 'assessor'; no implicit 'superior' person who must assess, no authoritarian figure with the automatic right to assess. Within the clinical setting, therefore, it is an open question as to whether the role of 'assessor' is fulfilled by the clinical educator, university staff, an external examiner or a fellow student or colleague.

Thirdly, the adjective 'assiduous' can be applied to both students and clinical educators. The word conjures up a picture of hardworking, conscientious students, diligently applying themselves to their clinical education. However, the adjective might also be applied to the 'assessor', and such an application carries with it the charge to perform the task of assessing with diligence and integrity.

6.2.1 ASSESSMENT IN THE CONTEXT OF ADULT LEARNING

In a statement summarizing the outcomes of a national study in the UK funded by the Council for National Academic Awards (Oxford Centre for Staff Development, 1992), the observation was made that the assessment system is the most significant influence on the quality of student learning and that without changes to assessment, changes in a student learning will not be reinforced. Pletts (1981) makes a similar observation, specifically within the context of clinical education: 'the evaluation of the student is also a vital part of the whole teaching process. It is useful, when setting out on a journey, to know the destination; to plan the route, and finally, be able to recognize when one has arrived' (p. 131).

It is clear, then, that when considering facilitating students' clinical learning, it is necessary to take a long hard look at the whole area of assessment and to consider its place within the sphere of adult learning philosophy and practice. Indeed, one of the indicators of 'good' teaching is that an explanation is given early in the course of how learning will be tested. Further, assessment must be congruent with, and must reflect, teaching and learning objectives. These indicators follow naturally on the heels of two others – good course organization and a clear definition of what has to be learned (Eastcott & Farmer, 1991).

Reference has already been made in this book to Kolb's learning cycle (see Chapters 2 and 4) involving experimentation, experience, reflection and conceptualization (Kolb, 1984). Nowhere is this cycle more applicable than within clinical education; the phases implied in Kolb's model help move the student from one stage to the next in a sequential spiral. Each spiral represents a stage in clinical development which, it could be argued, can be assessed before the student moves to the next stage.

For example, the student might plan an intervention session for a client (experimentation), then implement this plan while being observed by a clinical educator (experience). The third stage would be the student's self-evaluation of the session (reflection) and the fourth stage would be making sense of what occurred in the light of the clinical educator's feedback and his or her own theoretical knowledge (conceptualization). The student then proceeds to the next 'loop' in the developmental spiral and plans the following session with accumulated wisdom and constructive criticisms from this most recent assessment. This example may be regarded as an over-simplification of the whole process, but it serves to underline the principle that the assessment procedure is an integral part of the learning experience and can be absorbed naturally within the whole process.

6.2.2 LEARNING STYLES

Within the context of adult learning it is important to consider not only the stages and processes involved, as described in Kolb's learning cycle, but also the learning styles of individual students (see Chapter 1). Different learning styles will affect the way in which students learn within the clinical situation, but they also affect the way in which students anticipate assessment, respond to criticism, react to failure and benefit from feedback. It is important for clinical educators to be aware of the varied reactions which the assessment process might arouse. Indeed, it could be argued that the better acquainted clinical educators are with students, the more sensitive they will be able to be to that individual's learning style, and the more easily they will be able to adapt the feedback to ensure maximum benefit and progress, as opposed to increasing anxiety, anger and frustration.

For example, 'activist' learners (Honey & Mumford, 1986) may respond in a very positive manner to assessment and welcome suggestions for a change of approach, perhaps without reflecting enough on the rationale behind the criticism; 'reflectors' may prefer to think through the implications of specific criticisms and produce their own solutions; 'theorists' may feel threatened and wounded initially by criticism, but after further consideration may think through to a logical conclusion and a new approach; 'pragmatists' may not feel personally implicated by the critical comments and may greet with enthusiasm new ideas for future management.

6.2.3 STUDENT GROWTH

As students grow in their clinical skills and professional competence, what is assessed and how it is assessed should change. Beginning level students have been found to be anxious about their ability to perform basic clinical procedures, such as writing session plans for therapy with clients (Chan, Carter & McAllister, 1994) (see Chapter 3). Students at this stage are often self-focused as they concentrate their attention on developing clinical skills. Assessment of such students would appropriately focus on their mastery of basic clinical procedures. Beginning students may need feedback designed to prompt them to think of the client holistically and to build self-confidence to enable the shift of focus to the client. Advanced level students have been shown to feel confident about their clinical skills but anxious about their emergent professional personae (Chan, Carter & McAllister, 1994) (see Chapter 3). Such students would benefit from assessment and feedback designed to promote the growth of professionalism and confidence in their professional selves. As well as end-point assessment needed for certification or licensure, self-assessment and peer assessment should be emphasized, in preparation for the real world of evaluation in professional practice.

6.3 WHY ASSESS?

According to Harris and Bell (1994) the rationales for assessing students are seven-fold:

- mastery
- increasing the motivation of learners
- prediction of an individual' s potential
- diagnosis of learning
- diagnosis of teaching
- evidence of competence or attainment
- accreditation, classification and comparison with other learners.

These reasons for assessment apply in the clinical setting within various health professions.

The student's mastery of the clinical situation is an obvious target and reason for assessment to take place. This mastery will require evaluation at various stages throughout the educational programme. Early assessments provide opportunities to identify learning needs and to support the growth of clinical skills, while exit point assessment ensures that professional standards have been attained.

Motivation of the student is an essential element of assessment. Positive reinforcement, reassurance that progress is being made and encouragement that further development will occur are key reasons behind the assessment process. In relation to formative assessment (i.e. assessment for the purpose of providing feedback), the nature and mechanism of the feedback following assessment is vitally important to the continuing motivation of the student. Prediction of the individual student's potential is primarily the responsibility of the clinical educator and is an integral part of that role. However, students also must be able to view their potential in an objective way through the process. Occasionally, an appropriately-timed assessment may give a negative prognosis for developing as a clinician, and in the ideal world it should be the student who recognizes this and with guidance from the clinical educator perhaps makes the decision to withdraw from further clinical education. On the other hand, a well-timed assessment with positive reassurance of good clinical potential at a time when the student' s morale is flagging will provide motivation.

Assessment will undoubtedly focus to some extent on what has been learned. This is a major reason for periodic testing of theory and skills. The use of the term 'diagnostic' implies that the student and the assessor will recognize the strengths and weakness of the knowledge and skill base and plan future study and practice accordingly.

It is not only the student's learning which is the focus of assessment. Directly or indirectly, the assessment process should also help to identify and review the amount, nature and effectiveness of the teaching which has taken place. Further, changes in content, style or emphasis of teaching may be a desirable outcome of assessment.

When a student reaches the end of a period of study and clinical education, it becomes essential that evidence of competence is presented.

Implicit in this aspect of the rationale is an understanding of the concept of competence which should be explicitly defined for both students and clinical educators.

The final reason for assessment on the Harris and Bell list is the need to certify that students are fit for practice – that they are eligible for the awards of the educational establishment and the professional body, and that they compare satisfactorily to other graduating students within the same field. Thus assessment provides students, clinical educators and the educational programme with evidence that the defined end-point standards have been met, and that a required level of professional competence has been attained.

6.3.1 ASSESS FOR WHOM?

Implicit within the question 'Why assess?' is a second question 'For whom is the assessment?' As implied above, several people are directly affected by, or involved in the assessment process.

Firstly, consider the students. They are the major focus of this collaboration. The system exists to facilitate their development. As the focus of this collaboration they are subject to some extent to the whims and demands of the other participants – the clinical educator, university staff and perhaps also at some point, an external assessor. In many programmes this triad of assessors writes the regulations, defines the standards and, at least to some extent, dictates the procedures. On the other hand, students can demonstrate knowledge, skills and mastery of the clinical situation through, perhaps, choice of client, assessment procedure or treatment technique, or the setting of achievable sessional goals. It is important that the assessment process provides some degree of choice, so that students retain some control.

Secondly, consider the clinical educator, either as external assessor from the university or as on-site clinical educator. However much they may appear to be 'in control' in the assessment process, there is an element of self-assessment which they themselves bring to the process. Their teaching standards are exposed to scrutiny; they have to recognize and adhere to the demands of external assessors and statutory bodies. They must be the gatekeepers to the profession, which means that they have the burden of decision-making and justifying such decisions to both external bodies and students alike. Theirs also is the responsibility of judging fairly and without prejudice.

Finally, consider the external forces involved in the assessment process. To a great extent they can be regarded as the 'overlords' of the whole system. These external forces to be reckoned with are the overseers of the educational system, the outside adjudicators checking comparability of standards, and the awarders and rubber stampers of certificates to practise. They too must be regarded as collaborators in the assessment system. As bodies which award credentials to programmes, they can at most only 'sample' the assessment process – they can observe, examine and/or evaluate a small proportion of the students, the clinical educators, the teaching, the techniques, the competencies or the standards. They uphold the standards of the profession or an institution and yet they cannot assess every professional. Accreditation of an individual, a course or an institution must always, to some extent, be taken on trust.

6.3.2 THE STUDENT'S VIEW OF ASSESSMENT

It is probably true to say that most of the decision-making regarding methods, timing and feedback mechanisms of student clinical assessment is undertaken by the academic or academic plus clinical team designing the course. Students, in most instances, would have very little input into such planning, yet they are central to the whole exercise. Their perceptions of the validity and fairness of the assessment process are vital to their valuing of the results of the assessment. If the assessment outcome matches what students feel inwardly, it will give them confidence to take upon themselves the role of self-assessor. On the other hand, if the mismatch is too great or if students do not trust the assessment system, they may be seriously hindered in their professional career, lacking the confidence to monitor their own performance.

Stackhouse and Furnham (1983) suggest that students need to develop a confidence within themselves and not just meet external criteria in order to feel an inward competence with which to meet the world of clients: 'The recognition that clinical competence is as much dependent on inner satisfaction (Ward & Webster, 1965), self-awareness (Kaplan & Dreyer, 1974), and interpersonal skills (Klevans & Volz, 1978), as on meeting prescribed academic standards has resulted in self-awareness as well as sensitivity to others being important goals in clinical teaching' (p. 171). Stackhouse and Furnham further observe that: 'unilateral assessment, i.e. by supervisors alone, will result in extrinsic based learning, such as for examination purposes or attempting to please supervisors, rather than more intrinsically motivated factors such as curiosity, discovery, and personal satisfaction' (p. 172). These concepts were also discussed in Chapter 1 with regard to deep versus surface approaches to learning. If it is agreed that the ultimate goal of clinical supervision is to produce a clinician capable of self-supervision (Dowling & Shank, 1981) then the balance must be struck between a supervisory 'stranglehold' on assessment (Heron, 1988) and a student-dominated system which is equally undesirable.

In a survey of final-year speech therapy students in the United Kingdom, one author sought their views on the clinical assessment procedures they had experienced during their course (Robertson, 1995). Fifty per cent of the respondents (n = 212) felt very positive about the methods of clinical assessment used; 35 per cent were non-committal and 15 per cent felt their clinical assessment was unsatisfactory and inappropriate. The optimist might interpret this data as indicating that students were reasonably happy with the assessment process. However, the more critical reader would recognize that approximately half of the students had some misgivings about the fairness of the system.

Further analysis of the methods of clinical assessment reviewed in the Robertson survey indicates that 95 per cent of the students had experienced assessment by visiting university staff and, of this number, 64 per cent found the visits to be very/extremely valuable. Thirteen per cent did not find these visits valuable and 23 per cent were non-committal. Clinical educators' report forms, a nationwide method of evaluating students, were considered by 79 per cent of the students to be a very/extremely valued method of assessment.

A definite trend emerged from this data which was confirmed by a question which asked how valuable was the contribution of university staff, clinical educator and combined university staff/clinical educator to the assessment of students' clinical work. The responses are displayed in Table 6.1. Students perceived clinical educators' input to assessment as important, adding value and fairness to the whole procedure. In any model of clinical assessment, therefore, it is important to ensure that the clinician with whom the student has been working over a period of time is an integral part of the assessment process.

Table 6.1 Students' perceptions of the contribution to the assessment of students' clinical work by university tutor, clinical educator and combined university tutor/clinical educator (Robertson, 1995)

Tutor	Very valuable	57%
	Non-committal	28%
	Not valuable	15%
Clinical educator	Very valuable	91%
	Non-committal	8%
	Not valuable	1%
Tutor/Clinical educator	Very valuable	82%
	Non-committal	14%
	Not valuable	4%

6.4 WHAT IS TO BE ASSESSED?

In Chapter 1 reference was made to the goals of clinical education as being much broader than discipline-specific clinical skills. The need to develop competence and capability for professional practice were emphasized. If these broader goals are to be pursued, the focus of assessment will need to change.

6.4.1 CLINICAL OR PROFESSIONAL COMPETENCE?

In her development of a model of professional practice, Stengelhofen (1993) commented: 'If we are to prepare students adequately for professional work then we need to consider what is involved in the practice of the profession' (p. 11). She suggests that professionals typically recognize three elements of professional practice, which are knowledge, skills and attitudes. Stengelhofen considers that what is important is not simply to see these as individual elements of professionalism, but rather to consider their inter-relationship. She proposes a model (see Table 6.2) which shows the gradual integration of the elements of knowledge and attitudes with skills to produce a whole, which is professional competence.

Table 6.2 A model of the elements of professional competence (Stengelhofen, 1993)

Surface level	Techniques and procedures	
First deep level	Knowledge and understanding and Knowledge awareness	Relationship with employing authority	All levels are influenced by: Life experiences Pre-registration learning Work experience Continuing education Work context (e.g., hospital, school, clinic, private practice, etc.)
Second deep level	Attitudes Giving meaning to what is done and influencing use of knowledge, technique and procedures	

At the surface level, it may be possible for students to pick up skills through practice and at this level to appear to be clinically able. However, for students to prove that they are professionally competent, then the deeper levels of knowledge and understanding as well as professional attitude must also be evident. It is not sufficient to assess only the knowledge base of students. Nor is it enough to view the acquisition and demonstration of clinical techniques as an indication of competence, since these may be utilized at an efficient but mechanical and superficial level.

The third attribute at the deepest level of professionalism is the most difficult to define, the most elusive to address within a course of study and the most intangible to assess, yet *attitude* is at the very heart of professionalism and we neglect it at our peril. Stengelhofen (1993) describes attitude as 'the driving force for effective practice'. It certainly encompasses notions of ethical, moral and considerate behaviour towards clients and colleagues, seeing clients holistically and working with colleagues to achieve holistic management of clients. It is in these aspects of professional practice that marginal students often experience greatest difficulty (see Chapter 7).

Genuinely mature professional practitioners will recognize that the knowledge, clinical skills and professional attitude discussed above must continue to develop throughout their professional career. However, these elements must begin to show integration at the student education stage so that the idea of competence becomes holistic and internally conceptualized, leading to professional maturity. It is this holistic integration of knowledge, skills and attributes which allows for the inclusion of educationally as well as professionally sound, competency-based curricula in higher education (see Chapter 1) and for competency-based assessment, which is discussed further later in this chapter. Graduation and certification or licensure are the first rungs of the professional ladder. However, progression from ground level to that first rung is an enormously important step and each of the three elements must already be showing definite signs of growth and internalization. These elements must be viable and capable of surviving with minimal support once the student graduates.

If the most important outcome of the clinical learning experience is that students demonstrate 'professional competence', then competency-based assessment is an appropriate method of assessment in clinical education.

6.4.2 COMPETENCY-BASED ASSESSMENT

'Competency-based assessment is the assessment of a person's competence against prescribed standards of performance' (Gonczi, Hager & Athanasou, 1993, p. 5). It contrasts with norm-referenced assessment in that it is based on prescribed standards rather than on a set of norms or the normal distribution. It is based on the inference of competence from performance with consideration being given to the context of the performance. Characteristically, it uses a variety of assessment methods in order to gather adequate evidence of competence. Competency-based assessment is a form of judgemental assessment rather than scientific measurement. That is not to say that it is any less valid or reliable than traditional scientific measurement techniques, but it is based on cognitive theories of human functioning which reflect the complex combinations of abilities, skills and knowledge that are not fixed and finite.

Competency-based assessment, as is made clear by Gonczi, Hager and Athanasou (1993), can use all existing forms of assessment such as questioning, direct observation and evidence of prior learning. The difference lies in how the forms of assessment are used and interpreted. A competency-based approach to assessment needs to have an emphasis on performance and on integrated or holistic methods of assessment if it is to be valid and effective. Ideally, assessment is carried out in the workplace by direct observation, but in practice this is not always practical nor possible because of time constraints.

At present, competency-based assessments are used in some tertiary and further education institutions, but there is potential for far greater use of this type of assessment especially in undergraduate and postgraduate education of health professionals (see Appendix 6.1). Case Study 6.1 describes the structure of the competency-based occupational standards developed by the speech therapy profession in Australia, to be used to assess overseas applicants for membership of the Speech Pathology Association of Australia.[1]

Case Study 6.1 Competency-based occupational standards: An example from the speech therapy profession in Australia

In 1994 the Speech Pathology Association of Australia, then known as the Australian Association of Speech and Hearing (AASH), published the Competency-based Occupational Standards for entry level speech pathologists in Australia, now commonly known as the C-BOS. This provided the profession with the criteria against which to assess candidates for entry to the profession using a competency-based assessment (see Appendix 6.1).

Briefly these standards describe the skills, knowledge and attitudes of speech therapists in terms of units, elements and performance criteria. They start with a key purpose statement for the profession. It also includes a range indicator statement that outlines the contexts and areas of responsibility covered by the profession at entry level. An example is the first range indicator which states that 'if requested, the speech pathologist must be able to demonstrate competence in any unit in both paediatric and adult practice in the areas of speech, language, swallowing, voice and fluency' (p. 7).

To facilitate the description of the complex total competency of the entry level speech therapist, the standards are divided into seven *units* which describe broad areas of professional activity:

---

[1] Formerly known as the Australian Association of Speech and Hearing (AASH).

Unit 1: Assessment of the client

Unit 2: Description and/or diagnosis of the client's communication and/or swallowing problem and determination of the likely outcome or prognosis

Unit 3: Planning client management

Unit 4: Implementation of speech pathology management of the client

Unit 5: Planning, maintaining and developing speech pathology service

Unit 6: Professional, group and community education

Unit 7: Professional development.

Each unit is further broken down into *elements* that describe specific activities carried out to achieve the unit. For example, Unit 1, Assessment of the client, contains six elements, which are:

1.1   Interviews and takes case history

1.2   Identifies the speech pathology areas requiring investigation and the most suitable manner in which to do this

1.3   Administers the speech pathology assessment to obtain the information required

1.4   Analyzes and interprets speech pathology assessment data

1.5   Provides feedback on results of speech pathology assessments to the client and/or significant other and referral sources, and discusses management

1.6   Writes report.

Each element is elaborated by *performance criteria* that specify the evidence that is required for the element to be carried out competently. As an example from Unit 1, the five performance criteria for Element 1, Interviews and takes case history, are:

1.1a   The clients and/or significant other's description and perception of the communication and/or swallowing difficulty is identified so that the nature of the problem is clarified and its impact established

1.1b   Information required for speech pathology assessment, diagnosis and intervention is elicited by using an appropriate interview process and collection of data

1.1c   Information that is pertinent to the communication and/or swallowing problem is identified to ensure that the necessary information for speech pathology management is gathered

1.1d   Information gathered is not released without the informed consent of the client or guardian, and every effort is made to maintain confidentiality at all times in accordance with the Australian Association of Speech and Hearing Code of Ethics and Freedom of Information Acts

1.1e   Information is recorded accurately, systematically and in English, according to speech pathology and the service provider's requirements.

Further information on what is required for some performance criteria is supplied in the cues for assessors. These are examples or illustrations of the behaviour or items referred to within the performance criterion to which they are attached and are neither inclusive nor exclusive.

6.5 HOW DO WE ASSESS?

'We believe that decisions relating to assessing can make or break a learning situation'. This is the strongly held view of Harris and Bell (1994, p.96) who outline many routes through the minefield of assessment. They suggest that there are many types of assessment available, from informal and casual observations, through teacher organized and marked questions, standardized tests, to assessment of criteria devised and used by students. They suggest that each mode of assessing can be located within bipolar continua (see Figure 6.1). Although these constructs are listed as bipolar, it is not necessary to assume that a given mode of assessing contains elements of only one pole. Indeed, in the clinical situation, it is quite possible, for example, that we could utilize assessments which contain both formative and summative elements. Nor should we regard the selection of one of these constructs, for example, process/product, to preclude application of any of the other constructs.

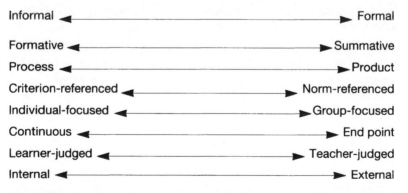

Figure 6.1 Bipolar continua for each mode of assessment (Harris & Bell, 1994)

Pletts (1981) reminds us that 'when attempting to measure clinical skills the number of variables that must be accounted for makes the task daunting. Even more difficult to measure are the attitudes and interpersonal skills so essential to successful clinical work' (p. 131). This comment reminds us once again of the necessity to assess the three major components – knowledge, skills and attitudes. Each of these components probably requires a different method of assessment. For instance, although it may be possible to link a test of skills with a test of knowledge, it is difficult to conceive that this could also incorporate an evaluation of attitude. Therefore, the methods of assessment must vary in accordance with the focus of the component to be assessed. Let us briefly consider the Harris and Bell aspects of assessment and note their relevance to clinical assessment.

6.5.1 INFORMAL-FORMAL

It is impossible to imagine a clinical situation in which informal assessment does not take place. Clinical educators are constantly observing a wide range of student behaviours every time they watch students in action in the clinic. Similarly, students are also making constant informal judgements of the clinician and of themselves. To reinforce the value of such observations, it is probably helpful to introduce a more formal element into the proceedings. For instance, at the end of each therapy session or clinical day, it is important to hold a debriefing period. In this way, students and clinical educators may be encouraged to focus on specific areas which can be varied from session to session, so that learning can be enhanced over a period of time.

6.5.2 FORMATIVE-SUMMATIVE

Stengelhofen (1993) describes 'formative assessment' as the 'feedback process' and encourages us to view 'summative assessment' as developing naturally from this process. 'The student's self assessment, together with assessment by clinical tutors preceded by and followed by setting objectives and working towards achieving them, again receiving feedback and making further progress, is all part of continuous assessment' (p. 180).

The concept of summative assessment and a discussion of its relevance to assessment within clinically-based courses is crucial to our subject. The term 'summative assessment' describes an appraisal of various aspects of student clinical performance; numeric values are assigned to each of these aspects, and the values are added together to provide an overall rating of current clinical skill. Note that in summative assessment there is an implicit assumption that the parts add up to the whole – that is, the component aspects which are assessed do indeed comprise a rounded picture of clinical performance. An example of a summative assessment tool is found in Figure 6.2 and discussion of its development is found in Case Study 6.2.

The University of Sydney
Faculty of Health Sciences

CLINICAL EDUCATION: MARKING GRID
School of Communication Disorders
Speech Pathology Clinical Subjects

Name of Student: _____ Clinical Educator: _____

Period of Training: Year of Course _____ Clinic: _____
                     Semester _____
                     Mid or End (Circle one)
                     Adult or Child (Circle one)

Weightings*	Shows no skill in this area	Shows a little skill in this area	Shows some skill in this area but not to expected level	Satis-factory	Shows above average skill in this area	Shows consistent excellence in this area
Rapport with client						
Rapport with relative/caregiver						
Rapport with other clinicians, staff and outside agencies						
Knowledge of Clinical Procedure: Preparation						
Investigation and evaluation speech and language						
Investigation and evaluation of contributing factors						
Therapeutic procedure						
Theoretical background						
Writing up and reporting						
Clinical management						
Clinical behaviour as demonstrated in: Awareness of factors influencing client's behaviour						
Adaptability						
Interest in client's total rehabilitation needs						

Recommendation & Comments

_____

_____

_____

Year 2:   Number of client contacts:
Year 3/4:   No of days present: Signature: _____
Year 3/4:   No of days absent:
Year 3/4:   No of absent days made up: Date: _____
Year 4:   No. of on-campus client contacts:
*   Assign each behaviour item a weighting between 0 and 25. Only one weighting of 0 and 25 may be assigned. Weightings must total 100.

Figure 6.2 The Grid: A summative assessment protocol devised in the School of Communication Disorders, The University of Sydney (see Case Study 6.2)

Case Study 6.2 The Grid: An example of a summative assessment tool

For our explanation and discussion of summative assessment we use as an example a summative assessment protocol which was devised in the School of Communication Disorders at The University of Sydney. This assessment protocol, which is shown in Figure 6.2, became familiarly known among staff and students as *The Grid*. The Grid was developed over a number of years with input from the many clinical educators and students who used it, found its problems, and made suggestions as to how it could work better. In basing our discussion of summative assessment on the Grid we in no way suggest that it is the ideal summative instrument for all programmes. However, consideration of aspects of the Grid will help the reader to appreciate the decisions to be made in developing a summative instrument.

Parameters to be assessed

One axis of a summative assessment protocol lists the parameters of student clinical performance which are assessed. In the Grid these parameters are listed on the left side, beginning with 'Rapport with client'. How, it may be asked, are these parameters determined? How can the user be sure that all important aspects of clinical performance are included? How can overlap between parameters be avoided?

Developers of assessment protocols do not reinvent their particular wheel! Published protocols and protocols used in similar settings provide multiple resources for selecting suitable parameter descriptors. In the case of the Grid, initially 14 parameters were chosen: in addition to those shown, a category 'Self confidence in therapeutic role' was included. After some time of trial use of the Grid in a variety of settings, clinical educators were asked to evaluate its parameters. In a brainstorming session clinical educators reported comfort with assessing all parameters except this 'self confidence ...'; they believed it overlapped with other parameters and was indeed to a certain extent an outcome of performance in other parameters. As a result of these considerations 'self confidence ...' was dropped as a parameter, to the evident satisfaction of users.

Brainstorming sessions among experienced clinical educators, as mentioned above, are an important tool in development of a summative assessment protocol. Consultation with users, both clinical educators and students, can provide an impetus for changes leading to improvements in validity and reliability of the instrument. An example will demonstrate the use of brainstorming sessions to improve reliability of the Grid.

During the years of use of the Grid it became evident that, not surprisingly, all clinical educators did not necessarily consider the same behaviours in assessing a particular parameter. Further, less experienced clinical educators expressed lack of confidence in their evaluation of particular parameters, such as 'Rapport with relative/caregiver'. Students expressed a wish for a clearer delineation of what was being assessed. It thus became apparent that the parameter labels alone did not provide sufficient information for users. Several brainstorming sessions held with clinical educators were used to develop lists of behaviours to be considered within each parameter. Some of the more than 50 behaviours listed for 'Rapport with relative/caregiver' included:

- respects caregiver's privacy rights and maintains confidentiality
- explains purposes of tests used
- checks out that 'messages' are received, re-explains where necessary
- responds appropriately to verbal and behavioural cues provided by caregiver
- maintains caregiver's optimal involvement in therapy.

Clearly, not all the listed behaviours would be expected of a beginning student. Therefore, again by a process of consultation with clinical educators, the behaviours were assigned to levels of the education programme at which they should be expected. Some behaviours, like 'smiles, uses friendly voice' would be expected at early stages of student practicum; other behaviours would be expected only of students near to graduation. In addition, certain behaviours, such as those involving confidentiality were highlighted as prerequisites for passing any clinical placement.

Since each parameter on the Grid was now associated with two or more explanatory pages of component behaviours, a booklet of these guidelines was printed for use with the instrument. The booklet was provided to all clinical educators, with the aim of maximizing uniformity and hence reliability in the use of the instrument.

Method of assigning marks

The second axis of a summative assessment protocol provides the skill level descriptors to be used by the assessing clinical educator. It is possible simply to use a numerical range such as 1–7, or a percentage scale, or verbal descriptors, or a combination of these. In developing the Grid, the decision was made to use verbal descriptors, which could subsequently be converted to numerical marks by administrative staff. This decision was based on the consideration that there would be more agreement among users if asked to rate performance on a particular parameter with a verbal description such as 'shows some skill in this area but not to expected level' than if asked to rate it with a numerical mark such as 4 out of 10. The actual values assigned to the verbal descriptors were, however, made known to both clinical educators and students (they were a numerical range 0–10).

An additional essential consideration in assigning marks is the relative weighting to be given to each parameter in the total. It is unlikely that each parameter will be of equal importance in the overall picture of clinical performance. In the case of the Grid, it could be argued that 'Therapeutic procedure' is more important to overall clinical performance than is 'Rapport with other clinicians, staff and outside agencies'. Admittedly, the converse could also be argued – fuel for an interesting debate on clinical effectiveness! The first solution to this problem in the case of the Grid was to allocate weightings to each parameter. (For information for the mathematically inclined, the weightings totalled 100, and the assigned mark for each parameter became one tenth of the allocated weighting for that parameter, producing a total mark out of 100 which could be converted to a grade.)

This solution had its own problems, however, in that the fixed weightings allocated to parameters were not necessarily appropriate in diverse clinical settings. Some clinical settings, for example, provided relatively little opportunity for interaction with clients' relatives or caregivers; in other settings such interaction was an important part of the clinical process. This particular problem was highlighted by student input to discussions of the Grid. It was resolved by requiring clinical educators at each placement to allocate their own weightings to each parameter, based on their knowledge of the demands and nature of the setting. The weightings were still to total 100, with parameters allocated a weighting between 0 and 25, although each extreme weighting could be applied to no more than one parameter. Student and clinical educator response indicated perceptions that this 'individualized weighting' system increased the validity of the Grid as a summative instrument.

It is clear that a summative assessment instrument, such as the one described, needs flexibility in its development. It is unlikely to remain unchanged. It benefits from contributions both from those who use it and from those whose performance is assessed. In addition, those who are to use it benefit from induction into its use.

6.5.3 PROCESS-PRODUCT

On first consideration it would appear that clinical performance is more amenable to process assessment than product assessment. In most clinical situations students will be judged on a sequence of events, such as the preparation, management and evaluation of a therapy session, or the gradual development of a relationship with a new client. However, on further consideration, it is possible to select specific 'products', to isolate target tasks and to judge the result. This 'product assessment' could apply to evaluation of a student's ability to score a standardized test, or to write a report or letter for a particular purpose, or to design and produce a piece of equipment for a client.

6.5.4 CRITERION REFERENCED-NORM REFERENCED

According to Harris and Bell (1994) 'norm-referenced assessing aims to compare the achievements of the learner with those of other learners' (p. 101). While it may be helpful to students during their clinical education to have some indication of their progress clinically in comparison with their peers, ultimately it is imperative that their work is measured against clearly defined standards for entry into the profession. Thus we must aim for criterion-referenced assessment which assesses the learner by comparison with some predetermined or negotiated criteria. Most clinical education programmes will provide for students a detailed list of expected professional competencies developed according to established criteria, which must be met by the time students are due to graduate. Intermediate criteria should be set at various key points throughout the programme, so that students have a useful and achievable reference point. Consistent with adult learning approaches, the ultimate goals and criteria must be communicated to the students early in the programme.

6.5.5 INDIVIDUAL FOCUSED-GROUP FOCUSED

Within a clinical education programme leading to a professional qualification it is clearly inappropriate to consider anything other than an individual-focused assessment. An assessment of group performance, although having its uses perhaps in some areas of the learning process, is not relevant to the acquisition of clinical skills and techniques, since learning in this area must take account of individual needs, strengths and weaknesses. However, a compilation of clinical assessment profiles of a cohort of students may be of value to the educational institution. Such a compilation could indicate deficits in the educational programme which prepares students for and supports their clinical practice. Or it might reveal areas of clinical practice to which students have inadequate exposure. A responsive educational institution would seek to make appropriate curriculum changes.

6.5.6 CONTINUOUS-END POINT

Continuous assessment is a two-edged sword. On the one hand, it would seem to be the ideal learning situation for the student in a clinical education programme since it allows for immediate and constant feedback by the clinical educator who is able to monitor each stage in development. This may also relax the tension normally associated with assessment. On the other hand, some students report that they feel constantly under scrutiny and pressure and feel they are never able to make mistakes in private.

Continuous assessment is most suitable for the clinical educator responsible for the day-to-day practicum of a student placement. As Stengel-hofen (1993) suggests, this situation is conducive to the use of continuous assessment, which may be the least invasive in relation to the ongoing work of the student. This will have benefits for client care as well as student learning. However, it should be recognized that objectivity in assessment is sometimes compromised because of the personal interactions between clinical educator and student in the clinical setting.

A valuable type of assessment which captures both the concept of continuous assessment by the clinical educator and regular self-evaluation by the student is the checklist. Figure 6.3 provides an example of a checklist adapted from one originally designed to be used by a teacher after a teaching session.

	Very well	Satisfactory	Not very well	Not applicable
How well did I ...				
plan this session?	......	......	......	......
introduce this session?	......	......	......	......
make the aims clear to the client?	......	......	......	......
present the materials?	......	......	......	......
pace the session?	......	......	......	......
interact with the client?	......	......	......	......
use reinforcement?	......	......	......	......
handle problems of inattention/distraction?	......	......	......	......
handle the client's questions?	......	......	......	......
record the client's questions?	......	......	......	......
build up the client's confidence?	......	......	......	......
round off the session?	......	......	......	......

Figure 6.3 Example of a self-evaluation checklist to be used after a therapy session by the student, which could also be completed by the tutor and used as a basis for discussion (adapted from Eastcott & Farmer, 1991)

At the opposite pole of this aspect of assessment is 'end point' assessment. While it is probably important to assess students within a clinical setting just prior to their qualifying, it would seem to be extremely bad practice to judge the whole of a student' s clinical work on one final clinical examination. It may be felt necessary to have an 'end point' assessment for the purpose of certification or licensing, but where this exists it surely must be part of a wider assessment package.

6.5.7 LEARNER JUDGED-TEACHER JUDGED

A major metamorphosis that must occur in the student clinician is the transformation from dependent, non-skilled, apprenticed technician into an independent, responsible, skilled, self-evaluating professional. The ability to evaluate oneself is a skill which individuals need in everyday professional life, so it must be nurtured during the embryonic stages of clinical education. Students must learn to recognize their strengths, and weaknesses, abilities and limitations, since recognition of these will be important throughout their working life. By learning to use effectively some of the self-assessing procedures already mentioned, (for example, the sessional checklist in Figure 6.3), students will eventually become skilled, reflective practitioners.

In the clinical situation, of course, assessment by the clinical educator is clearly necessary, but within the context of deep approaches to learning, this should not be a unilateral judgement. As previously discussed in the Robertson (1995) study, students value particularly the judgement of the clinical educator.

6.5.8 INTERNAL-EXTERNAL

Internal assessing is widely accepted in higher education. It involves all those participating in the learning/teaching process having control over the assessment – student, peer group, university staff and clinical educator. They should all be involved and utilize the relevant forms of assessment already discussed.

In addition, however, in an education process leading to a professional qualification, it is entirely appropriate, and may even be a statutory requirement, that an external examiner is also involved. It is normally not possible for the external examiner to assess each student individually, so the role of this external person may be to scrutinize the assessment process and possibly to examine a sample of the students in order to evaluate and moderate the fairness of the internal judgements made.

In preparation for future professional work, the involvement of internal and external judges is important, since the work of the clinician on a daily basis is constantly under scrutiny. As a professional, the clinician is accountable to the clients and to the employing body to maintain high standards of client care.

6.5.9 STUDENT SELF-ASSESSMENT

The discussion above of the various continua in assessment has referred a number of times to self-assessment. What is the role of the student self-assessment in the evaluation of clinical skills? Falchikov and Boud (1989), highlighting the need for students to take more responsibility for their own learning, state: 'Life-long learning requires that individuals be able not only to work independently, but also to assess their own performance and progress (p. 395). Woolliscroft, Tentlaken, Smith and Calhonn (1993), describing the use and value of self-assessment in the training of medical students, underline the view that 'self-evaluation is central to the function of the clinician' (p. 290). They further suggest that individuals' views of themselves are 'constructed from repeated feedback from others as well as through introspection' (p. 290) and that it is multidimensional, combining the actual self, the potential self and the ideal self.

Students, therefore, who engage in self-assessment are not only looking at themselves as they are, but are trying to judge realistically what they could become, while at the same time holding in mind the vision of how they would like to be, perhaps modelled on observations of more experienced practitioners. Students are aware of the standards against which to measure themselves, or, as Woolliscroft *et al.* (1993) summarize, 'accurate professional self-assessment requires a self-representation of actual performance that is congruent with reality as it would be judged by other individuals using appropriately developed performance monitoring systems' (p. 290).

It is possible for discrepancies to exist between some students' views of themselves and the way they are viewed by clinical educators. Woolliscroft *et al.* (1993) were able to identify such cases by the administration of the questionnaire shown below to third-year medical students within the University of Michigan Medical School, comparing the responses with those of clinical educators. Early identification of students whose self-assessment is unrealistic may permit the introduction of remedial strategies, such as placement with clinical educators who could become strong clinical role models.

Boud (1992) considers the use of self-assessment schedules like the one devised by Woolliscroft *et al.* (1993) to be of great value, because schedules appear to prompt students 'to reflect on their learning and think about the application of ideas in their own situations' (p. 191). The self-assessment schedule which Boud himself describes incorporates four main headings: goals, criteria, judgements, and further action. He reports that 'although the exercise appears at first sight to be an intellectual one, it drew a number of students into their personal experiences, emotions and feelings' (p. 192). Students found the task both 'excruciating' and 'challenging', as well as useful. As one student reported: 'It highlighted the need to improve my discipline of keeping a portfolio regularly'; and another reported: 'What it added to my understanding and to my awareness of what learning had taken place was a sense of form' (p. 192).

Self-assessment by students: Questionnaire used in the Internal Medicine Clerkship, University of Michigan Medical School, USA, 1988–89
(Woolliscroft *et al.*, 1993)

Medical history/interview
1 I elicit an appropriate medical history.

Physical examination
2 I am able to detect the important physical findings.
3 I accurately interpret the significance of the physical findings.

Initial patient write-ups
4 I accurately document appropriate data in my initial patient write-ups, including all major and minor problems.

Daily patient progress
5 I am aware of my patients' daily developments.
6 I accurately document all patient developments in my daily progress notes.

Oral presentations
7 My oral presentations are logical and well organized.

Application of knowledge
8 I apply my knowledge base in a well-integrated manner to patient problems.

Problem list, assessment, and plan
9 I develop appropriate problem lists.
10 I develop complete differential diagnosis.
11 My diagnostic and therapeutic plans are well organized.

Self-education
12 I use independent self-learning to extend my medical knowledge base.
13 I require little direction to perform my patient care responsibilities.

Interpersonal interactions
14 I interact with patients and their families in a professional manner.
15 I interact with other members of the health care team in a professional manner.

(a) Limits to self-assessment

Should we assume that students are the best judges of their own performance and that, in appreciation of reflective learning, ultimately students should be their own assessors? Whilst it is an admirable aim that developing professionals should become responsible and well-equipped to monitor their work, we must remember that this, like many other skills students are developing, needs practice and training. The observations of Falchikov and Boud (1989) suggest that students at a more advanced stage of their studies are more accurate assessors than those in the beginning stages.

A further indication that students' untrained self-assessment may lack validity is provided by Stackhouse and Furnham (1983), who compared the ratings of speech therapy students' clinical skills by students themselves, clinical educators and university staff. The clinical educators tended to give the highest ratings of the students' skills, while the students gave themselves the lowest ratings. Stackhouse and Furnham (1983, p. 176) commented:

'Observations have shown high anxiety levels in students entering their first clinical placement and this, coupled with inexperience, results in unrealistic goals being set for themselves ... Another reason for students' harsh ratings of themselves may be artefactual. It is well known that self-raters may conform to social desirability factors and succumb to pressures of humility ... As the student's role as "learner" is clearly defined they may be unwilling to score high ratings as this would be inappropriate for their role at this time'.

Over the years a number of studies of student self-assessment have indicated that when evaluating themselves, students not only use different criteria to university staff or clinical educators, but when, for example, they view themselves on video they will look at and comment on different aspects of their own and the client's behaviour. This observation was made clearly by McGovern and colleagues in a series of studies of speech therapy students in Scotland in the early 1980s (McGovern & Davidson, 1982; 1983; McGovern, 1985; McGovern & Dean, 1991).

Three groups (students, university staff and clinical educators) watched video-taped recordings of other students' treatment sessions and made comments which were later transcribed and grouped into various categories: viewer orientation, therapist behaviour, content presentation, content stimuli, interaction, management of space, client behaviour and generalizations. The trends can be described as follows. The clinical educators as a group looked mainly at content presentation and rarely at client behaviour. The students as a group looked mostly at content presentation but also at client behaviour. They made few comments about therapist behaviour or management of space. The university staff as a group most frequently commented on interaction or content presentation, rarely on client behaviour and management of space.

The studies revealed wide discrepancies in the way that the three groups commented on the video. The authors therefore urge that clinical educators become aware of their own biases in allocating importance to different aspects of the clinical situation. Case Study 6.3 contrasts students' self-assessment before and after viewing a video of their treatment session.

The observation has been made that educational assessing is traditionally a unilateral activity controlled by the educators (Harris & Bell, 1994). They set the criteria, mark students' work and provide the feedback. A contrasting picture is that of independent learners who decide their own goals and criteria, manage their learning and monitor their progress towards the final outcome. These are the two poles of the continuum representing learner autonomy.

Case Study 6.3 Student self-evaluation: The usefulness of video replay (McGovern, 1985)

Eight beginning speech therapy students were videoed for a minimum of 15 minutes during an ongoing therapy session with a client. At the end of the session the students were asked to comment on their session. These comments were recorded. The students then viewed the video of their performance and were again asked to comment on the session and a tape recording of their comments was again made. The two tape recordings were transcribed and analyzed for the number, range and focus of comments made.

Comments made by students immediately following the session mainly related to the success or otherwise of the session plan they had prepared and their perceptions of their performance, for example, 'I'll need to spend a bit more time explaining how to do that'; 'He got all the words and he seemed to enjoy finding them' (p. 298). When the students were asked to comment on the same session after viewing a video of it, their observations were much broader and could be subdivided into three headings:

1 *Observations on personal factors affecting interaction*, for example, 'My voice wasn't particularly clear at times'; 'I wondered if I could possibly make more use of gestures' (p. 298)
2 *Criticisms of student therapist's response to client's performance*, for example, 'The task might have been too long. I should have changed to something else'; 'I could have got his attention more before trying to do certain things' (p. 298);
3 *New observations on client's performance*, for example, 'I was interested in the difference between his reading rate and his conversational rate'; 'She didn't understand "yours" and "mine" ... gives me a new lead into therapy' (p. 298).

Within the context of healthcare clinical education, neither of these extremes is appropriate. The first is undesirable because it is important for students to develop the skills of monitoring their own performance and taking responsibility for it in preparation for professional life. The other extreme is also inappropriate since there is a statutory duty on the part of the educational institution setting up and managing a professionally accredited course to examine the student and judge their fitness to practise. A balance between the two poles of assessment must therefore be found and such a model will no doubt contain elements of assessment which reflect several stages between *teacher-controlled assessment* and *learner-controlled assessment*. We conclude this discussion with an apt comment by Boud (1990): 'The challenge for all of us is to find meaningful ways of incorporating aspects of self-assessment within courses so that learning within the course is enhanced and students gain confidence in judging their own performance. This is most likely to occur when self-assessment is an integral part of learning activities and not an appendage or afterthought' (p. 110).

6.5.10 PEER ASSESSMENT

With the growth of programmes leading to a speech therapy qualification, there has been a corresponding trend for placement of more than one student at a time in clinical settings. Taking advantage of this situation, clinical educators have 'paired' students in clinical roles and functions which facilitate learning. Probably the most frequent mode of peer placement is one in which members of the pair treat a client together, alternating between being clinician and observer (Stengelhofen, 1993). This practice provides opportunity for students to give each other feedback. In the Robertson study (1995) cited earlier in this chapter, speech therapy students were asked for their views on peer placements. Sixty-nine per cent of students who had experienced paired placements considered them to be very valuable.

While the concept of peer or collaborative placements has been well documented (for example, Callan, O' Neill & McAllister 1993; Lincoln & McAllister, 1993; McFarlane & Hagler, 1993) (see Chapter 4), less has been recorded about the processes and results of peer assessment in clinical practice. Informal discussions with students confirm the impression that when carrying out clinical peer assessment students are supportive of each other, giving positive reinforcement and praise as well as honest, constructive criticism. The benefits of such a method of assessment are best experienced when the students concerned have worked closely with each other, probably during a joint placement, for some time. This allows them to build mutual trust, potentially leading to an evaluation which is both open and rigorous.

Harris and Bell (1994) propose that peer and self assessment are closely related. They point out that judgements made during self-assessment are responsive to feedback from peers, particularly when those peers are co-learners in the same educational situation. Peer assessment is in all senses a collaborative activity making equal demands on each student involved in the process. It not only allows the assessed partner to learn constructively from a colleague, but the requirement that students watch, question, criticize, praise and instruct their fellow students demands a high level of concentration, knowledge and skill on their parts.

6.6 CONCLUSION

Throughout this chapter we have emphasized our belief that assessment in clinical education can be congruent with the approaches and characteristics of adult learning. To achieve this congruence clinical educators need to be clear about the reasons for assessment and the constructs which underlie assessment procedures. For this reason, this chapter has discussed the topics of why assess?, what to assess?, who should be involved in assessment? and how might we might choose or construct assessment procedures?

APPENDIX 6.1: DEVELOPMENT OF COMPETENCY-BASED ASSESSMENT STRATEGIES (VICKIE DAWSON)

The Competency Based Occupational Standards (C-BOS) is a detailed, accurate and powerful document which has been developed with considerable consultation with the profession and is widely accepted as a valid reflection of the desired standards for entry level practice of speech pathology in Australia. Accordingly the profession desired to base the assessment of overseas-educated speech pathologists who wish to practise in Australia on the C-BOS. In order to do this it was necessary for the Speech Pathology Association of Australia[1] to set about developing competency-based strategies that could be used with the document.

In principle the project steering committee felt that the assessment of overseas-educated candidates for membership to the profession should be similar to, and no more stringent than, that imposed on Australian university graduates. It was therefore proposed that the professional association would work with the six Australian universities that provide undergraduate education for speech pathologists to achieve parity between the university assessments and the competency-based assessment strategies to be applied to overseas candidates.

Although, ideally, competency-based assessment takes place through direct observation in the workplace, in this case it was not a practical possibility. It is frequently found that such direct workplace involvement is impractical or impossible, and indirect observation using, for example, simulations, standardized cases and video, is used as a substitute. Many of the university departments use video presentation for various forms of assessment and it seemed appropriate that videoed performance in a student's final placement clinic or in the overseas-educated candidate's current clinic might well be an acceptable way to view and assess the competency of the candidate.

With this in mind, the first draft of the assessment strategies included as the forms and methods of assessment, indirect observation via video, pen and paper questioning through a modified essay and extended multiple-choice examination and recognition of prior learning through presentation of a portfolio. There was also some provision for areas of the

[1] Formerly known as the Australian Association of Speech and Hearing

standards, which are not easily evaluated outside the workplace, to be covered by a mentoring system of support rather than assessment.

PILOT PROJECT

Because so little is known about using video as an assessment tool, it was decided to carry out a pilot study on this method of assessment. As stated, the indirect observation method initially adopted was observation and assessment of videoed performance in clinic. The videos were to be made of the candidate working in clinic situations in his or her native country. For the pilot study, video tapes of a simulated candidate carrying out one assessment session and one treatment session in clinic were shown to panels of assessors. Documentation covering the plans, goals, results and conclusions of the candidate in relation to the two sessions was also given to the panels. The panels included university staff and non-university practising speech pathologists who were all asked to view the videos and review the documentation to assess the competence of the simulated candidate. Half of the panels had been given some training in assessment using the C-BOS and half had not.

There were four levels on which panel members were to assess the candidate's performance. These were: overall competency, competence in each of the two sessions (one assessment and one treatment), competence at the element level of the C-BOS and competence at the performance criteria level of the C-BOS. In order to achieve overall competency, the candidate had to be judged competent in both assessment and treatment. The hypotheses were that the videoed clinical performances and accompanying documentation submitted by the simulated candidate could be reliably evaluated using the C-BOS, that the university assessors would be more reliable than non-university assessors and that trained assessors would be more reliable than untrained assessors.

Inter-rater reliability analysis on the four levels demonstrated that the reliability of assessment was not adequate using video extracts of performance, even though all assessors came to the same conclusion about the overall competency of the candidate (i.e. that competency had not yet been achieved). Many of the assessors felt that the possibility of cheating in the production of the videos, for example by scripting and editing, made video unsuitable as an assessment method for overseas candidates. Problems also arose with the difficulty of standardizing the assessment when considering the enormous variety of clinic situations which could be presented. There were also major difficulties with candidates in their native countries having access to clients with whom they could work in English. With such a level of dissatisfaction it was necessary for the reference group to review their recommendations and make far reaching changes.

Consultation has been carried out throughout the project not only with the speech pathology profession but also with representatives of government employing bodies, unions, the Government's National Office of Overseas Skills Recognition and the universities, all of whom provided feedback which was used in the revision of the assessment strategies.

THE ASSESSMENT STRATEGIES

In the final form of the assessment strategies, the reference group maintained the pen and paper questioning and the portfolio for the recognition of prior learning, but adopted a much modified video section in two parts. The first part of the section involves standard video presentations made by the Association and viewed by the candidate, followed by a telephone interview between the assessor and the candidate based on the clinical situations presented on the videos. Because the areas of responsibility are so broad in speech pathology and the Association wished to sample the candidate's competency in a variety of areas, it was decided that a number of different videos were to be made by the Association. The videos would cover both adult and paediatric cases, and those involving speech, voice, language, fluency and swallowing problems. It was agreed that the candidate would be presented with the list of scenarios on video and be permitted to choose the first one, but the Association would choose the second one to ensure a variety of situations for assessment. A certain amount of documentation about each of the videos would also be given to the candidate who, following the interview, would be asked to write a report or letter about the clinical situation presented.

The reference group worked out that this method would cover many of the same elements of the C-BOS that had been the target of the previous video presentations. However, there were some elements that referred to the establishment of rapport and the manner in which a client is approached that were still not covered by any assessment. In a second part of the video section therefore, it was decided to ask the candidate to present a video of him or herself interacting with a client and to present a summary of the case for the assessors. This video would not be used for the assessment of clinical decision-making but purely to evaluate the interactive skills, attitudes and manner of the candidate with a client.

In the assessment strategies devised by this project, clinical decision-making, client management, planning and report-writing are assessed using the standard video cases with interviews and reports or letters. Interactive skills are assessed through observation of a video of interaction with a client and through the telephone interview. More extensive assessment of the knowledge base and its application to the management of speech pathology services, community education and professional development is carried out in the pen and paper examination. Extra qualifications and initial education are reviewed in the portfolio for the recognition of prior learning. In covering such a wide variety of assessment methods the assessment strategies comply with the principles of competency-based assessment and have face validity in that assessors should have considerable exposure to the various skill areas of the candidate.

CONCLUSION

The assessment strategies described are as yet untested as the Association is still developing the materials to be used in them. The Speech Pathology Association of Australia plans to use the new assessment concurrently with the existing assessment for a period before switching entirely to the new competency-based strategies. This will provide an opportunity to compare the performance of the new with the old, and allow for the fine tuning of the more extensive competency-based assessment. Following the results of the pilot study, it is thought it will be essential to train the assessors in the use of competency-based assessments and in the C-BOS before being able to rely on the strategies for accepting or rejecting candidates for membership to the profession.

Competency-based assessment is claimed to be a fairer and more realistic assessment of skills, knowledge and attitudes. It is not a quick and easy alternative to examinations of knowledge, but is thorough, time-consuming and requires a broader evaluation of performance within context. It is essentially a summative type of assessment, evaluating whether or not competency within a complex professional activity has been achieved.

REFERENCES

Australian Association of Speech and Hearing (1994). *Competency-based occupational standards for speech pathologists (1) Entry level, (2) Basic grade practising level.* Melbourne: AASH

Boud, D. (1990). Assessment and the promotion of academic values, *Studies in Higher Education*, **15**, 1, 101–11.

Boud, D. (1992). The use of self-assessment schedules in negotiated learning. *Studies in Higher Education*, **17**, 2, 185–200.

Callan, C., O'Neill, D. & McAllister, L. (1993). Adventures in two to one supervision: Two students can be better than one. *Supervision*, **18**, 1.

Chan, J., Carter, S. & McAllister, L. (1994). Sources of anxiety related to clinical education in undergraduate speech-language pathology students. *Australian Journal of Human Communication Disorders*, **22**, 1, 57–73.

Dowling, S. & Shank, K. (1981). A comparison of the effects of two supervising styles, conventional and teaching clinic, in the training of speech and language pathologists. *Journal of Communication Disorders*, **14**, 51–8.

Eastcott, D. & Farmer, S. (1991). Planning teaching for active learning. *Effective Learning in Higher Education*, Module 3. London: CVCP.

Falchikov, N. & Boud, D. (1989). Student self-assessment in higher education: A meta-analysis. *Review of Educational Research*, **59**, 4, 395–430.

Gonczi, A., Hager, P. & Athanasou, J. (1993). The development of competency-based assessment strategies for the professions. National Office of Overseas Skills Recognition, Research Paper No. 8. Canberra: Australian Government Publishing Service.

Harris, D. & Bell, C. (1994). *Evaluating and assessing for learning* (Rev. ed.). London: Kogan Page.

Heron, J. (1988). Assessment revisited. In D. Boud (Ed.). *Developing student autonomy in learning* (2nd ed.) (pp 77–90). London: Kogan Page.

Honey, P. & Mumford, A. (1986). *The manual of learning styles*. Berkshire: author.

Kaplan, N. & Dreyer, D. (1974). The effect of self-awareness training on student speech pathologist-client relationships. *Journal of Communication Disorders*, **7**, 329–42.

Klevens, D. R. & Volz, H. B. (1978). Interpersonal skill development for speech clinicians. *Journal of National Studies, Speech and Hearing Association*, December, 63–9.

Kolb, D. (1984). *Experimental learning*. New Jersey: Prentice Hall

Lincoln, M. A. & McAllister, L. (1993). Peer learning in clinical education. *Medical Teacher*, **15**, 17–25.

Maxwell, M. (1995). Problems associated with the clinical education of physiotherapy students: A Delphi study. *Physiotherapy*, **81**, 582–7.

McFarlane, L. & Hagler, P. (1993). Collaborative treatment and learning in a university clinic. *Supervision*, **18**, 13–14.

McGovern, M. & Davidson, J. (1982). Appraisal of therapeutic performance. *British Journal of Disorders of Communication*, **17**, 23–31.

McGovern, M. & Davidson, J. (1983). Student perception of performance. *British Journal of Disorders of Communication*, **18**, 181–5.

McGovern, M. (1985). The use of video in the self evaluation of speech therapy students. *British Journal of Disorders of Communication*, **30**, 297–300.

McGovern, M. & Dean, E. C. (1991). Clinical education: The supervisory process. *British Journal of Communication Disorders*, **26**, 373–81.

Oxford Centre for Staff Development (1992). *Improving student learning: Project report*. Oxford: Oxford Polytechnic/CNAA. 1–4 March.

Pletts, M. (1981). Principles and practice of clinical teaching. *British Journal of Disorders of Communication*, **16**, 129–34.

Robertson, S. J. (1995). *Clinical education in speech and language therapy*. Unpublished data.

Stackhouse, J. & Furnham, A. (1983). A student-centred approach to the evaluation of clinical skills. *British Journal of Disorders of Communication*, **18**, 171–9.

Stengelhofen, J. (1993). *Teaching students in clinical settings*. Cheltenham: Stanley Thornes (Publishers) Ltd.

Ward, L. M. & Webster, E. S. (1965). The training of clinical personnel I: Issues in conceptualisation. *Asha*, **7**, 38–40.

Woolliscroft, J. O., Tentlaken, J., Smith, J. & Calhonn, J. G. (1993). Medical student's clinical self-assessments: Comparisons with external measures of performance and the students' self-assessments of overall performance and effort. *Academic Medicine*, **68**, 285–94.

Students experiencing problems learning in clinical settings

7

Diana Maloney
School of Communication Disorders,
The University of Sydney, Australia

Diana Carmody
Department of Social Work,
New Children's Hospital, Australia

Eva Nemeth
School of Communication Disorders,
The University of Sydney, Australia

7.1 CHAPTER OVERVIEW

This chapter discusses students experiencing difficulties with clinical learning. The chapter begins by exploring theoretical information about approaches to learning, locus of control, life cycle, life context and moral and intellectual development, so the reader gains some insights about the nature and context of the problems students may experience. We then propose a four-stage approach to the management of students experiencing problems which is grounded in adult learning theory. Within this approach to management, important issues, such as possible indicators of distress in participants in clinical interactions and failure in academic and clinical subjects, are discussed. Finally, we suggest problem management strategies which facilitate successful learning by the student and clinical educator.

Postcard 7

Dear All

What a day we had yesterday (Wednesday)! On Tuesday, we talked about planning to see this family 4 hours walk away. The team didn't have their assessment plan ready by the end of the day, but assured me they'd do it that night. Stupid me, I should have insisted we do it before we went home. So Wednesday morning we walked 4 hours in mud up to our calves, under umbrellas (this monsoon season can be depressing!) to this family. No plan, no ideas, no suitable materials for assessment. After a wasted hour, we headed back, 3 hours down the mountain in the rain. I was so angry, that I cried on the way back. But I was mainly angry with myself for not insisting the day before that they get organized. I know this will strike you as pretty funny, given how hopelessly disorganized I used to be. You'll probably think it's justice, at last! Back then, when I was 'marginal' (used to laugh at that word! – I'd have said 'in the margins' or 'off the planet!'), I used to blame everybody and everything for my lack of organization and failure. Amazing how I've come to value organization in myself, and others. It's awful when you can't blame anybody for your failures but yourself!! Life's little lesson # 321,000.

love Sally

Fax reply to Postcard 7

Dear Sally,

Justice, retribution! I know them well! From time to time I ponder those things we put so much energy into fighting against, like structure and planning; when in fact they can make life so much easier. By the way, I never thought of you as 'marginal'.
Love, Di

This chapter contains transcripts and case studies that have been gathered from undergraduate speech therapy students and social work students who have been identified as either experiencing difficulties with their clinical work or who are perceived to be gifted student clinicians. One of the authors has collected transcripts for research about how speech therapy students, who have difficulties with their clinical subjects, perceive, describe and account for these difficulties (Nemeth, 1996). Another of the writers has collected transcripts from students' journals about interactions between students and care givers (Maloney, 1994).

7.2 BACKGROUND

We refer to students experiencing problems in clinical settings as *marginal students*. These are students who do not consistently meet the required level of competence for their expected stage in the clinical programme. Some writers describe these students as 'challenging' or 'problem students' (Best & Rose, 1996). In our view, marginal students include those students who have failed or are failing in clinical subjects and also those who, whilst not failing, show a pattern of inconsistent clinical performance. These students require 'extra' attention to assist them to achieve their full potential.

We have, by the nature of our particular skills and job specialization, worked with many students identified as being marginal students. Our experience has been that clinical educators spend considerably more time with students with problems than they spend with students without problems. We have therefore developed management strategies that enhance marginal students' learning, whilst not detracting from the provision of learning opportunities for students at all levels of competence.

A general goal of clinical educators is to provide a learning climate that increases students' options for learning from their experiences (Egan, 1990). Being able to determine at an early stage which students are at risk of having difficulties in clinical placements, due to a learning barrier, may ensure that students are directed to appropriate services before a pattern of 'failure' develops. Should appropriate support be warranted, students can be offered assistance to deal with their particular barriers to learning so that they can attempt to move towards being interdependent and competent in their chosen profession (see Chapter 1).

It would be incongruent with adult learning theory to have a textbook 'recipe' that provides an exhaustive and comprehensive appraisal of barriers to clinical learning. The principles of adult learning (see Chapter 1) value individual experience and knowledge and therefore students who experience difficulties need to be allowed to tell their own stories (Knowles, 1990). Intelligence, sensitivity, understanding and insight are needed when dealing with these students. We believe it is counterproductive to approach students presenting with difficulties with a narrow, prescribed description or explanation of their behaviour. Nonetheless, in this first section of the chapter we address some of the barriers to learning in clinical settings that have been discussed in the literature and that we have experienced with students. Whilst this material is by no means exhaustive, it will hopefully encourage the reader to approach each student's barrier to learning with greater understanding of the range of possible contributory circumstances.

7.3 CURRENT RESEARCH RELATED TO THEORIES OF STUDENT LEARNING AND POSSIBLE BARRIERS

There is considerable literature on student learning styles (see Chapter 1) and the attributes necessary for academic success. Examining the way students approach learning in clinical situations is one way clinical educators can seek to understand the problems students experience. There is, however, considerably less information on the skills necessary for the application of knowledge to clinical work (see Chapter 5). Theories about students' approaches to learning (including Coles, 1990), locus of control, life context, life cycle and moral and intellectual development provide possible insights into the nature of the problems students experience.

7.3.1 APPROACHES TO LEARNING

Coles (1990) questioned the deep and surface processing stance (see Chapter 1) as being too simplistic in explaining how medical and other health professional students learn, suggesting that students adopt one of four approaches: restricted, adequate, clinical or elaborated approaches. According to Coles, the elaborative approach is the most effective for applying theoretical material to clinical settings.

(a) Restricted approach

Coles (1990) reported that students using a restricted approach feel cynical, overloaded, unmotivated and want to give up. They work in order to pass exams and typically fear failure. These students also tend to approach learning by memorizing, are disorganized and lack understanding of the material being taught. Case Study 7.1 gives an example of a student who takes a restricted approach to learning.

(b) Adequate approach

Students adopting the adequate approach tend to pay great attention to understanding the meaning, but see little application or its relevance to client management. Their motivation tends to be extrinsic and dependent upon academic results. These students are disappointed with less than excellent grades. Their learning is good in the short term, but retrieval of material learned early is limited. Case Study 7.2 is an example of a student who utilized the adequate approach and this ultimately contributed to clinical learning difficulties.

Case Study 7.1 An example of a student taking a restricted approach to learning

Rosemary was in her first year of clinical education when she experienced difficulties. Her description of her approach to learning appears typical of the restricted approach. She reported that she was poorly organized, lazy and periodically questioned the value of her chosen profession. The following quote exemplifies the restricted approach:

'At school you do your maths or biology and its easy. It's not actually learning but memorizing which is quite different to applying things to clinical work. So I was having some difficulties and my clinical educator said, "You have to make an effort otherwise you're not going to pass". And that was probably the best thing she could have said to me. Like, if you don't do some work you're going to fail. And that really helped me get my act together and get through.'

Case Study 7.2 An example of a student taking an adequate approach to learning

Chris was a final year speech therapy student who experienced problems in her last clinical placement. Throughout her undergraduate training, she had some difficulties passing some academic subjects. She reported that she was slower than her peers in processing information, and retrieving information that had been covered academically, even when she had passed the corresponding academic course. Her own words further highlight her use of the adequate approach.

'A lot of things my clinical educator asked me related to courses done in first and second year and I just thought, "I have no idea. I can't remember." There was this dread of not remembering things, that ran throughout the whole placement.'

(c) Clinical approach

For students who take the clinical approach, clinical experiences assist their understanding of the theoretical and abstract information taught. However, they may become so immersed in the clinical picture that they miss the opportunity to read textbooks or re-examine previous coursework. Case Study 7.3 gives an example of a student who takes a clinical approach to learning.

Case Study 7.3 An example of a student taking a clinical approach to learning

Anna was an enthusiastic social work student in her second clinical place-ment. In her spare time, she did voluntary work with families of children with cancer. She revelled in her clinical work, was tireless in following up treat-ment plans for her client families, but found difficulty in relating the university theory to practice.

'Work is so much more interesting than lectures, which just seem irrele-vant and boring, and I never have time to get all the reading done that they give us!'

Fortunately, there was still plenty of time left in her course for further integra-tion of theory with practice, and poor marks on some of her assignments made her turn back to her textbooks and pay enough attention to lectures to see the relevance of theory to practice.

(d) Elaborated approach

The elaborated approach enables students to perform successfully by relating the knowledge they are acquiring to clinical examples and inte-grating theoretical concerns. Students taking this approach can retrieve information easily and tend not to have gaps in their knowledge, like those using the clinical approach may have. The quote in Case Study 7.4 was col-lected from a student who was deemed to be a gifted student clinician. It embodies the essence of successful utilization of the elaborated approach.

Case Study 7.4 A quote from a student using an elaborated approach to learning

'I have a good memory which helps. I've got a good theoretical basis and applying it isn't hard. I'm lucky 'cause I catch onto things easily and I can learn really quickly from clinical experiences and from my clinical educa-tors. I can adapt those things quite readily as well. I understand how things work and fit together and how to apply that.'

Locus of control theory is another area of theoretical knowledge which may provide insight into students' difficulties.

7.3.2 LOCUS OF CONTROL

Rotter (1966) described a construct of internal versus external control of reinforcement. This construct provides some insight into perceptions of causality and control. The internal/external locus of control is defined as follows:

> 'When a reinforcement is perceived by the subject as following some action of his own but not being entirely contingent upon his action, then, in our culture, it is typically perceived as the result of luck, chance, fate, or under the control of powerful others, or as unpredictable because of the great complexity of the forces surrounding him. When the event is interpreted in this way by an individual, we have labelled this a belief in external control. If the person perceives that the event is contingent upon his own behaviour or his own relatively permanent characteristics, we have termed this a belief in internal control.' (Rotter, 1966, p. 1)

Rotter (1966) discussed locus of control theory in the context of clinical education and suggested that students who apportion blame or responsibility regarding their learning to external factors are less successful learners and potentially less responsible clinicians. Egan (1990) also makes reference to 'problem ownership' and the difficulties clinicians can experience in trying to facilitate change when the goals are not truly owned by the student or client involved in the learning process. Case Study 7.5 gives an example of a student who apportions responsibility for clinical learning difficulties to factors external to herself.

Case Study 7.5 A quote from a student with an external locus of control

'My clinical educator wasn't very good. That's not just me, because I have spoken to a lot of people and they feel the same way, including a lot of professionals outside. I think she's a little bit rigid and she really got my back up. Anyway, she said I'm a very disorganized person which I am, and I hadn't prepared for this client and she was really cranky about it. She said she thought I had changed and stuff like that. I was sitting there and going "Yeah, yeah" and in my head I was saying "I hate you, I hate you!" She really picked on me. I really denied that it had anything to do with me.'

Students who have an internal locus of control function as though outcomes of their learning and those related to client care are largely a result of their own efforts, or lack thereof, and are consequently more likely to accept responsibility for their actions. Using an internal locus of control may well enhance other aspects of clinical practice. For example, student nurses who were found to have a tendency toward internal locus of control used a higher proportion of complex decision-making processes than those tending to use external locus of control (Tschikota, 1993).

On the other hand, those students who believe in external control, see little relationship between what they do and outcomes that occur. They view the responsibility for their learning and clinical work, as being a result of external factors. The internal/external locus of control paradigm can be a useful framework for understanding students' attribution of causality when difficulties arise with their clinical work. It may help clinical educators understand why some students have difficulty being responsible for their learning and client management.

Rotter (1975) warned there are limitations to the internal-external control concept which need to be considered. He suggested that locus of control can be used effectively to describe specific expectancies, but has limitations when used to describe generalized expectancies because it fails to account for other possible extraneous variables. It is tempting to align acceptance or non-acceptance of responsibility to either an internal or external locus of control. However, various other factors could well account for a particular behaviour. For example, a student who values academic achievement greater than clinical achievement may appear to have an external locus of control, in the clinical setting. In this case the student could have an internal locus of control but is responding strategically to the competing demands of academic and clinical work.

We discuss the internal/external locus of control paradigm again later in this chapter, when exploring possible indicators of distress in marginal students. The next sections address some of the other factors which impact on students' abilities to learn in clinic.

7.3.3 LIFE CONTEXT

The historical and socio-cultural background of an individual constitutes an important backdrop to any learning (Finger, 1988). Thus, it would seem to be essential to have some understanding of the background of students who experience barriers to learning in clinical work. Mezirow's (1991) 'perspective transformation' describes how adults operate within meaning structures which are defined as personal beliefs and values, perceived societal norms, and personal and significant others' expectations. These function as filters through which all experiences are interpreted and given meaning. Giving some consideration to students' meaning structures could also assist in illuminating some barriers to learning. Case Study 7.6 highlights the importance of having a comprehensive appreciation of a student's background. This student experienced difficulties with clinical work which could be largely attributed to her life context, including her value system, and significant others' expectations and influences. We believe that without this understanding, it would have been difficult to access appropriate intervention which in this case involved professional counselling.

Case Study 7.6 An example of the impact of life context on clinical performance

Rita was the second last child of a large family. During her early years, she relied heavily on friendships and more particularly on being part of 'the group', being liked and being involved with peers. On the one hand, having friends and being a member of a group was important to her, but on the other hand, Rita took great delight in defying group behaviour.

After finishing school, Rita enrolled in a degree at an interstate university and lived on the university campus. The freedom here, in comparison to her previous life and boarding school, was unprecedented. She had a 'wild time for about six months. I was drunk the whole time'. Consequently she failed her academic subjects. 'I was very depressed 'cause I couldn't believe I failed and then I hated the whole theme of college life'. She lived with a family member, but felt isolated, bored and lonely and broke up with her boyfriend. She began experiencing feelings of depression, 'You know when you're depressed you sleep so much. It's the worst feeling. Like you just like you feel you're dead. I'd never felt dead before'.

Rita moved out and flatted with a friend. During this period she allowed herself to be coerced into taking various drugs. This occurred toward the latter part of Rita's first year of clinical experience. Not surprisingly, with her socio-cultural background and current life context, Rita's clinical work began to suffer. Her clinical educator told her that she had poor organizational skills and came to clinic unprepared. 'I had no idea of anything, I didn't have the skills at all. Couldn't even develop them'. These life context factors began to affect her overall cognitive functioning, and emotional well-being. Consequently she was directed to seek professional counselling.

This case study encapsulates the impact historical and socio-cultural background can have on an individual's learning. We believe, whilst seemingly very difficult or destructive for the individual at the time, given the appropriate assistance, they can gain much insight and learning which can assist them in their clinical practice.

7.3.4 LIFE CYCLE

In Australia and the United Kingdom students may begin the clinical education component of their degrees one year after completing high school. Consequently it is helpful to have some understanding of the life context surrounding adolescence. In our experience the 'adolescent stage' is protracted, long past school-leaving age by some students. Knowledge of life stages may be helpful too in understanding mature age students presenting with problems in clinical practice. Awareness of movement in and out of life stages can provide a useful structure for assisting marginal students. Some life cycle approaches will be discussed later in this chapter.

Erikson (1971) described eight stages of development through life. Individuals come to each stage's ascendance, meet its crisis and find its lasting solution towards the end of the stage. Adolescence is Erikson's fifth stage of development. The crisis of adolescence is one of identity versus role confusion. In this stage, adolescents are preoccupied by their appearance in the eyes of others, rather than how they feel. The task of establishing an individual identity is the major task of adolescence. Thus, choosing the 'right' occupational identity in late adolescence is identified by most young people as an integral component of this task. This has implications for all undergraduate students and may contribute to difficulties that some students experience with their clinical learning. Case Study 7.7 reflects some of these adolescent preoccupations.

Case Study 7.7 Adolescence

Jane stood out from her peers in both lectures and around the clinic because she always appeared excessively well-dressed and groomed. She said that her friends from school were all in 'glamorous jobs, meeting interesting people and had all the time in the world to have lots of fun', whilst she felt she had to study and work hard all the time.

'I went through a stage where I wanted to drop out of uni, like every semester I did ... all first and second year. So I wanted to drop out of uni and get away. I didn't have time to meet people and I didn't feel I fitted with the other students. I wasn't sure that after all the hard work I wanted this type of profession at the end.'

This case study encapsulates some of the dilemmas that can be faced by students when they do not identify with their chosen occupational group and they are attempting to develop close and meaningful relationships.

During adolescence intimate relationships with others are established. This issue is observed quite frequently with students whose social life, including developing intimate relationships, takes precedence over their study and clinical work. Client care is consequently compromised due to competing life stage events which can result in poor student performance.

7.3.5 MORAL AND INTELLECTUAL DEVELOPMENT

Theories about moral and intellectual development may also provide insight into how and why students function in a way that hinders their clinical growth. Perry (1970) outlines nine stages, or as he designates them 'positions', which describe attitudes to knowledge and authority and stance as learners in male, American university students. Perry noted a progression from dualistic, black or white thinking to an appreciation of relativism. That is, that knowledge is not fixed, right or wrong, but is relative to the context. His first position describes students viewing the world in extremes, with 'we-right-good' at one pole and 'other-wrong-bad' at the other pole. Knowledge and goodness are absolute and therefore it is teachers' responsibility to impart this perceived absolute authority. For students at this stage the acquisition of knowledge is achieved through hard work and obedience.

In Perry's second stage, students perceive the possibility of a diversity in opinion, but they account for this diversity as unnecessary confusion. Students may believe teachers are withholding 'the answers'. Clinical educators will recognize this in the student who seeks the clinical educator's 'prescription' so as to 'be clear about exactly what I have to do'. Perry (1970) suggests that students' moral and ethical development gradually progresses until they can tolerate legitimate uncertainty and multiplicity of opinion. Dualistic right-wrong dichotomies are reserved for special cases. Students eventually consciously commit themselves to a set of values or career, and begin to explore the implications of their commitment and the issues surrounding responsibility. The last stage allows for the affirmation of a commitment which is held consciously and yet with flexibility. There is also an awareness that future growth is part of an experience which expresses 'life' (Perry, 1970).

It should be remembered that Perry based his work on young, male, American university students. The development of female students appears to be different. Blenky, Clinchy, Goldberger and Tarule (1986) found that females experienced similar stages of development to those described by Perry, but that the development was less linear and more dependent on context. Gender differences were also found in studies of moral reasoning conducted on males (Kohlberg, 1984) and on females (Gilligan, 1982).

Attitudes to knowledge and authority can be influenced by culture (Ballard & Clancy, 1991). Students from different cultures may approach teachers, learning, knowledge and the development of academic skills in different ways. We should not assume that 'everyone thinks like us' or holds similar values about education. Case Study 7.8 contains an example of a different attitude to knowledge.

Case Study 7.8 An example of a different attitude to knowledge

An overseas student viewed the world as 'black and white'. Consequently, there was only one correct way of 'doing' clinical work and she was constantly searching for ways to find it. She was dependent on the clinical educator and latched onto inappropriate therapy approaches discussed in textbooks or published articles. As a result, she found applying theory to the clinical setting impossible because she was incapable of adapting ideas to suit individual clients and situations. Considerable time was spent talking with her clinical educator about diversity. Together they analyzed the clinical setting and clients' needs and selected appropriate strategies to assist her clients and broaden her views about knowledge.

Although determining students' stages of moral and intellectual development may elucidate where barriers to effective learning originate, this information needs to be integrated with all of the other theoretical considerations which were discussed earlier.

This section has discussed theoretical material which is pertinent to understanding why some students experience difficulties in clinical education. The next section discusses management strategies for marginal students.

7.4 IDENTIFICATION OF MARGINAL STUDENTS

We are indebted to all those students and colleagues who have consulted with us about problems in clinical education. They have provided an ongoing opportunity for us to learn from our peers and caused us to ponder on the short- and long-term outcomes of our interventions. They have provided much of the material for this section.

While reading this section of the chapter it is important to remember that some of the behaviours exhibited by marginal students are seen in most students at some time during their clinical experience. However, the difference lies in the degree and extent of interruption to clinical learning experienced by marginal students. This is evident in their response to feedback. Marginal students do not respond appropriately to constructive feedback and appear unable to make changes in response to feedback, consequently their clinical skills do not improve. Students who present with occasional problems, but are not marginal students, are those who respond and learn from their clinical educators' feedback. Marginal students present with constantly occurring clusters of behaviours, including poor preparation, poor organizational skills, limited interactional skills and poor communication skills. The marginal student may experience continual poor health, feel depressed, angry, uncommitted, withdrawn, sad, emotionally labile, tired or listless.

How then do clinical educators assist marginal students? The following is a four-stage approach to the management of marginal students in clinical settings:

1 *Identification of students experiencing problems.* Students experiencing problems may be identified by themselves or any member of the university or clinical staff.
2 *Exploration of the identified problems.* During this stage the clinical educator, director of clinical education or counsellor explores the background and cause of problems with students. Students' indicators of distress often provide the starting point for problem exploration.
3 *Consideration of possible management strategies.* During this stage the clinical educator decides on strategies to use during future interactions with the student experiencing problems.
4 *Outcome.* The aim of all the strategies discussed is to help the student confront the factors contributing to their problems and begin the process of taking control of their own learning.

This appears to be a linear approach to understanding and facilitating marginal students' learning in clinical settings; however, we have found that we move through the stages in cycles, often returning to earlier stages to assist the student gain clarification about a perceived problem (Egan, 1990).

7.4.1 IDENTIFICATION OF STUDENTS EXPERIENCING PROBLEMS

(a) Identification by students

Some marginal students will accept that they are having problems learning in a particular clinical setting after constructive feedback from clinical educators. A number of these will consider the possible causes of the identified problems and take responsibility for accessing the assistance needed to make the required changes in their behaviour or in the placement.

(b) Identification by others

Marginal students may also be identified by any member of staff of the university, clinic, department or family. Sometimes the very nature of their behaviour is a cry for help. They may be unable to request assistance for themselves in the usual manner.

Parents may be aware that the student is unhappy and feel that he or she needs access to more assistance than family support. Administrators of departments and clinics and professional colleagues may identify a student with problems because of unacceptable behaviour patterns in complying with administrative requirements. Clinical educators identify a student with problems in learning when the student does not show positive change following expanded opportunities for discussion about client management and clinical issues. These students do not appear to be able to learn from the feedback process (see Chapter 3). Clients also may identify students who are having problems with client management. Clients who are managed routinely by students provide helpful information about how they or their family member is being treated by a student clinician. However, other regular clients may 'protect' a new student or conversely fail to attend for appointments if they are dissatisfied with the service. In large teaching units or clinics, clinical educators find that clients are often experienced at identifying students' strengths and weaknesses. (See Chapter 3 on client feedback.)

7.4.2 EXPLORATION OF THE IDENTIFIED PROBLEMS

The detailed exploration of problems will be facilitated by clinical educators, the director of clinical education and/or the university counselling service. Clinical educators observe students' interpersonal communication skills when they interact with clients, peers and clinic staff. The clinical educator is usually the first person involved in exploration of students' problems. The setting of boundaries (see Chapter 3) will assist the marginal student to feel in control of discussions about perceived problems in his or her clinical placement. The level of this exploration by the clinical educator will depend on the boundaries previously agreed on by the student and clinical educator during the placement.

The director of clinical education or coordinator of clinical placements generally has policies and procedures for management of marginal students. Directors may choose to explore the problems with the student. Additionally, a university student counsellor is generally available for all students. Some students choose to seek assistance from staff outside their immediate department or school through this service. Our experience, however, is that many marginal students do not seek counselling assistance unless they are referred by clinical educators because of problems identified in clinical placements that would impede continuation in the clinical programme.

Metheny and Carline (1991) suggest that the most frequent problems for students in clinical settings are an inability to focus on what is important, possession of a poor fund of knowledge, disorganization, poor integration skills and excessive shyness, and inappropriate assertiveness. The next section discusses issues which may increase clinical educators' awareness of marginal students' problems. In our experience, problem exploration may encompass one or several of the following issues: career choice, continual ill health, non-compliant behaviour, self defeating patterns of behaviour, organizational skills, non-verbal behaviour, excellence and failure. Students invariably provide 'indicators' that identify from which area the problems stem.

(a) Issues related to career choice

School leavers may have a very clear idea that their desired career lies in the health science field. Other students are less sure and may even have tried other courses before their present one. Some students have no difficulty acting on the realization that they have made a wrong career choice. They are able to access appropriate information and assistance so that they can consider all the options open to them. However, other students presenting with problems in clinical education indicate that they need counselling to help them make decisions about their chosen course. These students appear unable to access the information and assistance they need to help them make informed career choices.

One overt indicator of students' distress is repeated discussion of withdrawing from courses. Students' abilities to verbalize thoughts and feelings about making a career change may vary depending on their sense of control over their life decisions (Rotter, 1975). In many courses students may not have the opportunity to experience face-to-face work with clients until the second or third year of their course. They may feel that, having already committed considerable time, money and energy to the course, they are 'stuck'. These factors may impact on their ability to contemplate the possibility that they have made a wrong career choice. These students provide a dilemma for clinical educators, especially as some excel in academic work. As well, they tend to be critical of the profession rather than of themselves and this may challenge the clinical educators' own belief in their chosen field.

We have divided the following section into career choice issues for school-leavers (those students who completed high school and immediately started undergraduate courses) and mature age students, because different issues arise for each of these groups.

School-leavers

Students who enter a chosen field immediately after school may feel they have had their career decisions made for them by their parents or others (for example, their university entry mark gaining them a place in a highly competitive course). Careers with a vocational strand may be seen by parents and career advisers as being very desirable for many reasons: a strong possibility of employment on graduation, 'doing good' for the world, a socially acceptable profession or above average remuneration.

Case Study 7.9 contains an example of a school-leaver facing a career dilemma.

Case Study 7.9 An example of a school-leaver facing a career dilemma

The country parent of a year 1 student rang the director of clinical education. The director first ascertained that the parent had the student's permission to speak to her about her daughter's concerns. The director learned that the student felt that she couldn't contact a staff member herself for fear they would tell her it 'was a great job and why wouldn't she like it'! Further, the student felt she would be jeopardizing her position in the course if she let her doubts be known. The parent said the family did not mind what the student decided, but she felt the student needed assistance to consider her options and come to a decision about her career. The clinical director provided information about who the student could contact, both within the department and the university counselling service.

As discussed earlier in this chapter, the importance of role identification during adolescence may result in distress related to choice of career. Consideration of this seems very important when managing school-leavers in crisis.

Mature age students

At the other end of the career choice continuum are mature age students who have made a career change, often at considerable financial and emotional cost to themselves. They may place unrealistic expectations on the chosen new career and put stress on themselves to believe that this career switch will fulfil all the needs that were not being met in their life before. The reality is that they may be confronted by situations in their clinical education experience that make them reconsider aspects of their life and this may impact on their ability to make objective, appropriate and effective decisions. Case Study 7.10 contains an example of a mature age student with unrealistic career expectations.

(b) Students with continual ill health

Students can show their distress in clinical settings by having continual poor health. They may have a poor clinical attendance record due to valid medical reasons for their non-attendance. On the other hand some students will attend the clinic even though they are obviously ill. Many students live away from home, support themselves through university by

> **Case Study 7.10** Unrealistic career expectations
>
> David had been a primary teacher for five years. He decided to return to university and study social work. In his second clinical placement, he often referred to 'performance anxiety' when working with clients and preferred to read reference books and search out resources rather than working with clients. He disliked supervision and seemed to avoid his clinical educator, and any interaction with her colleagues in the department. The seemingly 'safe world' of one-to-one interactions with a client, compared to the blackboard jungle of the classroom, was no longer as safe as he had expected.

working and are in the process of learning general life skills related to economics and effective time management, and feel they cannot 'afford to be ill'. As suggested by Best and Rose (1996) it is worth checking that these students are having adequate nutrition, rest and exercise.

Some students, especially those from overseas and from different cultures may feel so unhappy that they unconsciously see being ill as the only way for them to escape. In this case, depression presents as physical illness. Other students are not able to manage in their clinical placements because they are too exhausted after suffering a long-term debilitating illness that has left them physically and emotionally 'wrung out'.

(c) Non-compliant behaviour

Clinical education settings provide students with the opportunity to develop understanding of themselves in relation to authority figures. We believe that the ability to be non-compliant is a healthy part of normal student life-stage development and is related to developing a sense of self and their own individuality. Students will test the rules of the system as part of learning the reason for specific 'rules'. However, students who are not coping in clinical settings may carry non-compliance to unacceptable lengths. These students may test all the limits related to clinical management of time, dress, appearance, policies, procedures and ethical practice.

(d) Self-defeating patterns of behaviour

Another indication that a student is having problems is continued demonstration of self-defeating patterns of behaviour. These patterns of behaviour may occur in the student's life outside the clinic as well (see Case Study 7.6, for an example). The behaviour patterns may also occur within the clinic and impact on the ability of the student to work successfully with clients, despite continued teaching and assistance from the clinical educator.

The self-defeating behaviours may relate to aspects of: clinical administration (for example, appointments not kept, incomplete files), interpersonal skills (for example, failure to listen to the client and continuing provision of information that the client either does not understand or cannot apply), or responsibility for client management (for example, not following up contacts with other relevant professionals involved in the client's management).

These are obviously not clear cut areas and each may impact on the other. Students' behaviours may be overt and obvious (for example, failing to attend for client appointments or appointments with the clinical educator) or the behaviours may be covert and insidious (for example, commencing a client session without telling the clinical educator where the session will take place or 'forgetting' to turn the video camera on so the clinical educator can observe the session).

(e) Poor organizational skills

Students' disorganized behaviours show in every aspect of their performance. They are disorganized with required paperwork, often not providing the clinical educator with necessary information at the required time, and thus endangering client management. They fail to prepare themselves thoroughly for new clients, placements and experiences. These students tend to be late with reports and are often well known to the clerical staff of clinics who comment on the disruption they cause in the clinic administration. These students will have a clinic room that looks chaotic, lacks appropriate furniture and is distracting for the client.

We have found that early confrontation of such problem behaviours is beneficial to students in clinical settings. They can be given extra assistance before the behaviours become habitual. For example, one practical strategy is for the clinical educator and student jointly to develop a checklist for room preparation to assist the disorganized student.

(f) Non-verbal behaviours

Students may provide the clinical educator with non-verbal indications of distress. These students may comply with all requests, they attend conference group sessions, hand in written session plans on time and carry out all the administrative requirements but their distress shows in the 'robotic' manner in which they carry out the requirements. This effect in most cases will also show in their interpersonal communications with clients. Their behaviour lacks 'realness' and they appear to be somewhat puppet-like in the way they interact with clients, peers and clinical educators. A few of these students may in fact be clinically depressed and in need of urgent referral for appropriate assistance.

(g) Excellence

Clinical educators enjoy the challenge of excellent students. However, they may present as being 'at risk' rather than marginal, because their desire and need for perfection may interfere with their ability to learn in clinical settings. They may be so self-critical that this impedes their ability to establish effective working relationships with some clients. These students may demand the same high standards from their clients as they do from themselves. As beginning student clinicians they believe they should have their clinical skills perfected, that it should all come naturally and that if they make a mistake they have failed. These students vary on the dependent/independent continuum (see Chapter 3). However, they often have a very strong sense of responsibility and, in our experience, those who present with problems tend to cluster more at the dependent end of the scale, because it seems they are overly fearful of causing harm to the clients in their care.

(h) Failure

Some students learn from the experience of failure and go on to achieve success. To put it another way, they are able to seek out and understand the 'how come' of the failure and use this to make positive change in their life. The locus of control (Rotter, 1975) is internalized and the student takes responsibility for his or her own actions. Case Study 7.11 is an example of a student who learned from failure.

Case Study 7.11 Learning from the experience of failure

A university medical lecturer was surprised when approached at a social function by a confident young woman, who had recently been making her name in art design. She thanked him for helping her to make 'the most important decision of her life!' To his baffled enquiries, she told him that his 'help' had been failing her in a first-year medical subject, and taking the time to discuss her failure with her. She realized that she had in fact only done medicine because of her high university academic entrance mark and not through deep commitment. The result made her rethink her future, and decide to follow her real area of interest and skill. Thus this failure was a very effective part of her learning.

Failure is not a positive experience for many students and for the clinical educators who work with them. For some students, failure is a devastating experience and can appear to be a scar they carry throughout life. The authors have participated in clinical education workshops with various professional groups where members will allude to a failure they had as student in some clinical setting, apparently anticipating that the university staff member will recall this failure. We rarely do. This is a salutary experience and one that shows the impact of past failure and how it is carried.

Failure in academic subjects

Whilst our prime focus in this section is on those students who have failed or are failing in clinical subjects, mention must be made of students who have failed in academic subjects and the impact this can have on their learning in clinical settings. When the failed subject is a prerequisite for entry to the clinical education programme, the student will be 'out of step' with his or her peer group and may lose opportunities for peer learning (see Chapter 4). When the failed subject is not a pre-requisite for entry to the clinical programmeme, the student may carry over subjects and have a heavier academic load whilst in the clinical education programme.

Failure in an academic subject can impact on students' confidence in their ability to understand and meet the requirements of the course and this reduction of confidence can affect their performance in clinical settings. In our experience, some students who fail university subjects have never experienced academic failure before and have always achieved excellent grades. Their confidence about themselves as a person has been linked to their achievement of excellent grades. These students say 'I have failed' rather than 'I failed a subject'.

Failure in clinical subjects

We have found that whilst some students contemplate or choose withdrawal from a course as a way of managing a problem, other students appear to have to fail before they can consider problem identification and management. These students externalize the locus of control (Rotter, 1966) saying 'I was failed' rather than 'I failed because ... '. They perceive the cause of their failure to rest outside their control and as long as they 'blame' externals, be they the administration, the clinical educator or the client, they do not take responsibility for their own learning.

Other students, when told they are failing, will at first react with sadness and anger and then later be quite relieved. They often have felt insecure about their level of clinical abilities in previous placements in relation to their clinical education and client management. Students have told us 'It's so good not to pretend, now I feel I can say when I don't know and extend my learning and increase my clinical skills'.

Many clinical educators find failing a student very challenging and often will avoid this responsibility when the student is new to the clinical education programme hoping that, given time, the student will improve. Therefore clinical educators are encouraged to identify and explore problems with the student and access at an early stage the options of assistance available to both of them with appropriate members of the university staff.

The effects of student failure on clinical educators

We developed the list of behaviours and feelings described below, from the experiences clinical educators have shared in workshops. The list explains how clinical educators feel about themselves when they have a student who is failing in their clinical setting:

- frustrated with students' lack of positive change and resentful and angry about the demands the student places on them
- concerned that their own skills are inadequate for a specific student's needs
- ambivalent about their commitment to the dual role of clinician and clinical educator
- resistant to recognizing serious learning difficulties because they want the student to succeed
- anxious that their own expectations may be unrealistic for the student's stage of learning
- fearful that the student's failure reflects badly on themselves as a clinician and clinical educator.

Clinical educators, we believe, need to have many options available for managing individual student's learning needs in the specific clinical setting. The management strategies discussed in the next section are applicable to all students and clinical educators and represent a range of options for dealing flexibly with marginal students.

7.4.3 CONSIDERATION OF POSSIBLE MANAGEMENT STRATEGIES

This section considers some management strategies that clinical educators can use with students experiencing problems at any stage of the clinical education programme. These are grounded in the principles of communication (Pickering, 1995) that were discussed in Chapter 3.

Clinical educators, remembering that a range of options provides for flexibility and creative solutions, may elect to use one or several of the following: adopting a counselling role, referral to another professional, active listening, collaboration with the student, identification of communication difficulties between the clinical educator and student, immediacy (using the supervisory relationship to facilitate student learning), group learning.

(a) Counselling role

Clinical educators may take on a counselling role with marginal students (see Chapter 2). In instances where the taking of this role conflicts with the need to be judge or examiner of the student's clinical performance, negotiation between clinical educator and director of the clinical programme to provide an alternative assessment is required.

However the counsellor role in the management of marginal students is not necessarily a comfortable position for all clinical educators. Those educators may choose to refer students presenting with a problem to professional counsellors (Turney *et al.*, 1982).

(b) Referral

There are a variety of reasons why marginal students may need assistance from someone other than their current clinical educator. Some possible reasons for referral include:

- A student appears unable to apply knowledge in the current clinic setting.
- A student consistently does not accept responsibility for learning.
- A student consistently avoids discussion with the clinical educator.
- A student's behaviour is symptomatic of emotional illness.
- The clinical educator feels that the student needs specialized counselling or educational intervention.
- The clinical educator and student jointly feel that the student would learn from the opportunity to discuss problems with a professional from another field (for example, medical, educational or psychological).

The referral may be either within the clinic or department, for example to a more senior colleague or outside, to another practitioner. The marginal student's need for referral to another professional, whilst obvious to the clinical educator, may be less apparent or acceptable to the student. A referral is more likely to have a successful outcome if the following factors are present in the interaction between student and clinical educator:

- The clinical educator gives a clear explanation to the student about the reason for referral.
- The clinical educator gives the student information about the service provided by the professional to whom he or she will be referred.
- The clinical educator actively listens to the student's concerns about accepting the referral.
- When necessary the clinical educator may facilitate making the appointment and continue to meet with the student until the referral has been satisfactorily negotiated.

(c) Active listening

Another possible management strategy is to use active listening with marginal students. Active listening skills provide a climate in which problems can be identified and acknowledged by the clinical educator and student, leading to the exploration of possible management options. Students report that the experience of 'being heard' increases their feeling of being in charge of their own learning. The skills used in active listening include:

- keeping the total focus of the interaction on the student
- paraphrasing the content and giving feedback about the feelings that the student is expressing
- reflecting the content and feelings expressed so the student feels understood from his or her frame of reference and can hear and understand him/herself
- allowing silences in the conversation to provide time for reflection.

(d) Collaboration

Clinical educators may collaborate with students to develop creative and appropriate ways of handling management strategies for the student's identified problems. Collaboration provides a learning environment that promotes the student's sense of responsibility for changing unsuccessful behaviours. For example, when discussing a student's history of poor achievement in previous clinical placements, the student identifies that report writing has been an on-going difficulty for her. The clinical educator and student brainstorm about possible methods of improving report writing skills (for example, computerized report writing aids, looking at reports by other clinicians, allowing sufficient time so several drafts can be submitted for feedback from the clinical educator). The student identifies the strategies to be implemented and contracts with the clinical educator about expectations of the clinical educator's role in the achieving of these goals. Through collaboration the clinical educator and student have developed a workable plan for managing a clinical problem. Marginal students may need extra assistance in learning the skills involved in successful collaboration.

(e) Identifying communication difficulties between clinical educators and students

Various student behaviours, such as defensiveness, can be viewed as symptoms of communication blocks between students and clinical educators. One possible explanation for such blocks may be differing learning styles (see Chapter 1). A flexible way of managing this problem is for clinical educators and students to compare learning styles when they are seemingly at cross purposes in planning client management.

Communication breakdown may also result from a mismatch between the style or level of clinical education being given and the student's perceived level of independence on the supervisory continuum (Anderson, 1988) discussed in Chapter 2. Marginal students often need more assistance understanding clinical educators' roles. They benefit from jointly marking their position on the continuum with clinical educators (Anderson, 1988). This activity provides a starting point for discussion about both the student's and the clinical educator's perceived expectations about level and style of supervision. Moreover, mismatch between the clinical educator's expectations in the placement and the student's learning stage, aptitude or ability to apply theory to specific aspects of the placement may occur and need to be recognized and acknowledged.

(f) Immediacy

Another strategy which clinical educators may find effective in helping marginal students focus on problem areas is termed immediacy. Immediacy or 'direct mutual talk' between clinical educators and students uses the supervisory relationship as the focus of learning (Egan, 1990, p. 224). Examples of immediacy include:

- statements about oneself that are in the present tense and are a personal response to a student's work with a client. For example, a clinical educator says 'I liked how you began the session but I noticed that you went over the allotted time for this client'
- statements about the clinical educator–student relationship so that what is actually happening between them is examined. For example, a clinical educator says to a student 'You seem to be avoiding our joint planning sessions by double booking or forgetting the time. I wonder what is happening between us to cause this behaviour'
- statements of immediacy in the 'here and now' of any given interpersonal communication between clinical educators and students. For example, a clinical educator says to a student 'You seem angry and upset about the comment I just made to you about your last session'.

(g) Group learning

Specialist tutorial groups, external to the clinic placement and in addition to normal course requirements, can provide marginal students with a non-threatening environment where they can examine and share their problems about learning in clinical settings. When run on the mutual aid model (Schulman, 1984), such a group provides members with reassurance that they are not the only ones with problems or fearing failure and also with a framework for sharing strategies and strengths. In such groups members bring their varied learning styles and life experience into the group so that each member may benefit from mutual contributions (Kolb, 1984). For example, a refresher course for social workers, who had either trained overseas or been out of the field for some time, successfully used such tutorial groups to deal with the anxiety around clinical practice, updating of theoretical knowledge and integration of the professional self with life skills and experience (Studdy, Cooper, Carmody & Cohen, 1994).

On the other hand, some marginal students experience difficulties participating in groups. As group and team interactions are expected of health professionals, these students may need individual assistance in developing these skills. The aim for these students is to practise the skills they have gained with the clinical educator in group conference sessions.

(h) Identifying students' strengths

Marginal students sometimes have difficulty acknowledging their areas of strength and tend to focus only on areas of weakness. This can result in unrealistic expectations for themselves and for their clients. For example these students may say 'I can *never* get children to complete *all* the tasks I have planned'. Clinical educators may respond by reframing this comment into 'You have really great ideas for therapy, lets consider how you can change your management so that the tasks are completed and the client achieves success'.

Students can be assisted to see their strengths and to set more realistic goals by reviewing those tasks they have completed successfully and the interpersonal skills they demonstrate with clients. This management strategy encourages students to utilize their strengths to assist them to improve their areas of weakness.

7.4.4 OUTCOMES

It is hoped that through the use of appropriate strategies with marginal students, clinical educators will have assisted them to gain a clear understanding of the factors contributing to their non-achievement in the clinical setting. Providing the opportunity for individual students to explore their perceived reasons for failure gives clinical educators increased opportunities to also learn from students' experiences. As Pickering (1989–1990) says 'the supervisory process is a time of intense personal growth for many supervisors and supervisees' (p. 18).

Once the marginal student has accepted responsibility for managing his or her difficulties, the clinical educator needs to adopt a flexible approach to problem management. A flexible approach may include advising students of other learning opportunities which could facilitate their professional development. For example, encouraging them to participate in assertiveness or other skills training programmemes; providing students with information on interpersonal skills training programmemes available outside of the university, or giving information about available language proficiency courses for those students from another culture who have difficulty understanding and being understood by clients.

There will be realistic limits to the extra time and number of courses students will be prepared to undertake, or will be able to afford. When faced with the reality of either failing the course or perhaps scraping through and not being able to get a job, marginal students may feel participation in extra courses could be a viable extra option.

7.4.5 SOME FINAL COMMENTS

In the closure of this chapter we propose the following 'absolutes' for clinical educators working with marginal students and encourage readers to add to these from their own experience.

(a) Clear and open communication

It is imperative that clear and open communication about a marginal student's current learning status is achieved between the clinical director, student and clinical educator. Many writers on communication (Gordon, 1974; Pickering, 1987) provide important information on the skills required to achieve effective interpersonal communication. An essential aspect of this clear communication is the ability of the listener to check that they have accurately heard the message given by the speaker. This reduces the opportunity for miscommunication and problems arising from participants making assumptions about each other's knowledge.

(b) No categorizing or labelling of students

Labelling students as 'problem students' (Best & Rose, 1996) can have dual negative effects on both the student and the clinical educator with whom the student is being placed. The student is likely to feel that he or she is the problem rather than experiencing difficulties with an aspect of his or her learning. This will reduce confidence and will probably inhibit the ability to use existing skills, resulting in further loss of self esteem and compounding the existing problems. The clinical educator, moreover, may commence the placement with a stereotyped view of a 'problem student'. Such situations may be avoided if the student is supported through the process of giving clear information about his or her view of their past difficulties in clinical learning

(c) Flexibility and adaptability of approach

Flexibility is based on the clinical educator's knowledge of the student's theoretical level at the time of placement, the level of clinical expectation of the student in the placement, the individual students' demonstrated skills and deficits in the placement, and a range of possible 'best fit' strategies to deal with difficulties experienced in the placement.

(d) Extra support or supervision opportunities for the clinical educator

In writing about individual supervision Williams (1995) talks about ways to develop 'clinical wisdom'. He says that 'super-vision' is a vision offered by the supervisor as a 'second time around' view of the process in which the other person has been involved, be they student or clinical educator. It is not an imposition of the supervisor's philosophical or theoretical viewpoint. We believe that students benefit when they are placed with clinical educators who have access to supervision of their own work with students. We advocate that supervision should also be available for clinical educators who mentor other clinical educators or those who regularly work with marginal students.

It is also important for clinical educators to have the opportunity to be active members of professional groups whose prime focus is on student learning in clinical settings and particularly those students who present challenges. With the help of an experienced facilitator, these groups serve an important function in providing a forum for discussion of the needs of clinical educators. Such groups can also provide opportunities for ongoing learning and discussion about research questions in clinical education (see Chapter 8).

7.5 CONCLUSION

This chapter began by exploring some theoretical constructs which may help clinical educators develop insight into the problems some students experience when learning in clinical settings. A four-stage approach to the management of marginal students was then described in detail. The chapter concludes by giving four 'absolutes' about the management of marginal students.

REFERENCES

Anderson, J. L. (1988). *The supervisory process in speech language pathology and audiology*. Boston: College Hill Press.

Ballard, B. & Clancy, J. (1991). *Teaching students from overseas: A brief guide for lecturers and supervisors*. Melbourne: Longman Cheshire.

Best, D. & Rose, M. (1996). *Quality supervision, theory and practice for clinical supervisors*. London: W. B. Saunders.

Blenky M., Clinchy B., Goldberger N. & Tarule J. (1986). *Women's ways of knowing: The development of self, voice and mind.* New York: Basic Books.

Coles, C. R. (1990). Elaborated learning in undergraduate medical education. *Medical Education*, **24**, 14–22.

Crago, M. B. & Pickering, M. (1987). *Supervision in human communication disorders perspectives on a process.* Boston: College-Hill.

Egan, G. (1990). *The skilled helper a systematic approach to effective helping* (4th ed.). Pacific Grove, CA: Brooks/Cole.

Erikson, E. (1971). *Identity: Youth and crisis.* Whitsable, USA: Latimar Trend.

Finger, M. (1988). The biographical method in adult education research. *Studies in Continuing Education*, **10**, 33–4.

Gilligan, C. (1982). *In a different voice: Psychological theory and women's development.* Cambridge, MA; Harvard University Press.

Gordon, T. (1974). *Teaching effectiveness training.* New York: P. H. Wyden.

Hughes, L., Heycox, K. and Eisenberg, M. (1994). Fear of failing: Field teachers and the assessment of marginal students in field education. *Advances in Social Welfare Education.* Melbourne: Melbourne University.

Knowles, M. (1990). *The adult learner: A neglected species.* Houston, Texas: Gulf Publishing Company.

Kohlberg L. (1984). *The psychology of moral development.* San Francisco: Harper & Row.

Kolb, D. (1984). *Experiential learning: Experience as the source of learning and development.* London: Prentice-Hall.

Maloney, D. (1994). *Client centred student journaling: A descriptive study.* Proceedings of the Council of Supervisors in Speech-Language Pathology and Audiology (CSSPA) International and Interdisciplinary Conference on Clinical Supervision (pp 191–5). 19–22 May, Cape Cod, USA.

Metheny, W. & Carline, J. (1991). The problem student: A comparison of student and physician's views. *Teaching and Learning in Medicine*, **3**, 133–7.

Mezirow, J. (1991). *Transformative dimensions in adult learning.* San Francisco: Jossey-Bass.

Nemeth, E. (1996). Students experiencing difficulties in clinical education: Their perspective (unpublished Masters thesis in progress).

Perry, W. G. (1970). *Forms of intellectual and ethical development in the college years.* New York: Holt, Rinehart & Winston.

Pickering, M. (1987). Supervision: A person-focused process. In M. Crago & M. Pickering (Eds). *Supervision in human communication disorders: Perspectives on a process.* San Diego, CA: College Hill Press.

Pickering, M. (1989–1990). The supervisory process: An experience of interpersonal relationships and personal growth. *National Student Speech Language Hearing Association Journal*, **17**, 17–28.

Pickering, M. (1995, June). Supervision in communication disorders: Examining the process and learning the skills. Annual clinical education workshop. Sydney: The University of Sydney.

Rotter, J. B. (1966). Generalised expectancies for internal versus external control of reinforcement. *Psychological Monograph*, **80**, 1–8

Rotter, J. B. (1975). Some problems and misconceptions as related to the construct of internal versus external locus of control of reinforcement. *Journal of Consulting Clinical Psychology*, **43**, 56–67

Schulman, L. (1984). *The skills of helping individuals and groups.* Illinois: F.E. Peacock.

Studdy, L., Cooper, L., Carmody, D. & Cohen, P. (1994). Recycling social workers: Implementation of an adult learning model in a refresher course for social workers. *Advances in Social Welfare Eduction*, **January**, 17–18.

Tschikota, S. (1993). The clinical decision making process of students nurses. *Journal of Nursing Education*, **32**, 389–98.

Turney, C., Cairns, I., Eltis, K., Hatton, N., Thew, D., Towler, J. & Wright, R. (1982). *Supervision development programmes: Role handbook*. Sydney: Sydney University Press.

Williams, A. (1995). *Visual and active supervision*. New York: W. W. Norton.

Directions in clinical education research

8

Paul Hagler
*Centre for Studies in Clinical Education,
University of Alberta, Canada*

Lu-Anne McFarlane
*Department of Speech Pathology and Audiology, University of
Alberta, Canada*

Lindy McAllister
*School of Communication Disorders,
The University of Sydney, Australia*

Postcard 8

Dear All

The mindmapping exercises to teach how to think about program planning
has been moderately successful for some of the team. I'd love to get inside
the team's minds and figure out how they think and feel about the work they
are doing, so we had a better idea about how to help them learn this stuff.
I'd also like someone to come and analyze the hilarious cross-cultural
communication breakdowns that still happen on a regular basis. Now that
I've been here for two months many of the locals know me and I get asked in
for tea or a meal quite often when I'm walking home (30 minutes up the
mountain). I cherish these times; the people who have made me so welcome in
their homes.

love S

Fax reply to Postcard 8

Dear Sally

A quick response from all of us about your comment in the last postcard about 'getting inside the minds of the team members' so you have a better idea about how to facilitate their learning. There are two things we think you could consider:

1) Thinking about your own and the team members' learning styles. Are you adapting the learning task to suite their preferred learning style?

2) Would encouraging the team members to engage in self-evaluation about their own performance and learning needs help you gain their perspective on things? Perhaps this type of disclosure on a one-to-one basis may be difficult for them, so perhaps a group session would work better.

Best wishes

Lindy, Michelle, Sharynne and Di

8.1 CHAPTER OVERVIEW

This chapter has one overriding purpose – to encourage research in clinical education. Before clinicians skip this chapter thinking, 'This chapter is not intended for me', let us say that we have designed this chapter for clinicians. To encourage clinical professionals to consider clinical education research as part of their professional lives we will:

- present a review of qualitative and quantitative approaches to research in clinical education
- suggest a research agenda intended to move clinical education from an intuitive process to one that combines intuition with more scientific ways of knowing
- accomplish the first two objectives in a readable and thought-provoking way.

The chapter begins by reviewing types of scholarly activity in clinical education. We conclude that while much has been written about clinical education, few areas have been researched. This leads to a discussion of quantitative and qualitative research methods in clinical education. Potential areas of research such as clinical educator–student relationships, curriculum design, the efficacy of models of clinical education, predictors of success in clinical education, assessment tools and the economics of clinical education are discussed.

8.2 RESEARCH ABOUT CLINICAL EDUCATION

Educators have always studied students. In fact, research is one of the roles that Farmer and Farmer (1989) and Rassi and McElroy (1992) advocated for clinical educators (see Chapter 2). Educators have always wanted to know whether learning was taking place and how best to measure it. They have always suspected that good teaching methods contributed to good learning. Testing students was, and still is, the most popular means of measuring learning. Of course, popularity is by no means a guarantee of validity. Testing students with objectivity in the classroom is hard enough, but testing them with objectivity in the clinic may be next to impossible. Clinical education is an excellent example of an area in which learning cannot easily be measured and in which even minimal levels of objectivity may be unattainable. Instead, learning must be judged, not tested, and it must be judged in reference to as many different standards for performance as there are clinical educators doing the educating and judging.

Those most interested in studying clinical education were and still are, for the most part, more clinicians than researchers. Because of the nature of their education, clinicians tend not to possess the expertise with which to do research independently and often do not view research as part of their role as professionals. Acknowledging this phenomenon and appreciating the importance of better understanding it, Pain, Hagler and Warren (1996) developed a survey tool with which to assess clinicians' orientation to the role of research in their clinical practices. This interdisciplinary tool revealed differences among clinicians grouped according to their research involvement. Highly involved clinicians were found to recognize the value of being good consumers of research and the benefits of applying research findings in their clinical work significantly more than their minimally-involved colleagues. No difference was found between the groups in their desire to pursue new information (St Jacques, 1994). Clearly, those clinicians involved in research have a greater appreciation of its importance and applicability. Perhaps to know it is to love it.

In order to present a direction for the future of clinical education research and to provide a framework for discussing research options, it is appropriate to survey where we have been and the types of scholarly activity that led us there. A research agenda must be viewed from the context of current knowledge and beliefs. Alfonso and Firth (1990) described the related literature in education as consisting of three areas. The first area is adulation writings. Adulation writings stress the importance and value of clinical education in education programmes. The other categories are prescriptive writings, listing essential tasks and competencies and pronouncements of what should occur in clinical education practice, and descriptive writings, detailing what takes place in the process of clinical education. A review of the literature in the health sciences confirms the divisions noted in education. These divisions will form the basis of a quick review of clinical education literature in the health science disciplines.

8.2.1 ADULATION PUBLICATIONS

Clinical education literature began because of belief in the importance of education in clinical settings. Publications have described clinical educators as 'gatekeepers' of the professions, stating that they 'hold the key to the future of our professions' (McPherson, 1994, p. 5) and have complete control of who will become practitioners. Publications which stress the unique and valuable contribution of clinical training to the preparation of new professionals can perhaps be credited with providing impetus for creation of special interest groups and the recognition of clinical education as a unique area of expertise and study.

8.2.2 PRESCRIPTIVE PUBLICATIONS

Included in this general heading are publications which detail models of clinical education (see Chapter 2) and propose essential tasks and competencies. Development of this literature base is a logical progression from adulation publications. Once you have determined that a process is important, any sensible scholar will attempt to devise a model for the process or to divide the process into its component parts. Despite the relatively high numbers of such publications, scholars still support further clarification of the models and beliefs that support clinical education. Opacich (1995) sees the current pressures surrounding clinical education as providing impetus for a re-examination of the philosophies and guiding principles surrounding it. Development of a guiding 'educational philosophy' is seen as an important precursor to efficacy studies.

Early supervision theory came largely from social work (Brannon, 1985; Freeman, 1985; Goldstein & Sorcher, 1974; Sundel & Sundel, 1975) and education (Cogan, 1973; Goldhammer, 1969). The era and its then popular beliefs provided a markedly behavioural slant on teaching and learning. At the time, even principles of adult learning were believed to be embodied in behavioural theory. A discussion by Brannon (1985) provides an excellent example of that view. In the construction of 'models of clinical education', two authors were instrumental not only in their own field, education, but also in speech therapy and eventually the other health sciences professions. They were Cogan (1973) and Goldhammer (1969). These authors took a much less behavioural view of clinical education. They focused on clinical education as a process having component parts occurring in a logical and identifiable order. They observed that supervisory interactions traditionally had only the most tenuous relationship to objective evidence and emphasized the importance of having data on which to base clinical educator feedback. Cogan (1973) introduced the concept of collegiality between clinical educator and student, a phenomenon that was rarely appreciated and almost never observed in the process of clinical education. The good news is that it has increasingly influenced our thinking in the intervening 20 years.

Although adulation and prescriptive publications are scholarly work, they are not research. They are not research, because they represent the personal beliefs of the authors rather than the knowledge or insight that accrues from recognized methods of doing science. To paraphrase DePoy and Gitlin (1994), research publications reflect what has been learned from the implementation of systematic strategies for the generation of confirmable knowledge.

8.2.3 DESCRIPTIVE PUBLICATIONS

The section on research design and statistics (Section 8.4) will describe the remaining categories of descriptive writings and effectiveness writings, both of which qualify as research. However, before describing these last two categories of research publications, it will be helpful to compare and contrast two fundamentally different, but equally legitimate, approaches to science. These two approaches to science differ not only in their methods and terminology, but also in their philosophical underpinnings.

8.3 INTRODUCTION TO TYPES OF RESEARCH

This section cannot possibly teach all one needs to know about research. Rather it is a review of basic principles and methods in research. For those with previous education into research, it will serve as a review. For research-phobics and others naive about the process, it will serve as a basic introduction. On finishing this section, these readers will be able to identify expertise and other resources needed to design and complete a clinical education research project.

8.3.1 TWO APPROACHES TO THE RESEARCH GAME

A simplistic[1] distinction may be made between two major approaches to research: quantitative research and qualitative research. *Quantitative research* has its roots in positivism and a belief that a single objective reality exists in the natural world, which can be observed, measured and studied

---

[1] The distinction made in this section between qualitative and quantitative research is knowingly simplistic, for ease of reading as an introductory overview. This section does not discuss paradigms, nor does it account for additional research approaches such as critical and action research. It also does not account for the differences within the qualitative paradigm.

by a value free, detached researcher. *Qualitative research* has its origins in the philosophical tradition of phenomenology, which holds that as reality is socially constructed by individuals, there will be multiple realities and not one single objective truth which can be measured out of context. Qualitative researchers seek to describe, explain, interpret and understand the meaning of social phenomena as experienced by individuals in their context. 'Research with people, rather than on people, is the goal' (Dickson, 1995, p. 415). Hence, the people who participate in qualitative studies are known as informants, participants or collaborators, rather than as subjects.

This is in marked contrast to the purpose of quantitative research which seeks to test and verify the relationships between discrete variables, which have been operationalized for ease of measurement. Except in its simplest form which is the one-group descriptive design, quantitative research sets out to prove a theory or test a hypothesis, to establish a causal relationship or predict outcomes. Theory is established a priori. In contrast, qualitative studies seek to discover and describe theories that emerge from the data and are grounded in the data. In mixed method studies, variables identified in a grounded theory study may be operationalized for empirical (positivist) testing in a large group study.

The designs used in quantitative studies are generally experimental or quasi experimental, yielding numbers which lend themselves to statistical analysis. The most common designs utilized in the qualitative approach are phenomenology (both a method and a philosophical tradition), ethnography, historical study, grounded theory and case study. The data in qualitative approaches are usually words, recorded from interviews, located in existing documents, or written in the field notes of observations. The most common data collection strategies are observation and interviewing. The qualitative researcher becomes a participant observer, engaging in intensive and prolonged social interaction with participants. Interviews range along a continuum, from highly structured interviews to unstructured interviews and conversations. Data collected are logged in the form of field notes from the time spent observing in the field, methodological logs or memos which record the details of the conduct of the study, personal logs which record the researcher's reflections on feelings, ideas, experiences arising during the study, and theoretical memos which record ideas arising from preliminary data analysis.

Methods of data analysis used in qualitative studies are many and a discussion of these is well beyond the scope of this chapter. Tesch (1990) has provided a very lucid outline of analysis techniques which fit with the different research purposes. One of the most common techniques, according to Mariano (1995) is that of thematic analysis. In broad terms, this involves a careful reading of all the assembled data, identification and coding of units of meaning, leading to the creation of categories, which must fit the data, not the researcher's preconceived ideas. A category has been created when its attributes and characteristics have been identified, its boundaries have been defined, and it has a name. The researcher will then seek the interrelationships between the categories, looking for themes and patterns. The development of categories and relationships is a process of constant comparison between units of the data and between emerging categories and themes. It is a highly reflective, inductive and creative process, one which must be recorded in detail in analytic and theoretical memos, in order to establish trustworthiness of the study.

Both quantitative and qualitative research approaches are concerned with scientific rigour. In quantitative approaches, rigorous efforts are made to establish construct, internal and face validity, test-retest reliability, intra- and inter-rater reliability. Similar degrees of scientific rigour are used in qualitative studies, defying what Ely (1991) calls the myth that 'qualitative research is soft, unscientific, atheoretical, without substance. It is "touchy-feely" messing about, and at best, seeks unsubstantiated opinion rather than facts. Anyone can do it' (p. 102). The hallmark of a rigorous qualitative study is what Lincoln and Guba (1985) have called *trustworthiness*. Trustworthiness is a concept embracing credibility, transferability, dependability and confirmability.

To achieve trustworthiness qualitative researchers provide great detail of the methods used in their studies, and of the decisions made about the conduct of the study in progress, and of thoughts (analytic notes or memos) about the emerging data and its patterns and themes. Using this documentation, other researchers using the same methods on the same data or similar informant groups could yield similar findings. Data are collected over long periods of time. Researchers spend many hours in the field, observing their informants, making field notes, conducting interviews, and clarifying points as they arise. Triangulation is frequently used. This refers to the process of using multiple methods of data collection, multiple data types and data sources, and sometimes multiple data gatherers. Confirmation of findings from more than one source lends confidence to the interpretations made of the data.

Data collection and analysis are usually done concurrently in qualitative studies, the preliminary analyses and findings shaping the subsequent selection of informants and the type of data collection used. Informants can be selected to test out emerging themes or (grounded) theories; interviews can be structured to allow the collection of data that will expand on or clarify emerging concepts. The reports from qualitative studies typically contain thick description, excerpts of the phrases and words used by the informants to describe their experiences. These allow readers to derive for themselves the meaning of the experience for the informants. This device provides a check that the researchers have not allowed their own position or bias to unduly influence their interpretation of the data. The device of respondent validation, in which informants comment on the researchers' interpretations of their experiences or write ups of the study, also provides a further check against the presentation of researcher opinion and bias.

The research process, like the process of clinical education, has a logical sequence. This sequence is similar in both research approaches although the order, terminology and details differ. Knowing the steps in the sequence and taking them in order is important. Taking steps out of sequence and failing to take advantage of opportunities along the way creates unnecessary complications or an incomplete picture or understanding of the phenomenon under investigation.

Conducting applied, quantitative research is a bit like playing Mah Jong. Players know, before they start, exactly what their objective is, and all follow the same basic rules of play. A sequence of dice-rolling protocols contributes to randomness, guiding the process as players draw tiles from the Great Wall of China, just as researchers draw subjects from a population. Each player can use any of a host of strategies, several of which might reasonably be expected to achieve their objective, but they commit, near the beginning, to the one they believe most viable in their particular circumstances. Tiles are grouped and played in prescribed ways. Players try, sometimes without much success, to minimize extraneous influences or confounding variables by disclosing only what is required by the rules of fair play. Once the goal is achieved, there is an intricate counting protocol that quantifies the final results. The clarity of hindsight usually brings out a few self-recriminations for poorly executed strategies or opportunities missed, but a game well played always ends with much amiable discussion in a lively, multiple-participant forum.

Conducting qualitative research is a bit like playing Cluedo (Clue). At the start, none of the players has the whole picture or knows the answer. All players have to listen very carefully to each other, tailoring their questions to build on previous responses, making preliminary forays into different rooms of the house, testing out emerging theories about the meaning of the mystery, tracking down the possible participants in, motives for, instruments of and location of the deed in question. Following is an introduction to the basics of the research 'game'.

8.3.2 QUANTITATIVE RESEARCH: PROPOSING RESEARCH (RULES OF PLAY)

(a) Step 1: Object of the game (Asking a good question)

Proposing a research project is like learning a board game; you start with understanding the purpose. In research, this means understanding and articulating your question. A good question will provide at least three important pieces of information. It will indicate who is being studied, the conditions under which they are being studied, and what outcomes are of interest. 'Who' refers to subjects. 'Conditions' refer to independent variables. 'Outcomes' refer to dependent variables. A fourth piece of information, often but not always included, is a reference to the nature of the study itself, the research design.

Let's look at the following question: 'How can a student be so good in the classroom and so bad in the clinic?' This is a good question, because it addresses an important issue. However, it is not a good research question. A better version might be, 'What student characteristics combine with academic learning to predict clinical performance?' The subjects are obviously students who can be defined in terms of such things as programme of study and level of education, giving them a very specific identity. The independent variables are predictors, academic and other student characteristics. What these mean and how they are measured would be defined later by the researcher. The dependent variable is clinical performance. The research design is predictive in nature. Note that all of this information is contained in the question.

(b) Step 2: Pick your playing pieces (Defining variables)

Let's take a closer look at variables. The variables of interest will be either independent or dependent. Know which is which! Independent variables are the ones the investigator controls – if you're in control, you're independent. This is most obviously the case when the investigator is doing an experiment, that is manipulating what happens to the subjects. For example, when a clinical educator is providing two types of feedback, feedback type is the independent variable, having two levels, Type A and Type B. Other types of independent variables are grouping variables and predictor variables. A grouping variable could be student experience, with three levels: early placement, intermediate placement and late placement. Note that such groups pre-exist and are not created by investigator manipulation. The last category, predictor variables, are immediately measurable things that may relate to something of interest that is measurable concurrently or in the future. Student characteristics and academic learning, referred to above in the sample research question, are predictor variables. So independent variables are those that fall (in some way) under the control of the investigator. Control freaks will be happy to know that there can be several independent variables in the same study.

Dependent variables are the things one measures. They are the outcomes of the investigative process. Whether the independent variable is an experimental variable (for example, feedback type) or a grouping variable (for example, gender), the dependent variable is the one expected to change differentially as a function of the two feedback conditions. Perhaps this could be amount of student talk. If the independent variable is predictive (for example, student characteristics and academic learning), the dependent variable is called a criterion variable and measures characteristics of current or future interest (for example, clinical performance). Each study can have one or several dependent variables. Be judicious. Picking too many will complicate the issue and reduce the investigator's chances of being able to demonstrate a difference.

(c) Step 3: Picking teams (Selecting a research design)

Selecting a design that matches the research question clarifies purpose, suggests how subjects and tools will be managed and leads directly to appropriate methods of data analysis. The basic design categories are descriptive, relational, experimental, and causal-comparative. These designs and their various subtypes are discussed later in the section on research design and statistics.

(d) Step 4: Learning the rules (Deciding on methodology)

The rules of the research game define who can play (subjects), what pieces of equipment are needed (materials/instruments), how the game progresses (procedures) and who the winner is (data analysis). Subjects can be defined both by inclusion criteria (level of training, health discipline, etc.) as well as exclusion criteria (progressing satisfactorily in previous clinical placements, etc.). Materials and instruments include such things as questionnaires, tests, interaction analysis tools, and devices such as timers and recorders. Procedures determine what will be done to the subjects or with the data. Finally, data analysis tools must be selected to fit the design, which was selected to fit the question. See why order is important?

(e) Step 5: Ensure fair play (Considering ethical matters)

All research involving human subjects must meet certain expectations regarding ethics, and ethics committees usually review research proposals to ensure that these expectations are met. Ethics committees consider three basic issues. The first issue is whether the work is fundamentally worthwhile, and the second is whether the question can be answered with the proposed methodology. The third issue is that of informed consent. An informed consent document is almost always needed in prospective research, that is research about to be carried out and for which subjects' cooperation is required. Informed consent should address five aspects of the study:

- details of participation including purpose, nature and duration
- potential risks, inconveniences and benefits to the subjects

- any standard services to be withheld during the course of the subjects' participation
- subjects' freedom to withdraw without consequences
- assurance of confidentiality and subjects' anonymity.

The reading level of the informed consent document must correspond with the education level of the participants. Clinical education research typically involves university-educated students and professionals, so the reading level can be correspondingly high. If the research is to include clients, consideration must be given not only to reading level but to the individuals' competence to consent for themselves. Committees that review research proposals usually examine them with the above issues in mind. These committees perform three important functions:

- They ensure that researchers understand and are prepared to protect the rights and welfare of their human subjects.
- They often suggest methodological refinements and other improvements to the proposed work.
- They offer the researcher some protection, albeit limited, from vexatious complaints by subjects.

(f) Step 6: Play the game (Conducting the research)

Now that it's all organized, all that remains is to put the project in written form, following the headings above. Once a project is approved by a human ethics review panel, it is played out as precisely as possible, according to the rules of the game, the methodology. Finally, and perhaps most importantly, the results are shared with other potential players. First come oral presentations at conferences. In this venue, the researcher obtains thoughtful feedback from colleagues who attend because of their own interest and expertise in the same area. Wise researchers will use this opportunity for stimulating dialogue to improve their own thinking and subsequently the discussion and conclusions sections of a final written report of the research project. They will then submit this refined work for publication.

8.4 RESEARCH DESIGNS AND STATISTICS

As discussed earlier, the research design is determined by the research question. The following section will describe the variety of common quantitative research designs.

8.4.1 DESCRIPTIVE DESIGNS

Descriptive studies describe phenomena in the process of clinical education. Descriptive studies usually involve groups of subjects, but may examine a single subject, in which case they are referred to as case studies. Descriptive studies are best suited for early exploration of a new area of interest in an attempt to understand it better. Much of the early work in clinical education research was descriptive in nature. Descriptive studies have examined perceptions of the process of clinical education (Blumberg, 1980; Brasseur & Anderson, 1983; Caracciolo, Rigrodsky & Morrison, 1978; Dowling & Wittkop, 1982; Oratio, Sugarman & Prass, 1981; Smith & Anderson, 1982a), interpersonal variables in the supervisory conference (McCrea, 1980; Martin, Goodyear & Newton, 1987; Pickering, 1984), and supervisory conference content (Hatten, 1966; Underwood, 1973; Culatta & Seltzer, 1976, 1977; Dowling, Sbaschnig & Williams, 1982; Roberts & Smith, 1982; Smith & Anderson, 1982b) to name just a few.

Data analysis for descriptive studies can usually be conducted with a pocket calculator. Relevant statistical procedures include mean, median, mode, standard deviation and range. These are familiar and meaningful, even to non-researchers. A sophisticated form of descriptive analysis is factor analysis. This statistical tool is useful when many different measures are all taken on each member of a group of subjects (Norman & Streiner, 1986). Factor analysis determines whether these measures reflect smaller subsets of underlying constructs. It does this by exploring their interrelationships. For example, Smith and Anderson (1982) developed the Individual Supervisory Conference Rating Scale, consisting of 16 items. Factor analysis of subjects' responses to these items revealed three underlying constructs or factors: direct supervisory behaviour, passive clinician behaviour, and indirect supervisory behaviour. Factor analysis provided an organized, mathematical set of criteria to guide the investigators' understanding of how their subjects viewed the issues placed before them by the investigators. Before factor analysis, the investigators knew only that they had included in their tool references to aspects of the conference that they personally believed to be important and that they had worded their references in ways meaningful to them. After factor analysis, the investigators knew exactly what constructs were represented in their new tool and that it was a valid index of those aspects of the supervisory conference.

8.4.2 RELATIONAL DESIGNS

Relational studies include correlational and predictive designs. Correlational designs look for a relationship between two or more unlike variables measured at approximately the same point in time. Correlational applications in clinical education have examined the relationship between students' demographic variables and their various supervisory conference behaviours (Ghitter, 1987; 1989; McFarlane & Hagler, 1992b).

The data analysis method of choice for correlational designs will depend upon the type of data being analyzed. There are four types of data:

nominal, ordinal, interval and ratio. Nominal data represent an unordered categorization into which cases or subjects may fall, such as a pass or fail mark for the clinical placement and style of clinical education (direct/indirect/combination). Ordinal data represent ordered categorizations into which cases or subjects may fall, such as practicum grade (A–F), clinical education effectiveness (high, moderate, low), and most rating scales (1 = strongly disagree, 5 = strongly agree). Interval data represent ordered categorization based on the natural number system in which multiples are of known and equal amounts. On an interval scale, zero is either arbitrary or nonexistent. An interval scale enables the investigator to assign relative amount or value to each measure. A common example of interval data is the number of clients served by student clinicians in a specified period of time. Clients do not come in fractional parts, and although zero is not arbitrary, it does not occur in this variable for most students in most placements. The classic examples of interval levels of measurement are the two measures of temperature: Celsius and Fahrenheit. Each uses its own equal-sized intervals, that is, 40 degrees is twice as hot as 20 degrees, on both scales. They measure exactly the same thing, but zero is arbitrarily set on both scales. Finally, ratio data are real numbers with infinite and equal gradations between each number as well as a zero point which represents an absence of the variable being measured. Examples of ratio data are percentages of clinical educator or student behaviours, participant talk time and number of student self-evaluative comments during a specified period of time.

Nominal and ordinal data are analyzed with nonparametric procedures, which is a fancy way of referring to statistical analyses for data that aren't real (decimal) numbers. When one is looking for a relationship between two nominal variables, a contingency coefficient is used (Siegel, 1956). When one is looking for a relationship between two ordinal variables, a Spearman rank correlation coefficient or one of the Kendal rank correlations may be used (Siegel, 1956). Interval and ratio data are analyzed with parametric or inferential statistical procedures. Parameters are descriptive statistics for entire populations. The word inferential implies that one can infer things about the population from which the sample was drawn. Such inferences are contraindicated when using nonparametric procedures. When parameters such as the mean and standard deviation are meaningful descriptors for two variables, each represented by a data set, we can use parametric statistics such as the Pearson product-moment correlation coefficient to look for a relationship between the variables.

The other type of relational design is the predictive study. Remember that predictive studies look at the relationship between things immediately measurable and things that will be measured in the future. The first time, of course, this must be done with existing or historical data, but once a predictable relationship has been shown to exist in history, it can be applied to similar subjects in similar circumstances in the future. An ability to predict the future is enchanting to say the least. Predictive studies in clinical education have examined variables that influence future clinical and academic performance (Ghitter, 1987; 1989; Hagler, 1981).

Data analysis for predictive studies includes not only the procedures for simple correlation described above, but an even more fascinating tool called multiple regression analysis. Multiple regression analysis on a computer can manage large numbers of predictor variables (today's measures) of any type or level of measurement. The computer looks not only for relationships between each predictor variable and the criterion variables (outcome measure), but also for interrelationships among the predictor variables. In this way, it builds an optimal prediction equation containing only the best possible combination of predictors for the criterion or outcome of interest. It can even tell the investigator how much influence or weight to give each predictor in the equation. About the only constraint practiced by most investigators is that the criterion variable must be measured on an interval or ratio level scale. If the criterion variable happens to be categorical in nature, then other statistical tools may be more suitable. The two that are commonly used are logistic regression and discriminant function analysis.

8.4.3 EXPERIMENTAL DESIGNS

For the purposes of this chapter, experimental studies are divided into two sub-types: group comparison designs and single-subject experimental designs.

(a) Group comparison designs

Group comparison designs allow investigators to look for differences between two groups or among three or more groups in terms of a dependent variable. These groups are said to be 'independent groups' when each is made up of different people. This is also known as a 'between groups' design or comparison. Groups are said to be 'dependent groups' when they are made up of the same people being measured two or more times. Each time or measurement occasion constitutes a group of data that can be compared to another group of data. This also is commonly referred to as a 'within groups' or 'related groups' comparison or design. Some examples might help illustrate the difference. An example of an independent groups design would involve two groups of student clinician subjects, each group having different people in it. Each group would receive a different type of supervision and, at the end of their placements, they would be compared in terms of their satisfaction with the clinical education experience. Type of supervision would be the independent variable, and satisfaction would be the dependent variable. An example of a dependent groups design would involve one group of student clinician subjects, each receiving two different types of supervision and, at the end of each clinical education experience, being compared in terms of their satisfaction with supervision. Either type of group comparison study allows the researcher to determine the effects of the two supervisory methods on students' satisfaction. Group comparison studies in clinical education have examined effects of feedback to clinical educators (Cimorell-Strong & Ensley, 1982; Culatta & Seltzer, 1977; Hagler, 1986; Wellman, 1991), and effects of change in style or type of conference (Dowling & Shank, 1981; Dowling, 1983; McFarlane & Hagler, 1990, 1992a, b; Jans, Hagler & McFarlane, 1994).

Data analysis in group comparison designs differs according to the level of measurement. Nominal data may be analyzed with a Chi-square and ordinal data can be analyzed with the Wilcoxin matched-pairs signed-ranks test, the Mann-Whitney U test or the Friedman two-way analysis of variance (Siegel, 1956). Interval and ratio data are usually analyzed with t-tests and analyses of variance. The latter is often referred to as ANOVA. In all cases with parametric or nonparametric designs, the appropriate statistical procedure will depend on the number of groups being compared and whether there are multiple groups or multiple measures of the same group.

(b) Single-subject experimental designs

Single-subject experimental design, also known as single-case experimental design, involves manipulation of an intervention condition, the independent variable, in an attempt to drive up or down the frequency of occurrence of a student's target behaviour. This is not only a research design, it is perhaps one of the most useful forms of clinical accountability. The health sciences borrowed this methodology from experimental psychology in the late 1960s, and it is easy to see why. It is almost perfectly suited to tracking the effects of intervention by educators and health professionals. Clinical psychologists made their approach to science famous while demonstrating the power of behavioural principles, at first with rats, pigeons, dogs, and monkeys, and eventually with humans. Unfortunately, single-case experimental design dropped out of vogue, especially with clinicians during the 1970s, when behavioural principles were under indictment by Piaget, Chomsky and others who demonstrated that Skinnerian explanations for human learning were inadequate. The behavioural model of language learning was especially vulnerable to those new theorists. Two assumptions seemed evident among therapists. One was that, if behavioural principles failed to explain language acquisition, then behavioural principles should not be used to teach language. The other was that, if one was not using behavioural intervention, one would not track other styles of intervention with behavioural methods. In a sense, it was a matter of the baby being thrown out with the bath water. Single-case experimental design remains a viable method of tracking the response of subjects, clients or professionals, to intervention over time. The intervention need not be grounded in behavioural theory. There are many different sub-types of single-subject design, some very sophisticated in their complexity and purpose, but it is beyond the scope of this chapter to describe all of them. For a more thorough treatise on these variations and their unique purposes, refer to Barlow and Hersen (1984) and McReynolds and Kearns (1983). The purpose of this section is to acquaint readers with the fundamentals of single-case experimental design so they will recognize its potential and its limitations when considering its use in a proposed clinical education study.

There are four topics to be addressed in understanding single-case experimental design. They are:

- what a typical design looks like
- how to assess experimental or intervention effects
- ways of increasing confidence in the findings
- practical limitations.

Single-case experimental design always involves many measurements of one behaviour from a single subject over time. Some of these measurements are taken before intervention, and the remainder are taken during intervention. This is single-case experimental design in its simplest form. In its more complex forms, single-case experimental design may involve multiple subjects, multiple experimental conditions, and multiple target behaviours or outcome measures. An overview of these variations will be addressed below. Each measurement becomes a data point on a graph having time on its horizontal, or x, axis and frequency of occurrence of the target behaviour on its vertical, or y, axis. The time dimension is divided into at least two phases: Baseline or A phase and Treatment or B phase. Traditionally these phases are separated by a vertical dotted line, and the relationship between the phases is used to assess the effects of intervention.

Experimental or intervention effect is determined by comparing the A phase data points to the B phase data points. This comparison, by visually inspecting the graphed data, looks for a predictable difference between baseline and intervention conditions in terms of how frequently the target behaviour occurred. If the intervention was intended to cause a decrease in frequency of the target behaviour and the graphed data clearly indicate that it did, then the investigator can conclude that intervention was effective. In deciding whether there is an observable difference between the A and B phases, investigators may consider three characteristics of their graphed data: level, stability, and slope. If the general level or frequency of occurrence of the target behaviour is obviously higher or lower during the treatment phase than it was during the baseline phase, then intervention can be judged effective. If the data points are stable during both phases, then only a small change in level is required to observe a difference. However, if the data points scatter erratically during either phase, then a larger treatment effect must be evident in order to visualize an obvious difference. Slope is equally influential. For example, if the data show an upward trend over time in the baseline condition, then an intervention level that only continues rising to end higher than the baseline level is not enough. A more steep upward slope must be observed during intervention, and even that may be less than convincing. However, a slope reversal can be very convincing. Unfortunately, not all graphed data clearly demonstrate an effective treatment. That is to say, visual inspection of graphed data often leaves investigators scratching their heads and wondering whether their intervention worked or not.

There are some easy ways of increasing confidence in one's findings. These include increasing and controlling the number of subjects, behaviours, or conditions. A single-case experimental design actually can have more than one subject. When this is the case, baseline data are collected on all subjects. Introduction of the experimental condition to each subject at a different point in time enables the investigator to watch for treatment effects on a predictable schedule. Each time a subject responds in the same way to introduction of the intervention, the investigator becomes increasingly confident that it is the experimental condition causing the observed change in behaviour rather than some confounding variable outside the experimenter's control. Likewise, investigators may wish to track multiple behaviours or multiple conditions looking for predictable changes among target behaviours or predictable changes in a single target behaviour measured across a variety of conditions. Sometimes even these strategies do not provide a convincing picture of successful intervention. When this happens, single-case experimenters may turn to an array of statistical tools specially developed to help them sort out obscure or confusing treatment effects. It is not our intention to present these methods, but it is important that single-case researchers know they exist. Statistical tools for single-case experimental designs can be found in Barlow and Hersen (1984). Do not be intimidated by the fact that these tools are relatively unknown and little used; they tend to be easy to understand and implement.

There is one noteworthy limitation inherent in single-case experimental designs. The limitation is an almost complete lack of external validity. Put another way, one is on thin ice when trying to generalize the findings of a single-case experiment to other subjects, even when multiple subjects have been used. This limitation does not mitigate against doing single-case experimental studies; it simply means that investigators should be careful when making claims about the applications and implications of their work. Single-case experimental designs, like qualitative designs, are excellent strategies for discovery.

8.4.4 CAUSAL-COMPARATIVE DESIGNS

A variation on the comparative designs theme is the causal-comparative design. This is similar to comparative research except that the groups are existent rather than created or manipulated by the investigator. An example of a causal-comparative design is one in which students at three levels of experience (beginning, intermediate, advanced) are compared in terms of their ability to engage in accurate analysis of their sessions with clients. The independent variable is Level of Experience and the dependent variable is Analysis Ability. The investigator does not actually do an experiment on the subjects. Instead the investigator merely measures subjects' abilities to analyze their client sessions. They pre-exist in groups defined by the amount of experience they brought with them to the study.

Data analysis in causal-comparative designs is exactly like data analysis in comparative or experimental designs. The appropriate tool is determined by group composition and level of measurement. All of the same statistical options exist.

In summary this section has provided the reader with enough basic information to select an appropriate design and to determine which type of analysis is probably most appropriate. With this kind of 'know how', even naive investigators can enlist the expertise of a statistician or an academic who is facile with statistical tools and communicate effectively about their needs. Often research is carried out through collaboration between clinicians who are clinical educators and academics who are researchers. Such team work is practical and gratifying for a variety of reasons. The clinical educators know which questions to ask, because they regularly grapple with the issues, and the researchers know how to go about getting answers to those questions. Two heads are better than one, and more hands make less work. Complementary pairings like this make winning teams.

8.4.5 QUALITATIVE RESEARCH: PROPOSING RESEARCH (RULES OF PLAY)

(a) Step 1: Object of the game (Asking a good question)

The philosophical perspective held by the researcher will guide the type of question asked. A researcher who regards human behaviour as originating from multiple perspectives on the world is more likely to ask a question that will aim to understand and describe those perspectives. For example, a quantitative researcher might ask (as in section 8.3.2) 'What student char-

acteristics combine with academic education to predict clinical performance?', and a qualitative researcher might ask 'From their experience, what
personal characteristics or attributes do students believe lead to their successful clinical performance?' followed by 'How do they understand these
attributes to combine with academic education to predict successful clinical performance?' Asking questions in this way of a small group of student
informants should capture the individual variations in approaches to
learning which a large group study might mask. Knowing about these individual differences increases the likelihood of creating successful, individualized teaching and learning experiences for all students.

The purpose of the study will also shape the way in which the question
is asked. Dickson (1995) has described the major purposes to which qualitative research has been applied in nursing practice. These could be
adapted for clinical education as follows:

- to gain a different perspective on the process of clinical education.
  Much is written about how to optimize placements from the clinical
  educators' perspective; what of the students' perspective?
- to describe areas in which not much is known. For example, the
  experience of mature age practising nurses who return to university to
  upgrade their qualifications (Rather, 1992)
- to sensitize clinical educators to experiences outside their own. For
  example, the experience of failing a clinical placement; what do
  students think and feel during and after the process? (Nemeth &
  McAllister, 1995)
- to develop a research instrument. For example, following a qualitative
  study which observed and interviewed new nursing graduates about
  their work experiences, Kramer (1969) developed an instrument to
  measure nurses' responses to their first hospital job
- to create a theoretical explanatory model. For example, what are the
  stages that new clinical educators experience as they become
  socialized into their new role?
- to describe everyday experiences. For example, what is it really like to
  be a clinical educator? (McAllister, 1996).

Once the question has been refined, the qualitative researcher needs to
choose a design and methods which are philosophically congruent.

(b) Step 2: Choose your playing pieces

It is in this aspect that the two games of research differ markedly. In quantitative research, the players (researchers) get to pick ahead of time the
pieces they will move around the board; they define ahead of time the
variables they wish to manipulate. However, in qualitative research the
variables are not known ahead of time and the players do not seek to

manipulate them. Rather, they let the variables emerge from the data collected, without seeking to influence them; remember, qualitative research is about observing the variables in their natural state. Researches will deliberately try to find out more about the themes or patterns they see emerging from the preliminary data analyses, so that they can fully describe and understand their interplay. They do this by purposeful sampling and deciding who to observe or interview next, in order to clarify or test emerging categories. For example, they may look for a participant who will provide information which disconfirms the boundaries of the categories developed to date, forcing the researchers to look again at their data and perhaps collect even more data.

(c) Step 3: Picking teams (Selecting a research design)

In qualitative research, the researchers' philosophical stance will guide the framing of the question, which in turn guides the selection of appropriate designs, methods and data analysis techniques whose assumptions are congruent. All these stages of the project must be congruent for the study to establish trustworthiness.

(d) Step 4: Learning the rules (Deciding on method)

Qualitative research and quantitative research follow similar rules of play, in that decisions need to be made about who can play (although in qualitative research they are called informants or participants) and what their roles will be, and how the game will progress (the procedures of play). A major difference is in that the major instrument used in qualitative research is the researchers themselves. The researchers become participant observers in the field of their inquiry. Their knowledge of the field or phenomenon and of pertinent literature, combined with their intellectual and creative skills in collecting, analyzing and interpreting data are the tools of research. The qualitative researcher needs to be particularly aware of their preconceptions about the phenomenon or field of study and that procedures are in place to ensure these do not bias data interpretations. Video-recording is sometimes used to capture observation of the informants in their world for later analysis, and tape-recording of interviews for later transcription and analysis is routine.

Another major difference is that in qualitative research the participants often collaborate in the data analysis stages and write up stages, assisting with clarification and expansion of themes or theory emerging from the data analysis, and influencing the voice and shape of the final write up of the study. This is particularly the case in action research, and research grounded in women's studies or critical theory.

(e) Step 5: Ensure fair play (Considering ethical matters)

All research must be conducted in an ethical and sensitive manner. This is especially important in qualitative research studies where the people who act as informants are often socially vulnerable. Self-awareness and honesty as to who benefits from the research is required. Sensitivity needs to be exercised when approaching potential informants. For example, socially disadvantaged, minority, indigenous and developing world groups have been the recipients of so much 'exploitive' research attention and 'sensationalized' reporting that they are now increasingly wary of participating. Liaising with the gatekeepers for these groups is often the only way to gain access into their world.

Researchers will need to think through how they will manage feelings of distress, in themselves or in their informants, which may arise with the disclosure of emotionally laden material. They need to consider how they handle politically, ethically or legally sensitive information which may be revealed in the course of observations and conversations with informants. These and similar issues about who owns the data and publications, what data should be included and how data will be presented need to be negotiated prior to the study and re-negotiated during the life of the study. Researchers also need to plan for a sensitive withdrawal from the scene at the end of the project. They may well have spent hundreds of hours with socially disadvantaged or lonely people, becoming a 'friend' and confidant in the process, necessitating a graduated withdrawal (Minichiello, Aroni, Timewell & Alexander, 1990).

(f) Step 6: Playing the game (Conducting the research)

Unlike quantitative research studies, where if well planned the players can simply follow the rules, qualitative studies require the players to be flexible in their application and interpretation of the rules of play. Humans in their natural worlds don't always play by the rules, and so people observing them playing out their lives and talking to them about their games, may need to make up new rules as they go. This is quite acceptable in qualitative research, in fact it would be most unacceptable not to be flexible and to go with the flow. The 'rule' in these situations is to record all the changes in the game plan and the reasons for the changes. This will not only help with interpretation and write up of the data itself, but will address concerns about validity and reliability.

Writing up of the research is often a collaborative effort, between researchers and informants, and researchers and like minded colleagues. Data collection and analysis are concurrent activities in qualitative research. Early analyses suggest what data should be collected next. Many of the concepts which help sensitize the researcher to patterns or themes in the data, or allow discovery of the grounded theory, arise through ongoing discussion of preliminary data analyses, and their relationship to existing literature or other studies.

8.5 QUALITATIVE DESIGNS

Because of the flexible and recursive nature of qualitative research, there are many possible research designs. It is crucial to the credibility and trust-worthiness of the study that researchers' philosophies, choice of phenomenon for study, research questions, design and methods are all congruent. The terms design, approach and method are often used interchangeably in the qualitative research literature. What follows is a very brief description of four designs which have great potential for understanding the experience and processes of clinical education. More detailed descriptions of these and other designs can be found in Denzin and Lincoln (1994).

8.5.1 PHENOMENOLOGY

The literature around phenomenology can be quite confusing as phenomenology can be considered a philosophy, a theoretical framework, a methodology or a design. Husserl (1965) and Heidegger (1962) are generally credited with the development of phenomenology, which is concerned with the essences of human experience. Phenomenology seeks to uncover and describe the meaning of experience of a phenomenon as perceived by individual(s). The phenomenological designs and methods of Giorgi (1970), Colaizzi (1978) and van Manen (1990) have been used successfully in qualitative studies in psychology, education and nursing. In broad terms, phenomenological methods involve reading and 'dwelling' on all the descriptions (interview transcripts, field notes or other documents), extracting units of meaning (words and phrases) which pertain directly to the phenomenon, clustering these into themes with constant reference to the text to validate the themes and note discrepancies, and then synthesizing a detailed description of the experience framed around the themes. The descriptions generated in this manner are often shared with other researchers and the participants for validation. The researcher's role is to intuit, analyze, describe and validate the participants' descriptions of their experiences.

8.5.2 GROUNDED THEORY

Glaser, Strauss and their associates have outlined the grounded theory approach to the examination of the social context of human interaction (see Glaser & Strauss, 1967; Strauss & Corbin, 1990). Grounded theory is a procedure for systematically deriving a theory describing or explaining a phenomenon. Concepts and the relationships between concepts pertaining to a phenomenon are identified in an inductive manner, using constant comparative analysis of the data and theoretical sensitivity to the data. Data is collected until saturation occurs, that is, no new concepts emerge from the data analysis. The writing of analytic and theoretical memos as analysis proceeds is a key part of grounded theory analysis. The substantive or formal theory developed is said to be 'grounded' in the data.

8.5.3 ETHNOGRAPHY

Ethnography is a qualitative approach which collects and analyzes data about the ways in which people categorize meaning inherent in their culture. The focus is on the meaning of experiences within the cultural context. What results is a detailed description of the way of life of a group. The principal methods of ethnography are participant observation by living in the culture for a prolonged period, and extensive interviewing of key informants about the culture. The ethnographer looks for patterns, themes, rituals and relationships and the meaning these have for the people within the culture. The writings of Spradley (1979, 1980), Agar (1980) and Werner and Schoepfle (1987) have been influential in shaping ethnographic studies in education and health sciences.

8.5.4 CASE STUDY

Case studies are familiar to clinicians and clinical educators as teaching tools. They are potentially powerful as research tools because of the depth and breadth of detail offered with descriptive, exploratory, explanatory or causal intent. Yin (1989) suggests that their value lies in their ability to retain the holistic and meaningful characteristics of the case's real-life events, for example, the chronology of life events, the context and processes of change. The methods used in the development of case studies are interviews, observation and document analysis of, for example, files and other existing published literature.

Denzin (1978), and Fielding and Fielding (1986) suggest that qualitative and quantitative research methods can be combined to describe and explain phenomena, test theories and thus generate knowledge.

8.6 A RESEARCH AGENDA FOR CLINICAL EDUCATION

Clinical educators and health sciences professionals are beginning to produce quality research in clinical education, but the rapidly growing knowledge base that directs clinical practice in the health sciences disciplines does not yet exist for clinical education. It will be from just such research-based knowledge that we will learn how to implement effective and efficient methods of clinical education. During the past few years, researchers have spent considerable time answering microscopic questions in the hope of contributing to the big picture with a plethora of isolated facts, leaving for others the task of synthesizing them. Although it would be nice to have a better game plan, this approach is likely to yield some worthwhile information that eventually will help us understand what the big issues really are. In fact, a picture is already starting to form. By backing away, squinting and contemplating this incomplete jigsaw puzzle, we were able to see the basic shapes of some important parts of the bigger picture. In this section we, as producers and consumers of clinical education research, will discuss six areas of imminent need.

Why would a master plan be better than the plethora of isolated facts that currently typifies the knowledge base in clinical education? The answer is because we would get where we need to go sooner and with less frustration. Consider the game of 20 questions. In a room of 20 people, your conversational partner says, 'I'm thinking of someone in this room. Ask me questions until you determine who it is.' You could find out who your partner has in mind by pointing to each person and asking, 'Is it her?', 'Is it him?', and so forth, until you hit the right one. Or you could thoughtfully formulate more general questions that would help you eliminate the unlikely possibilities. You might ask, 'Is this person a male or a female?' thereby reducing the options by about 50 per cent. Next you might ask, 'Does this person have dark hair?' further reducing your possibilities. Perhaps with as few as three or four thoughtful questions, rather than 20 'shots in the dark', you will come up with the right answer. We need a master plan in clinical education research; we need a route map for our journey. Many important steps have already been taken on this journey, but they have been taken in the dark in largely uncharted territory. It is the authors' fondest hope that this work will be a pivotal step on this journey. Our agenda for clinical education research is outlined in the next section.

Our agenda for systematic study of the process of clinical education includes six areas of focus for future researchers. These areas are:

- clinical educator–student relationships
- curriculum design
- efficacy of models of clinical education
- predictors of success
- economics of clinical education
- student evaluation tools.

Their order does not reflect any assumptions about the relative importance of these areas to one another. All are important. All have received some attention by investigators in the health sciences disciplines, and each area seems to have piqued the curiosity of certain health sciences disciplines more than others. This is good, because the disciplines can learn much from one another. For example, much of what has been learned by speech therapy researchers about supervisory interaction in the conference context will be a valuable starting point for investigators in the other disciplines. Much of what has been learned by physiotherapy researchers about student evaluation tools likewise will be a valuable starting point for investigators in the other disciplines who wish to add to their own knowledge base. One caution seems appropriate here. We must not allow ourselves to be parochial in our thinking. There is a strong tendency to assume that our own profession is different and special, and therefore that the results of research in other disciplines have no applicability in our own. This is not so! Certainly it is dangerous to generalize findings from one set of subjects to an entire population of subjects who are identifiably different from the subjects originally studied. However, we can always be guided in the planning and execution of our own investigations by the theories, methods, findings and conclusions of investigations in other disciplines. To do otherwise is to do our students, our professions, ourselves and the research process itself an injustice.

At the end of each discussion of an area of research, there is one unrefined question related to that topic. With each question, try to do the following:

- Refine the preliminary question into a viable research question.
- Specify the independent and dependent variables.
- Select an appropriate design label.
- Sketch out the methodology in terms of the subjects, materials/instrumentation, procedure, and data analysis.
- Consider any pertinent ethical issues and how they might be addressed.

Do this for both a quantitative design and a qualitative design. By thinking through each problem and sketching out your strategy, you will teach yourself a great deal about research design. With any luck, you will finish this chapter with more than just new skills; you will have a new self concept. You will begin to think of yourself as a potential researcher in the area of clinical education. If you begin to do that, your natural curiosity about what makes the process work will turn into one exciting opportunity after another to ask and answer worthwhile questions. Every answer will have potential benefits for you, your students, your clients, your employer and your profession.

8.6.1 CLINICAL EDUCATOR–STUDENT RELATIONSHIPS

The first area of research to be considered in this section deals with the teaching dynamics between the individuals in clinical educator–student pairs. Unlike classroom teaching, most clinical teaching takes place in a dyadic information exchange. As a result, much of the current research, particularly in speech therapy, has focused on supervisory conference interactions between clinical educators and students. The results of these studies have revealed clinical education to be highly direct and in conflict with the stated goals of our accepted models of clinical education (see Chapter 1). Less direct teaching behaviours are more consistent with the teaching goals of student problem-solving and self-analysis. Another limitation of conferences appears to be their static nature. Results of comparative studies (Culatta & Seltzer, 1976; McCrea, 1980; Roberts & Smith, 1982; Tufts, 1984) indicate that clinical educators adopted content and interpersonal sets across all supervisory conferences and all students, irrespective of differing levels of experience and ability. Simply put, these studies told us what we are doing wrong or failing to do. Now we need to focus more on how to improve the situation.

Although we have a good start in the area of how to improve the situation, additional studies will be important. The first reason is that the research has focused almost exclusively on first-order effects, which are typically conference behaviours, as dependent variables. Alternative dependent variables might include second-order effects such as student clinical skills. Acquisition of more sophisticated clinical intervention strategies, particularly the ability to make modifications to techniques on-line can be seen as acquisition of problem-solving and independence and could be tied to conference interaction. As a third-order effect, research could explore changes in client progress as the ultimate measure of supervisory effectiveness.

Current theory in the health sciences professions supports a collaborative supervisory relationship in which critical thinking skills are developed. Rather than focusing on acquisition of specific instrumental knowledge, the teaching/learning process now seems to be focusing on helping the student acquire self-analytical and problem-solving abilities. Clinical education experiences which are designed to teach critical thinking skills can be referred to as 'reflective practica'. Supervisory behaviour in a reflective practicum would look quite unlike the supervisory interaction depicted in current descriptive studies. Students would do much of the problem-solving and decision-making, providing self-evaluations and justifications for them. The clinical educator would encourage critical thinking, asking the student to recognize and challenge assumptions, and to explore alternatives. Studies that compare outcomes of reflective practica compared to traditional practica are needed and form the second basic area of focus for clinical educator–student relationship research.

Learning Exercise 1: Designing a study of clinical educator–student relationships

Unrefined question: 'How can I get my student to take a more active role in the supervisory conference?'

8.6.2 CURRICULUM DESIGN

The next area of research need is that of curriculum structure. Many of our policies and practices have been born of a marriage of common sense and convenience. These arranged marriages are often good ones, but they are almost always consummated without the benefit of a good old get-acquainted courtship. Policies and practices are almost never empirically tested by systematically and scientifically comparing their benefits. Such practices characterize academic education programmes and clinical service facilities alike. Academic programmes typically make decisions about such things as the scheduling of placements, the temporal relationship of placements to academic coursework, the length of placements, the location of placements, and other such decisions in the absence of research-derived data. All of these aspects of the process of clinical education could be researched and decisions reached on the basis of empirical evidence. Unfortunately, once these convenient, common-sense policies and practices become a part of any institution, inertia tends to take over.

Occupational therapists are currently pursuing curriculum issues in their consideration of alternatives to the traditional beginning level clinical education experience (Zimmerman, 1995) and to the six-month advanced level clinical education experience (Phillips & Legaspi, 1995). Others are suggesting alternatives to the traditional one-to-one placement paradigm (Avi-Itzhak & Kellner, 1995) and to traditional types of placements (Griswold & Strassler, 1995). The American Occupational Therapy Association (1995) recently designated a position within their national office of Fieldwork Education Program Manager. That office is a repository for association information packets, guidelines on a variety of topics and products designed to make the process easier and more structured for all participants. The American Physical Therapy Association has a similar office, officer, and collection of support documents (Barr, Gwyer & Talmor, 1981; Barr, Gwyer & Talmor, 1982). Other models have been advocated in the physiotherapy literature as well (Perry, 1981), and physiotherapists have made suggestions about programme design (Deusinger, 1990; Windom, 1982). Rassi and McElroy (1992) devote an entire chapter to curriculum development in communication sciences and disorders programmes. They examine issues of selecting and specifying a type of programme (i.e., competency-based, experience-based, student-controlled, discovery-based and interdisciplinary), stating curriculum objectives, balancing professional standards with university dictates, and evaluating curricula.

Learning Exercise 2: Designing a study of curriculum design

Unrefined question: 'Will placement sites accept a new model for designating the nature of the clinical experiences they offer students?'

8.6.3 EFFICACY OF MODELS OF CLINICAL EDUCATION

The area of efficacy of models of clinical education is related to that of student–clinical educator relationships and also to the area of curriculum structure. Rather than focus on the interaction, or the general structure, this examines the models or structure of individual placements. With changes to health care delivery, new demands and challenges are faced by health care agencies and practitioners. At the same time, many professions are faced with decreases in availability of placement sites. Many options to promote effective and efficient placements have been suggested. One of the primary comparisons to be made is that between the demonstration style of placement more common to occupational and physiotherapy than to the model used in speech therapy, where minimal demonstration takes place. Speech therapy clinical education is more commonly characterized by the student clinician performing clinical functions under the observation of the clinical educator. In occupational therapy and physiotherapy, students and clinical educators are often working side-by-side with alternations of demonstration and observation of students' work. Other models of clinical education to be evaluated and compared are:

- the 2:1 student–clinical educator model (De Clute & Ladyshewski, 1993; Ladyshewski & Healey, 1990)
- split placement models, where more than one clinical educator is involved with the student
- non-traditional sites, where clinical education is done by someone other than a professional in the area in which the practicum is being offered, for example a psychiatric nurse supervizing an occupational therapy student on a psychiatric placement.

Comparative and perhaps even causal-comparative studies can examine the relative benefits of each of these models and assist in determining which model is most appropriate for specific student and clinic characteristics.

Learning Exercise 3: Designing a study of the efficacy of models of clinical education

Unrefined question: 'How can all these students be accommodated in so few placement sites?'

8.6.4 PREDICTORS OF SUCCESS

The next broad area of research need focuses on discovering predictors of success in the classroom and in the clinic. Students are typically selected on the basis of their previous academic performance. The extent to which such admission criteria select students destined for clinical proficiency is an important issue.

Several studies have investigated factors predictive of clinical achievement in speech therapy. Some studies found a relationship between academic performance and clinical achievement (Hagler, 1981; Shriberg *et al.*, 1975, 1977); however, continued study needs to explore other areas that may affect clinical performance. Similar studies in occupational and physiotherapy have confirmed the inadequacy of academic achievement as a predictor of clinical ability (Lind, 1970; Tidd & Conine, 1974). It seems evident that academic performance is not sufficient as the only indicator of performance in a clinical setting. What other variables may affect performance in this special setting? Hagler, Madill, Kampfe and Mitchell (1990) included locus of control and coping strategies, such as seeking social support, as predictor variables for clinical performance. The coping strategy seeking social support was found to have a direct relationship with clinical performance as measured by the Wisconsin procedure for appraisal of clinical competence (W-PACC) (Shriberg *et al.*, 1974). Age and marital status were also found to have predictive value when combined with grade point average (GPA) and endorsement of seeking social support as a coping strategy. Locus of control was not found to be related to clinical performance. The authors suggested that further investigation with other measures of locus of control should be pursued before discounting it as a predictive variable. Explanatory style has also been used as a predictor of behaviour and performance in psychology, education and business. Explanatory style describes the self-verbalizations that people use as causal attributes for success or failure in a given situation. Recent studies demonstrate that explanatory style is a predictor variable for achievement in the workplace (Seligman & Schulman, 1987), sports (Seligman, Nolen-Hoeksema, Thornton & Thornton, 1990) and academics (Peterson & Barrett, 1987; Kamen & Seligman, 1985).

Finally, many university programmes employ interviews as part of their admission procedures. These are typically done in the absence of empirical evidence to support their use. Exploration of all the possible variables and combinations of factors which impact clinical performance is essential. Determining the important factors will not only assist in selection of students with the highest potential but would also allow us to predict which students are at risk for clinical difficulties and provide specific and timely support.

Learning Exercise 4: Designing a study of predictors of success

Unrefined question: 'How can we pick the best students?'

8.6.5 ECONOMICS OF CLINICAL EDUCATION

Again, due to the changes in health care delivery and the emphasis on accountability, economics of clinical education is an important area for research. All health professions require clinical education in the training of new professionals. Placements are not necessarily viewed as beneficial to service facilities. There exists a belief among many clinicians and administrators that, when services are provided by students, there is a drain on the time of professional staff, concurrent reduction in services and decreased quality of service. Others believe that students increase both quantity and quality of direct client services. These differing perceptions are rarely supported with objective data but are voiced, nonetheless, with conviction. The physiotherapy profession has acknowledged the importance of this issue and offered constructive suggestions for cost reduction and support systems (Gandy & Sanders, 1990; Gwyer, 1990). Recent studies in physiotherapy have indicated that, in most areas of practice, students offer their practicum facilities a net gain in terms of client service (Bristow & Hagler, 1994; Bristow & Hagler, in press). A similar finding was obtained by Barrie and Ladyshewsky (1995) who developed the Clinical Education Quality Audit Tool (CEQA) for use by university clinical programme managers, clinical educators and students. The CEQA yields information on teaching and learning experiences, time invested, and satisfaction by stakeholders in the process of clinical education. The data can be compared from institution to institution, and Barrie and Ladyshewsky claim the CEQA has applicability across many disciplines.

A limitation of current research has been viewing the costs and benefits of clinical education from a cost or time basis. Meyers (1995) explored the costs and benefits involved in occupational therapy clinical education experiences. Using qualitative research methodology, Meyers looked at information from students, clinical educators, administrators and clients to learn what the costs and benefits were, as well as what their causes were. Results indicated the cost and benefits were diverse and divergent among the groups. Consistent with the results of Bristow and Hagler (1994), differences were also noted across service areas. Although there is some indication that student-provided services can be a positive addition to a clinic, further study is needed to determine how best to define 'quality' services and to determine the impact of variables such as service model, caseload, and student experience level on the economics of clinical education. The health issues are amount and quality of client care. Health service facilities and affiliated educational programmes need to know how services provided by students compare with services provided by qualified professionals and what impact participation may have on staff and clients. Administrators need to be able to make informed decisions about when and why to participate in the process of clinical education. More informed decisions might have secondary benefits, such as:

- an improved understanding of how to guard client care standards when students are involved
- strategies to improve participation by under-involved clinical service facilities or by certain programmes and disciplines within those facilities
- a generally more positive attitude toward the importance of on-site clinical education.

Learning Exercise 5: Designing a study in the area of economics of clinical education

Unrefined question: 'Are students an asset or a liability when they are on site?'

8.6.6 STUDENT EVALUATION TOOLS

Although not completely ignored as a viable area for research, student evaluation tools deserve more attention. The existing tools rarely have established reliability and validity. Perhaps the most noteworthy problem with student evaluation tools is the lack of consistency across training programmes. This lack of consistency also illustrates the importance of the health sciences and education professions having a master plan for research. The possibilities of cooperative research on student outcomes across training problems is complicated by the diversity of evaluation tools. The problem and the solution are best exemplified by events in physiotherapy in the United States. Clinical educators got so fed up with the number of different tools they were being asked to learn and implement that some even refused to take students whose academic programmes required the completion of an evaluation form they were not familiar with. More appropriately and more importantly, they complained to their professional association. Their complaints were heard and action was taken. The American Physical Therapy Association is in the process of developing separate evaluation tools for use with physiotherapy and physiotherapy assistant students. This work is being conducted with the kind of exacting standards and scientific rigour that should yield tools with known reliability and validity. The applications and limitations of these new tools will be carefully documented so they can be understood and adhered to by potential users. With any luck, these new student evaluation instruments will enjoy nearly universal acceptance by academic placement coordinators, clinical educators and students alike. The payoffs for this sort of research are monumental. They include instrument reliability and validity, the restored good will of the clinical educators who were once inundated with different forms, and universal indices of student performance. Consider the exciting possibilities that would be associated with a valid and reliable universal index of student performance. Academic programmes, clinical educators, researchers and employers would be able to make comparisons between individual students and across groups of students. So, if things are so well in hand, why do we list student evaluation tools as an area in need of research? Because in the other health science and education disciplines, the research processes, at least where student evaluation tools are concerned, have not yet taken this commendable turn of events. The reader will recall our earlier reference to the fact that the disciplines have much to offer one another. This is an area in which physiotherapy seems to have taken a leadership role. Their work can serve as a model for the other professions.

8.7 CONCLUSION

Clinical education research has been needed since the beginnings of formal training in the allied health disciplines, and it is needed more today than ever. One can understand why, during our developmental years as professions, we might have overlooked clinical education as an area of research. When our professions were in their infancies, toddling into their respective amorphous areas of practice and exploring their own boundaries, there were more pressing issues to study. We desperately wanted new diagnostic tools. We wanted to know which intervention methods were the most effective. To have ignored the study of clinical education practices in the face of these and other such pressing issues was understandable. To ignore it today seems somewhat less acceptable. The process

of clinical education is at the heart of our professional training programmes. It is at least as important as classroom education. Many would
argue more so. Educational programmes could double or triple their students' time in the classroom and never make clinical professionals of
them. Why is it we leave so much to chance where clinical education of
new professionals is concerned?

REFERENCES

Agar, M. H. (1980). *The professional stranger: An informal introduction to ethnography.*
New York: Academic Press.
Alfonso, R. & Firth, G. (1990). Supervision: Needed research. *Journal of Curriculum
and Supervision,* **5**, 181–8.
American Occupational Therapy Association (1995). The association. *American
Journal of Occupational Therapy,* **49**, 168–70.
Avi-Itzhak, T. & Kellner, H. (1995). Preliminary assessment of a fieldwork educa-
tion alternative: The fieldwork centers approach. *American Journal of Occupa-
tional Therapy,* **49**, 133–8.
Barlow, D. & Hersen, M. (1984) *Single case experimental designs: Strategies for study-
ing behaviour change.* New York: Pergamon Press.
Barr, J., Gwyer, J. & Talmor, Z. (1981). Standards for clinical education in physical
therapy: A manual for evaluation and selection of clinical education centers.
Washington, DC: American Physical Therapy Association.
Barr, J., Gwyer, J. & Talmor, Z. (1982). Evaluation of clinical education centers in
physical therapy. *Physical Therapy,* **62**, 850–61.
Barrie, S. & Ladyshewsky, R. (1995). Clinical education quality audit tool. Present-
ation at the Annual Meeting of the Australian Association of Speech and Hear-
ing, Brisbane, Queensland.
Blumberg, A. (1980). *Supervisors and teachers: A private cold war.* Berkeley, CA:
McCutchan Publishing Corporation.
Brannon, D. (1985). Adult learning principles and methods of enhancing the train-
ing role of supervisors. *The Clinical Supervisor,* **3**, 27–41.
Brasseur, J. & Anderson, J. (1983). Observed differences between direct, indirect,
and direct-indirect videotaped supervisory conferences. *Journal of Speech and
Hearing Research,* **26**, 349–55.
Bristow, D. & Hagler, P. (1994). Impact of physical therapy students on client ser-
vice delivery and professional staff time. *Physiotherapy Canada,* **46**, 275–80.
Bristow, D. & Hagler, P. (in press). Comparison of individual physical therapists'
productivity to that of combined physical therapist-student pairs. *Physiotherapy
Canada.*
Caracciolo, G., Rigrodsky, S. & Morrison, E. (1978). Perceived interpersonal condi-
tions and professional growth of masters level speech-language pathology stu-
dents during the supervisory process. *Asha,* **20**, 467–77.
Cimorell-Strong, J. & Ensley, K. (1982). Effects of student clinician feedback on the
supervisory conference. *Asha,* **24**, 23–9.
Cogan, M. (1973). *Clinical supervision.* Boston, MA: Houghton Mifflin.
Colaizzi, P. (1978). Psychological research as a phenomenologist views it. In R.
Valle & M. King (Eds). *Existential phenomenological alternatives for psychology.*
New York: Oxford University Press.

Culatta, R. & Seltzer, H. (1976). Content and sequence analysis of the supervisory session. *Asha*, **18**, 8–12.

Culatta, R. & Seltzer, H. (1977). Content and sequence analysis of the supervisory session: A report of clinical use. *Asha*, **19**, 523–6.

DeClute, J. & Ladyshewski, R. (1993). Enhancing clinical competence using a collaborative clinical education model. *Physical Therapy*, **73**, 683–97.

Denzin, N. & Lincoln, Y. (Eds) (1994). *Handbook of qualitative research*. Thousand Oaks, CA: Sage.

Denzin, N. (1978). *Sociological methods: A sourcebook*. Toronto, ON: McGraw-Hill.

DePoy, E. & Gitlin, L. (1994). *Intoduction to research: Multiple strategies for health and human services*. Toronto, ON: Mosby.

Deusinger, S. (1990). Establishing clinical education programmes: A practical guide. *Journal of Physical Therapy Education*, **4** (2), 58–61.

Dickson, G. (1995). Philosophical orientation of qualitative research. In L. Talbot (Ed.). *Principles and practices of nursing research*. St Louis, MO: Mosby.

Dowling, S. (1983). Teaching clinic conference participant interaction. *Journal of Communication Disorders*, **16**, 385–97.

Dowling, S., Sbaschnig, K. & Williams, C. (1982). Culatta and Seltzer content and sequence analysis of the supervisory session: Question of reliability and validity. *Journal of Communication Disorders*, **15**, 353–62.

Dowling, S. & Shank, K. (1981). A comparison of the effects of two supervisory styles, conventional and teaching clinic in the training of speech-language pathologists. *Journal of Communication Disorders*, **14**, 51–8.

Dowling, S. & Wittkop, M. (1982). Students' perceived supervisory needs. *Journal of Communication Disorders*, **15**, 319–28.

Ely, M. with Anzul, M., Friedman, T., Garner, D. & Steinmetz, A. (1991). *Doing qualitative research: Circles within circles*. London: Falmer.

Engnoth, G. (1974). A comparison of three approaches to supervision of speech clinicians in training. Doctoral dissertation, University of Kansas, 1973. *Dissertation Abstracts International*, **39**, 6261B.

Farmer, S. & Farmer, J. (1989). *Supervision in communication disorders*. Columbus: Merrill Publishing.

Fielding, N. & Fielding, J. (1986). *Linking data qualitative research methods* (Vol. 4). Beverly Hills, CA: Sage.

Finger, M. (1988). The biographical method in adult education research. *Studies in Continuing Education*, **10**, 3–42.

Freeman, E. (1985). The importance of feedback in clinical supervision: Implications for direct practice. *The Clinical Supervisor*, **3**, 5–26.

Gandy, J. & Sanders, B. (1990). Costs and benefits of clinical education. *Journal of Physical Therapy Education*, **4** (2), 70–5.

Ghitter, R. (1987). Relationship of interpersonal and background variables to supervisee clinical effectiveness. In S. Farmer (Ed.). *Proceedings of the national conference on supervision*. Jekyll Island, GA: Council of Supervisors in Speech-Language Pathology and Audiology.

Ghitter, R. (1989). Wonder why: Correlations for contemplation, discussion, and investigation. In D. Shapiro (Ed.). *Proceedings of the national conference on supervision*. Sonoma, CA: Council of Supervisors in Speech-Language Pathology and Audiology.

Giorgi, J. (1970). *Psychology as a human science: A phenomenologically based approach*. New York: Harper & Row.

Glaser, B. & Strauss, A. (1967). *The discovery of grounded theory: Strategies for qualitative research.* Chicago, IL: Aldine.

Goldhammer, R. (1969). *Clinical supervision.* New York: Holt, Rinehart & Winston.

Goldstein, A. & Sorcher, M. (1974). *Changing supervisory behaviour.* New York: Pergamon.

Griswold, L. & Strassler, B. (1995). Fieldwork in schools: A model for alternative settings. *American Journal of Occupational Therapy*, **49**, 127–32.

Gwyer, J. (1990). Resources for clinical education: Current status and future challenges. *Journal of Physical Therapy Education*, **4** (2), 55–8.

Hagler, P. (1981). Use of pre-programme academic achievement for prediction of performance in the B.Sc. programme in speech pathology and audiology at the University of Alberta. *Human Communication*, **6**, 41–53.

Hagler, P. (1986). Effects of verbal directives, data, and contingent social praise on amount of supervisor talk during speech-language pathology supervision conferencing. Unpublished dissertation, Indiana University, Bloomington, IN.

Hagler, P., Madill, H., Kampfe, C. & Mitchell, M. (1990). Students' coping strategies and prediction of practicum performance. Presentation at the Annual Meeting of the American Speech-Language-Hearing Association, Seattle, WA.

Hall, A. (1971). The effectiveness of videotape recordings as an adjunct to supervision in clinical practicum by speech pathologists. Doctoral dissertation, Ohio University, 1970. *Dissertation Abstracts International*, **32**, 612B.

Hatten, J. (1966). A descriptive and analytical investigation of speech therapy supervisor-therapist conferences. Doctoral dissertation, University of Wisconsin, 1965. *Dissertation Abstracts International*, **26**, 5595–6.

Heidegger, M. (1962). *Being and time* (J. Macquarrie & E. Robinson, Trans). New York: Harper Brothers.

Husserl, E. (1965). *Phenomenology and the crisis of philosophy.* New York: Harper & Row.

Jans, L., Hagler, P. & McFarlane, L. (1994). Effects of agenda use over time on participants' level of involvement in supervisory conferences. In M. Bruce (Ed.). *Proceedings of the national conference on supervision.* North Falmouth, MA: Council of Supervisors in Speech-Language Pathology and Audiology.

Kadushin, A. (1976). *Supervision in social work.* New York: Columbia University Press.

Kamen, L. & Seligman, M. (1985). Explanatory style predicts college grade point average. Unpublished manuscript reviewed in Tennen, H. & Herzberger, S. (1986). Attributional style questionnaires. *Test Critiques*, **4**, 20–32.

Kramer, M. (1969). Collegiate graduate nurses in medical center hospitals: Mutual challenge or duel. *Nursing Research*, **18** (3), 196–210.

Ladyshewski, R. & Healey, E. (1990). *The 2:1 teaching model in clinical education.* Toronto: University of Toronto Press.

Lincoln, Y. & Guba, E. (1985). *Naturalistic inquiry.* Beverly Hills, CA: Sage.

Lind, A. (1970). An exploratory study of predictive factors for success in the clinical affiliation experience. *American Journal of Occupational Therapy*, **24**, 222–6.

Mariano, C. (1995). The qualitative research process. In L. Talbot (Ed.). *Principles and practices of nursing research.* St Louis, MO: Mosby.

Martin, J., Goodyear, R. & Newton, F. (1987). Clinical supervision: An intensive case study. *Professional Psychology: Research and Practice*, **18**, 225–35.

McAllister, L. (1996). Clinical placements: A productive partnership for student learning and professionals' life long learning. Presentation at the Inaugural Conference of the New Zealand Speech-Language Therapists Association and the Australian Association of Speech and Hearing, Auckland New Zealand.

McCrea, M. (1980). Supervisee ability to self-explore and four facilitative dimensions of supervisor behaviour in individual conferences in speech-language pathology. Doctoral dissertation, Indiana University, 1980. *Dissertation Abstracts International*, **41**, 2134B.

McFarlane, L. & Hagler, P. (1990). Effects of peer supervision and supervisee-prepared conference agenda on conference interaction. Presentation at the Annual Meeting of the American Speech-Language-Hearing Association, Seattle, WA.

McFarlane, L. & Hagler, P. (1992a). An experimentally-based peer supervision component in a university clinic. In S. Dowling, *Proceedings of the national conference on supervision*. Nashville, TN: Council of Supervisors in Speech-Language Pathology and Audiology.

McFarlane, L. & Hagler, P. (1992b). Effects of a supervisee-prepared agenda on conference interaction. In S. Dowling, *Proceedings of the national conference on supervision*. Nashville, TN: Council of Supervisors in Speech-Language Pathology and Audiology.

McPherson, R. (1994). Softer foci: Broadening our understandings and uses of supervision. In M. Bruce (Ed.). *Proceedings of the 1994 international and interdisciplinary conference on clinical supervision: Toward the 21st century*. North Falmouth, MA: Council of Supervisors in Speech-Language Pathology.

McReynolds, L. & Kearns, K. (1983). *Single-subject experimental designs in communicative disorders*. Austin, TX: Pro-ed.

Meyers, S. (1995). Exploring the costs and benefits drivers of clinical education. *American Journal of Occupational Therapy*, **49**, 107–11.

Minichiello, V., Aroni, R., Timewell, E. & Alexander, L. (1990). *In-depth interviewing: Researching people*. Melbourne, Australia: Longman Cheshire.

Munson, C. (1983). *An introduction to clinical social work supervision*. New York: Haworth Press.

Nemeth, E. & McAllister, L. (1995). *Students' difficulties in clinical education: Their perspectives*. Presentation at the Annual Meeting of the Australian Association of Speech and Hearing, Brisbane, Queensland.

Norman, G. & Streiner, D. (1986). *PDQ statistics*. Toronto: B.C. Decker, Inc.

Opacich, K. (1995). Is an education philosophy missing from the fieldwork solution? *American Journal of Occupational Therapy*, **49**, 160–4.

Oratio, A. Sugarman, M. & Prass, M. (1981). A multivariate analysis of clinicians' perceptions of supervisory effectiveness. *Journal of Communication Disorders*, **14**, 31–42.

Pain, P., Hagler, P. & Warren S. (1996). Development of an instrument to evaluate the research orientation of clinical professionals. *Canadian Journal of Rehabilitation*, **9** (2), 93–100.

Perry, J. (1981). A model for designing clinical education. *Physical Therapy*, **61**, 1427–32.

Peterson, C. & Barrett, L. (1987). Explanatory style and academic performance among university freshman. *Journal of Personality and Social Psychology*, **53**, 603–7.

Phillips, E. & Legaspi, W. (1995). A 12-month internship model of level II fieldwork. *American Journal of Occupational Therapy*, **49**, 146–9.

Pickering, M. (1984). Interpersonal communication in speech-language pathology supervisory conferences: A qualitative study. *Journal of Speech and Hearing Disorders*, **49**, 189–95.

Rassi, J. & McElroy, M. (1992). *The education of audiologists and speech-language pathologists.* Timonium, MD: York Press.

Rather, M. (1992). 'Nursing as a way of thinking' – Heideggerian hermeneutic analysis of the lived experience of the returning RN. *Research in Nursing and Health,* **15,** 47–55.

Roberts, J. & Smith, K. (1982). Supervisor-supervisee role differences and consistency of behaviour in supervisory conferences. *Journal of Speech and Hearing Research,* **25,** 428–34.

Seligman, M., & Schulman, P. (1987). Explanatory style as a predictor of performance as a life insurance sales agent. *Journal of Personality and Social Psychology,* **50,** 974–98.

Seligman, M., Nolan-Hocksema, S., Thornton, N. & Thornton, K. (1990). Explanatory style as a mechanism of disappointing athletic performance. *Psychological Science,* **1,** 143–6.

Shapiro, D. & Anderson, J. (1989). One measure of supervisory effectiveness in speech-language pathology and audiology. *Journal of Speech and Language Disorders,* **54,** 549–57.

Sherstan, K., Hagler, P. & McFarlane, L. (1995). *Effects of supervisor presence on commitments made and carried out by students.* Paper presented at the 1995 Convention of the American Speech-Language-Hearing Association Convention, Orlando, Florida.

Shriberg, L., Filley, F., Hayes, D., Kwiatkowski, J., Schatz, J., Simmons, K. & Smith, M. (1974). *The Wisconsin procedure for appraisal of clinical competence (W-PACC).* Madison WI: Department of Communicative Disorders, University of Wisconsin-Madison.

Shriberg, L., Filley, F., Hayes, D., Kwiatkowski, J., Schatz, J., Simmons, K. & Smith, M. (1975). The Wisconsin procedure for appraisal of clinical competence: Model and data. *Asha,* **17,** 158–65.

Shriberg, L. D., Bless, D. M., Carlson, K. A., Filley, F. S., Kwiatkowski & J. Smith, M.E. (1977). Personality characteristics, academic performance and clinical competence in communication disorders majors. *Asha,* **19,** 311–21.

Siegel, S. (1956). *Non-parametric statistics for the behavioural sciences.* New York: McGraw-Hill.

Smith, K. & Anderson, J. (1982a). Relationship of perceived effectiveness to verbal interaction/content variables in supervisory conferences in speech-language pathology. *Journal of Speech and Hearing Research,* **25,** 252–9.

Smith, K. and Anderson, J. (1982b). Relationship of perceived effectiveness to content in supervisory conferences in speech-language pathology. *Journal of Speech and Hearing Research,* **25,** 243–51.

Spradley, J. (1979). *The ethnographic interview.* New York: Holt, Rinehart & Winston.

Spradley, J. (1980). *Participant observation.* New York: Holt, Rinehart & Winston.

St Jacques, E. (1994). Alberta speech-language pathologists: Involvment in clinical research. Unpublished masters' thesis, University of Alberta, Edmonton.

Starkweather, W. (1974). Behaviour modification in training speech clinicians: Procedures and implications. *Asha,* **16** (10), 607–11.

Strauss, A. & Corbin, J. (1990). *Basics of qualitative research: Grounded theory procedures and techniques.* Newbury Park, CA: Sage.

Sundel, M. & Sundel, S. (1975). *Behaviour modification in the human services: A systematic introduction to concepts and applications.* New York: John Wiley & Sons.

Tesch, R. (1990). *Qualitative research: Analysis types and software tools.* New York: Falmer.

Tidd, G. & Conine, T. (1974). Do better students perform better in the clinic? *Physical Therapy,* **54,** 500–5.

Tufts, L. (1984). A content analysis of supervisory conferences in communicative disorders and the relationship of the content analysis system to the clinical experience of supervisees. Doctoral Dissertation, Indiana University. *Dissertation Abstracts International,* **44,** 3048B.

Underwood, J. (1973). Interaction analysis between the supervisor and the speech and hearing clinician. Doctoral dissertation, University of Denver. *Dissertation Abstracts International,* **34,** 2995 B.

van Manen, M. (1990). *Researching lived experience: Human science for an action sensitive pedagogy.* London, Ontario, Canada: State University of New York Press.

Wellman, L. (1991). *Effects of supervisor self-exploration on supervisor and supervisee conferencing behaviour.* Unpublished Master's thesis, University of Alberta, Edmonton.

Werner, O. & Schoepfle, G. (1987). *Systematic field-work* (Vols 1 & 2). Newbury Park, CA: Sage.

Windom, P. (1982). Developing a clinical education programme from the clinician's perspective. *Physical Therapy,* **62,** 1604–9.

Yin, R. (1989). *Case study research design and methods.* Newbury Park, CA: Sage.

Zimmerman, S. (1995). Cooperative education: An alternative level I fieldwork. *American Journal of Occupational Therapy,* **49,** 153–5.

Clinical education and the future: An emerging mosaic of change, challenge and creativity

9

Marisue Pickering
Associate Vice-President for Academic Affairs, University of Maine, USA

Lindy McAllister
*School of Communication Disorders,
The University of Sydney, Australia*

Postcard 9

Dear All

This is the last postcard. In fact, you'll probably see me before the card arrives. The paediatrician at the hospital got Email this week. Amazing hey! Out here! If only he'd had it 2 months ago when I first arrived and felt like a fish out of water (or in too much water given it's done nothing but rain since I arrived)! I'll miss this place and the people. I feel like I've been able to make a useful contribution and I've learned so much – about the country, CBR and myself as well. It's been pretty challenging, especially the cross-cultural stuff. I realized only this week that some of the tension in my relationship with one of the team is about male/female role issues on top of cultural differences. I'm looking forward to coming home, drying out, thinking it all through. See you soon.

S.

9.1 CHAPTER OVERVIEW

This chapter discusses three areas of major change having an impact on clinical education: population changes, changes in higher education and changes in professional practice. In the context of these changes, three significant challenges confronting clinical educators are considered: the need to develop cross-cultural awareness and competence, to incorporate gender factors in education and practice and to recognize issues of global interconnectivity and social responsibility. Implications of these changes and challenges for clinical educators are noted throughout the chapter. Case studies that illustrate creative responses by clinical educators to these changes and challenges are provided.

9.2 BACKGROUND

This final chapter has taken a different direction than first planned. Originally the focus was to be on clinical education of students with unique needs, such as mature age students and foreign students, as well as on issues affecting students in special learning environments, such as in rural and remote sites. As we progressed in our thinking, broader issues emerged: the shifting foundations, changing priorities and ongoing challenges that constitute daily professional experience at the end of this century and of this millennium. It is as if the tectonic plates of professional work and cultural life are undergoing continual move-ment. Such movement or change creates numerous challenges for pro-fessionals. Clinical educators, by virtue of being educators of new generations of professionals, are and must be future-oriented. For the benefit of their students and clients, clinical educators must become adept at anticipating change, identifying issues and challenges and responding creatively.

For some readers, elements of this discussion will be familiar. Our deci-sion to craft the chapter the way we have is based on our desire to:

- show the pervasiveness of both change and challenge to clinical education across professions
- name clinical educators as professionals critically responsible for innovative leadership
- discuss issues that appear under-discussed in current clinical education professional literature
- share stories of creative responses by clinical educators and practitioners to the challenges they are facing.

An additional intent has been to present the information in a manner that illustrates the diversity of professional life. Thus, an ongoing, underlying construct for us as we wrote this chapter has been the view that the world is composed of both commonalties and differences. In particular, the world is composed of individuals whose interests and experiences reflect both commonalities and differences.

Another guiding construct for us is that the social, communicative and cultural boundaries between individuals and communities are sensitive and fraught with the potential for misinterpretations. We believe one way to minimize potential misunderstanding is for people to share their own biographies and also to identify places where their own biographies intersect with those of others. We think it important to know something about the context out of which people speak.

We begin then with a short introduction about ourselves to illustrate the similarities and differences in our own lives. Further, this introduction is intended to give readers an opportunity to make inferences about the influence of the cultural filters that guided our thinking as we researched and wrote.

Our introduction begins with the fact that we both are white women of Anglo-Celtic heritage, although one of us has a dose of French Huguenot in the mix. We are native English speakers and we write from a Western perspective and orientation. From this shared background, we diverge in terms of age, family situation, personal and professional experience, professional training and athletic ability. One of us is from the United States, the other from Australia. One of us currently has academic responsibility for a clinical education programme; one of us is a full-time higher education administrator.

We again converge in our strong backgrounds in clinical education in Communication Disorders, in sharing similar philosophical values and intellectual interests and in our desire to probe the influence of the macro on the micro and vice versa. Both of us are stimulated and enticed by the challenges of living and working in a globally interconnected world. Both of us have a wide range of international experiences and interests on which we have drawn in developing this chapter. Both of us continue to attempt to understand feminist issues and the impact of cultural diversity on our lives. We both are voracious and eclectic readers.

It is evident that our professional knowledge and experience is based in Communication Disorders. Nevertheless, we have tried to be sensitive to and inclusive of other fields. Similarly we included information about issues in countries other than our own. We believe that the changes, challenges and creative responses about which we have written are generalizable across professions and across societies; we hope readers will find this to be the case.

9.3 CHANGE

Change in all our lives and work is so pervasive as to be a truism. The discussion begins with a focus on change in three major areas that affect clinical education: population, higher education and professional practice.

9.3.1 CHANGE IN POPULATION

One of the most significant areas of change concerns who makes up a given population. Most professionals probably are well informed about the changing demographics of their particular countries. What perhaps is not known is that such change is occurring in many Western societies as a result of changed immigration laws and patterns, as well as changed birth rates. In many countries, there is increased cultural, ethnic, racial and linguistic diversity within the population. Societies, universities and clinical educators are needing to redefine who the 'we' are.

(a) Population diversity: The impact of immigration

Francese (1995), writing about 'America at Mid-Decade' states, 'America's households are diverse and diverging and so are their needs' (p. 24). In a country of about 262 million, between 1990 and 1994, 4.6 million immigrants arrived, the largest five-year total since the turn of the century. In 1994, about 1 in every 11 Americans was foreign-born; this is nearly double the percentage in 1970 (Hansen & Bachu, 1995). Mexico is the country of origin with the largest number of immigrants; the Philippines is second (Hansen & Bachu, 1995).

Growth is being seen also in the United States in the population usually referred to as minority, that is, American Indian, Asian American, African American and Hispanic American. This composite group constitutes about one in four of the United States population, having grown from one in five in 1980. The age concentration for minorities actually is in children; one-third of United States children in 1995 are reported to be black, Hispanic or Asian (Francese, 1995).

Canada, a country with a 1991 population of some 27 million, also has had a change in immigration laws and patterns. Like the United States, Canada, with the exception of its native or indigenous peoples, is a land of immigrants and their descendants. Although the percentage of foreign born has been about 16 per cent for 40 years, immigrants' countries of origin have changed. Until the 1960s, Canadian immigration was primarily from Europe (including the UK). By 1991, 75 per cent of all immigrants were coming from Asia, Central and South America, and Africa, thus impacting on Canada's racial heterogeneity. Furthermore, because of the shifts in countries of origin, neither of Canada's two official languages (English and French) is likely to be the native language of the new population of immigrants (Statistics Canada, 1993).

In Australia, migration patterns have changed from being predominantly Anglo-Celtic prior to World War II, to including significant non-English-speaking European migrants in the post-war years. The 1970s brought the beginning of significant Asian immigration. Australia in the 1990s is increasingly diverse: '75% of people are of British origin, almost 20% are of European origin and 4.5% are of Asian origin' (Lack & Templeton, 1995, p. xv). Noting the linguistic background of today's Australians may give an even truer picture of the country's diversity. In particular, the 1986 census in the state of Victoria, one of Australia's most ethnically diverse states, showed that '43.6% of the population of 4 million either spoke a language other than English, or came from NESB [non-English-speaking background] countries, or were exposed to other cultural influences due to their parent/s being migrants from NESB countries' (D'Cruz & Tham, 1993, p. 41).

(b) Population diversity: Not just a big city phenomenon

Although population diversity is most likely to be prevalent in a country's large cities and heavily populated regions, it is not limited to these areas. The state of Maine in the United States, a north-eastern, primarily white state, whose largest city has a population of 60,000, and whose state-wide population is 1.2 million, reports almost 90 different native languages other than English being used in the home by children in the state's schools (Berube, 1994). Further, the number of people of colour and of Hispanics is expected to increase and foreign immigrants are expected to continue moving into the state (Governor's Commission to Promote the Understanding of Diversity in Maine, 1994, p. 5).

An additional example comes from Australia's Northern Territory, a sparsely populated area that contains many isolated populations. This region, because of its proximity to south-east Asia, has a long history of Asian immigration. In addition, 24.5 per cent of the Territory's population is Aboriginal (Commonwealth Department of Health and Human Services, 1995). This is in contrast to Australia as a whole, where only 1.5 per cent of the total population identifies as a member of these two groups (Australian Bureau of Statistics, 1993).

(c) Population diversity: The impact of policy and social changes

Another change related to population has to do with governments taking increased notice and responsibility for the historic racial, ethnic and cultural diversity present in their societies. Examples abound. One comes from Australia's efforts to address the legal and social injustices endured by its Aboriginal and Torres Strait Islander populations. National actions such as the Native Title Act of 1993 and the Council for Aboriginal Reconciliation (1991) have paved the way for society as a whole to work toward redressing the loss of dignity and identity that followed the dispossession of Aboriginal and Torres Strait Islander lands. National initiatives also have promoted respect for and understanding of the knowledge inherent in both the dominant Australian cultures and in the cultures of the Aboriginal and Torres Strait Islander peoples.

(d) Population change: Impact on the client base

Changes involving a society's communities have a direct impact on a client base. First and most obviously, there are changes in who requests services. In Australia, for example, as social justice measures are put into place for Aboriginal and Torres Strait Islander peoples, the Australian professional communities can expect a greater demand for and participation in health, social and education services. Similar demands are being experienced in South Africa following the formal ending of apartheid. As a consequence, clinical educators will need to develop teaching strategies appropriate for students from indigenous communities and to participate in the delivery of services to these communities with both their indigenous and non-indigenous students.

Case Study 9.1 Increasing services to the under-served majority of the population: Community-based education for speech therapy and audiology students in South Africa

The University of Durban-Westville has committed itself to attracting a student population that reflects the ethnic distribution in the population of South Africa, preparing its students to work for the World Health Organization goal of *Health for All by 2000*, and being an agent of change in the transformation of the health service in South Africa (Jager, 1994).

Students from many health disciplines collaborated in a community-based and problem-based programme that integrates teaching, research, and service. The speech and hearing students spent one day per week in the final year of their programme of study in the peri-rural community of Kwa Dedangendlale, 40 kilometres from Durban. This community of 67,000 is described by Jager (1994) as mainly Zulu-speaking and impoverished. Although a highly successful public health programme has been in place since 1951, Jager reports there was little allied health service.

The programme for the speech and hearing students had three modules:

1 a research module where students designed and conducted a research project appropriate to the needs identified by the community
2 a seminar module that prepared the students for 'operating in Third World conditions' (Jager, 1994, p. 95), using public health care principles
3 a module that prepared and supported the students for work in the field.

One of the many challenges in this programme was to prepare students to work, with insight and sensitivity, in a language (Zulu) and a culture not their own. Examples of the research projects undertaken include: 'feasibility of an alternative hearing screening protocol for pre-schoolers in a black rural community; communication disorders: beliefs and practices in a Zulu community; acquired neurogenic communication disorders service needing identification using community health workers' (Jager, 1994, p. 101).

Jager includes in his project evaluation report student descriptions of their experience. The students' words speak powerfully of the positive effects of their experience, as the following extract shows:

'Whew! ... How do I begin to describe it?! A roller coaster ride: where I learnt about life, values, prejudice, politics, morals and about myself – up every hill, down every dip and around every hairpin bend on the route. I've learnt about community: the concept; and PHC [primary health care] – what that term does and does not encompass; I've acquired to a certain extent – cultural sensitivity and tolerance of others' values, lifestyles and practices. I've learnt about the essence and value of communication, and being an effective communicator. Most importantly – I've been forced to "see" what I've been "looking at".' (Jager, 1994, p. 102)

A second impact of population diversity on the client base concerns the differences in socialization experiences between client populations and professionals representing different races and ethnicities, as well as between clients from immigrant communities and clinicians and educators drawn from a country's citizenry. Socialization differences may be reflected though differing values, communication patterns, ways of viewing reality and the amount of information needed to make decisions. Hartley (1995a, 1995b), representing Communication Therapy International in the United Kingdom, discusses dilemmas involved in providing services across cultures, especially internationally. Hartley's ideas need not be limited to international experiences. Her point that not all groups have the same concept of what constitutes an impairment or a disability might be equally well applied to working with minority cultures within one's home country.

Another impact of population diversity concerns types of presenting problems. Evidence from Australia suggests that the health needs of non-English-speaking background (NESB) immigrant groups are different from those of English-speaking immigrants, possibly as a result of the stress of voluntary or refugee migration. Other factors include difficulties encountered in learning a new language and social mores, as well as in obtaining recognition of employment skills. D'Cruz and Tham (1993), in a study in the Australian state of Victoria, found the NESB migrant population to have a higher rate of admission to public hospitals. Similarly, Kayser (1994), looking at issues affecting multicultural populations in the United States, notes that 'economically disadvantaged populations are more likely to be predisposed to causes of disorders related to environmental, teratogenic ..., nutritional and traumatic factors than other groups' (p. 283). Shadden and Warnick (1994) report that the percentage of older adults in the United States who rate their overall health as fair or poor is much higher in the African American, Hispanic and Native American populations than in the white populations.

(e) Population change: The impact of ageing

Any consideration of changes in the population of industrialized countries must include ageing, which may be a particularly twentieth-century phenomenon (Jones, 1992). Writing about the United States, Lubinski and Masters (1994) state: 'Perhaps the fastest growing group of potential clients whom audiologists and speech-language pathologists will serve in the next 20 years are those above 65 years of age' (p. 150). In Canada also, the population clearly is getting older (Statistics Canada, 1993).

The demographics are similar in Australia. In 1961, 8.5 per cent of the population was over 65 years of age. By the year 2001, that figure is expected to be 10.6 per cent and to increase to 21.5 per cent by 2031 (Rowland, 1991). It is anticipated that one of the features of the ageing population in Australia in the next century will be location of a significant proportion in the outer suburbs of major cities, 'without satisfactory public transport and with poor access to shops, amenities and government services such as were available to previous generations of older people in the inner suburbs. Even though many of these older persons may drive cars, the majority will have their lives affected by the failure to locate essential public facilities close to their homes' (Sax, 1993, p. 21). The situation is not much different for the rural elderly in Australia. The drift of young people away from rural areas reduces the social support and caring network provided by families in the past (Millward, 1995).

An additional impact of an ageing population on health care delivery is that there will be increased service delivery options, such as domiciliary (home) care and palliative care. In addition, intervention services will need to include ongoing maintenance for particular populations, such as those with neurological conditions. Finally, an impact of an ageing population is that the professionals delivering the services will be older. Pannbacker, Middleton and Click (1995) discuss the implications for the ageing of the profession of Communication Disorders in the United States and point out the need to rethink professional development and the issues around an inter-generational workforce.

(f) Population change: The demand for services from new clinical populations

Advances in medical and nursing science and care technologies have led to an overall decrease in childhood mortality and an increase in childhood morbidity. Studies by McAllister, Masel, Tudehope, O'Callaghan, Mohay and Rogers (1993a; 1993b) point to the complex and ongoing educational, health and social needs of many children who survive neonatal intensive care. In a large longitudinal study conducted at a major Australian hospital, these researchers found that intellectual disability was present in 6 per cent of children in the cohort, sensory disability in 4 per cent and a major communication problem in 13 per cent of the children at three years of age. As the children grew older, the effect of medical variables decreased and family variables became more important. Results such as these indicate the need for new services, especially among high-risk infants and toddlers.

Case Study 9.2 Developing services for unique populations: Clinical education for nursing students in the United States

Advances in health care need to be matched with advances in the education of health care workers. Koch and Maserang (1994) describe a nursing education project that encourages students to identify, plan, and provide for health needs of new or underserviced populations in the community, such as babies born of crack-dependent mothers, migrant workers, mentally-ill homeless people and people in communities devastated by natural disasters. Early in the semester, students choose a population with which to work. They then develop specific personal learning objectives that relate to the general course goals. They plan the service they wish to develop and for the rest of the semester, they spend one day per week delivering their service in the community. Their supervisors visit them periodically in the community setting; these visits are combined with regular meetings on campus. Students keep a learning journal throughout the placement and are expected to share experiences and to engage in problem-solving with their peers. At the conclusion of the placement, students make an oral presentation that describes and evaluates the service.

With increased life spans, infant survival rates and infant morbidity rates, more people with disabilities require rehabilitation services. These needs are not limited to the Western world. Marfo and Walker (1986) estimate that by the year 2000, 80 per cent of people needing rehabilitation services will live in the 'developing nations' as opposed to the 'developed' nations'. Current indicators suggest, however, that these nations will be able to meet no more than 3 per cent of the demand (Pan American Health Organization, 1994). Clearly, creative models of appropriate service delivery are needed. Also required are different models of educating service providers.

Case Study 9.3 Training for and providing transdisciplinary services for African countries

Jelsma, Cortes-Meldrum, Moyo and Powell (1995) describe the development of a community-based, multidisciplinary children's rehabilitation unit in Harare, Zimbabwe, that serves as both a service and training facility. Children and their families may attend the centre in the capital city, but the aim is to educate the family and community members to continue the service in the community, be that within a town or a remote village. Services are provided in the towns and villages using a transdisciplinary model. The use of technology appropriate for the resource capacities of the country is emphasized. Few families can afford high-tech equipment which in any case is not viable in areas without regular electricity and access to maintenance.

(g) Population change: Rural and remote areas

The needs of under-served populations, such as those in remote areas, are not new. Greater importance is afforded them, however, in an era that respects diversity. Rural and remote communities often experience difficulties in having access to medical and allied health services. In countries like Australia, with its relatively small rural population scattered over vast geographic areas, the recruitment and retention of staff is an ongoing challenge. By necessity, providing services often involves professionals working transdisciplinarily. For example, at the time of writing this book, Wilcannia, a remote and isolated community of 1000 people in the far western section of the state of New South Wales, Australia, has been unable to attract a resident medical officer. Aboriginal people, who as a group have a significant number of health problems, make up the majority of the population in Wilcannia. The community's access to medical care is limited to the Royal Flying Doctor Service, which makes three visits per week and provides emergency evacuation services as necessary (Siegloff, 1995). Clinical educators need to consider how they might prepare students to work in such settings. They also need to consider the ways they might contribute to the attraction and retention of staff in such areas.

In reflecting on health care in remote areas, clinical educators need to examine closely their values about desirable places to work, about career paths and about the messages they may explicitly or implicitly pass on to students. They also need to provide students with positive learning experiences in rural and remote settings. If students receive early positive exposure to rural health issues and rural lifestyles, they are more likely to pursue rural careers after graduation (Kamien & Buttfield, 1990).

Case Study 9.4 Promoting rural health care careers: A government supported Australian effort

The Rural Careers Project for students at The University of Sydney started in 1991 with support from the government's Rural Health Support Education and Training fund. The project is managed by a committee of representatives from each professional preparation programme involved. Participation in the project is open to students from all 13 health and social work disciplines represented in the university.

The project has three major activities. Once or twice a semester students get to hear a guest speaker talk about the challenges and rewards of professional and personal life in their settings. Students are provided with positive role models of professionals who have made a career path and a fulfilling life in a rural setting. Once a year project staff and about 60 students from all disciplines spend a weekend in a rural centre, visiting local hospitals, community health centres, and private practices; attending seminars or discussion groups run by local professionals; visiting local industries; and participating in the social activities of the town. As many of Australia's Aboriginal populations live in rural areas, these visits provide a unique opportunity for students to meet and discuss issues with local Aboriginal people, as well as with their health and social welfare workers. Discussions also have covered farm safety issues, and industrial health and safety measures as part of a tour of a coal mine.

The project also provides financial support for students to undertake rural placements. Students obtain multidisciplinary contact and first-hand experience of learning, living and working in a rural or remote setting. Learning sometimes takes an unexpected twist as, for example, when three speech pathology students who went to Broken Hill in far western New South Wales came to realize that a drive of several hours to provide services to townships beyond Broken Hill might be less onerous than flying there with the Royal Flying Doctor Service and then being left behind 'if a patient needed [the speech therapist's seat on] a flight back to Broken Hill' (McAllister, Eadie & Hays, 1992).

This section has discussed changes in population and the enormous and challenging diversity seen in culture, language, age and disability. To enable future professionals to meet the health care needs of changing populations, clinical educators need to understand and respond to this diversity and its impact on health and welfare services, planning and delivery and on interactions with individual clients. The family-focused transitional care model proposed by Lipman and Deatrick (1994) to manage children's and families' needs across the continuum of care from hospital-based during the acute or early stages through to family or community-based care is an example of such a response. Clinical educators will need to understand and participate in new service models such as this, if they are to provide appropriate learning experiences for their students.

Clinical educators need to provide students with learning experiences that expose them to the diversity of clients and workplaces. They need to model cross-cultural awareness and competence for their students. Meeting the needs of emerging clinical populations, the ageing and rural and remote populations will demand of clinical educators a move from the 'expert', uni-disciplinary model of service delivery and education, into those models that emphasize primary health care and transdisciplinary collaboration and service delivery.

As momentous and pervasive as changes and needs are within the potential client base in the health sciences and education, they are not the only significant changes that clinical educators and their respective fields must consider. Change also is occurring worldwide in higher education itself. Such change has direct impact on the fields of health sciences and education and on clinical educators themselves.

9.3.2 CHANGE IN HIGHER EDUCATION

Throughout the world, higher education is either changing or being challenged to change. A major report on higher education in the United States states bluntly: 'Education is in trouble' (Wingspread Group on Higher Education, 1993, p. 1). The report identifies problems such as inadequate student preparation for higher education; insufficient knowledge, competence and skill upon university graduation; and a mismatch between what is needed from university curricula and what one receives.

In an effort to understand what is happening worldwide for higher education, Boyer, Altbach and Whitelaw (1994) surveyed academic staff in Australia, Brazil, Chile, Germany, Hong Kong, Israel, Japan, Korea, Mexico, the Netherlands, Russia, Sweden, the United Kingdom and the United States. As a result, they identified three critical issues expected to have an ongoing and significant influence on higher education: student access, institutional governance and the tension among teaching, research and service. The United Nations Educational, Scientific and Cultural Organization (1995) also studied higher education worldwide and notes three common developments:

- quantitative expansion as observed through growth in student enrolments

- diversification of structures, programmes and forms of study
- financial and resource constraints.

Changes in higher education affect clinical education programmes in deep and significant ways.

(a) Change in the structuring of higher education

Many countries are experiencing or have recently experienced major restructuring of their higher education systems. In 1992, the British system underwent a significant restructuring when 34 English polytechnics and five Scottish institutions had university status conferred on them. This almost doubled the number of British universities, from 47 to 88 (Hughes, 1995). Polytechnics historically offered many programmes at the level of a diploma or a professional qualification, rather than at the level of a bachelor's or higher degree. The restructuring set the stage for major changes in both governance and funding (Gaither, Nedwek & Neal, 1994). Rapid increases in enrolment also characterize British higher education in the 1990s; teaching larger classes and working longer hours are among the impacts of these changes.

Australian higher education also has seen significant restructuring. Beginning in 1991, universities, colleges of advanced education and institutes of technology were amalgamated into a unified system of 36 federally-funded universities. Simultaneous to these amalgamations, Australian universities also experienced significant increases in student enrolments, from 349,000 in 1983 to 584,000 in 1994 (IDP Education Australia, 1995). Rarely has this increase in student numbers and participation rate seen commensurate increases in resources and staffing levels. In Canada too enrolment in higher education institutions continues to show a steady increase (Gaither, Nedwek & Neal, 1994); nevertheless, the poor economic climate in Canada has reduced various revenues. Most of the funding comes from the provinces and they vary considerably in their economic health.

Changes in the structure of higher education are not limited to the English-speaking world. For example, Italian higher education, referred to as a 'System in Transition,' is moving from a system based on central control to one wherein universities have greater local autonomy; Italian higher education also is facing issues of financing and quality assessment (European Association for International Education, 1995).

(b) Change in higher education: The impact of policy and social changes

Changes in governments in Central and Eastern European countries in 1989 created numerous challenges for higher education in these countries.

A report on transition dilemmas in education in the social sciences in Bulgaria, for example, discusses the need for staff to offer both interdisciplinary and practical training, features not emphasized prior to the governmental changes of 1989 (Gotchev, 1993). Januszkiewicz (1991) discusses the important role needing to be played by educational institutions as the Polish people attempt to change their 'paradigms of thinking' in their new post-1989 society. Rinehart (1995) considers issues facing universities in the former German Democratic Republic as they move away from a 'centralized education system designed to further Marxist-Leninist social and political goals' (p. 15).

Nor is change limited to the industrialized world. African universities are facing numerous issues, including how to finance educational changes, disillusionment over the value of university education and a need for revitalization. Many of these issues result from the desire of African universities and governments to move from a colonial model of higher education to one more relevant to their environments (Sawadogo, 1994). China too is ready for a major transition in higher education, one from a system serving an elite to one serving the masses (Hayhoe, 1995). Resource issues are only one of the many needing to be faced.

(c) Change in higher education student cohorts

Student cohorts themselves also are changing. In the Western world, universities traditionally had students who were male, white and recent graduates of a secondary school. In the United States, students would live on the campus; in other countries, they might also have been able to live in the vicinity, in rooms or at home. They attended classes full-time and were expected to complete their degrees in a prescribed amount of time. The student body might contain a few overseas students. Women experienced limitations relative to career choice and many people were denied access to higher education.

The current reality is different. In the United States, there are approximately 3,600 institutions of higher learning, where more women than men are enrolled, where over 40 per cent of the population is over 25 (including 2.7 per cent over 50), where minority Americans constitute about 23 per cent of enrolments and where there is a significant number of part-time students (*The Chronicle of Higher Education Almanac*, 1995). Black women now make up 11.1 per cent of all female enrolment (Blacks in America, 1995). Further, since 1990, both Hispanic and Asian American groups have increased higher education enrolment by 26.3 per cent (Carter & Wilson, 1995, p. 3). As in other countries, the number and proportion of overseas students also have been increasing (Lambert, 1995).

Case Study 9.5 Responding to diversity in the student body: A programme in Communication Disorders at a university in the United States

In 1989 the School of Audiology and Speech-Language Pathology, at the University of Memphis in the state of Tennessee, began recruiting African American students into the master's level programme. In order to deal with anxiety which arose from 'uncertainty ... about strangers' attitudes, feelings, beliefs, values, and behaviour' (Gundykunst & Kim, 1992, p. 27), staff and students began to meet regularly. Their group, known as FASCE (Faculty and Student Cultural Exchange) met informally once a month for two hours in the home of either a staff member or a student. FASCE operated on the asset model, that is, valuing and appreciating cultural similarities and differences, rather than seeking to assimilate and fade difference. The goal was to empower students through sharing experiences and information, and recognizing learning and growth can occur in staff and students alike. Hillard, Tronolone, Mendel, Manning and Taylor (1994) report that the group came to recognize that many of the perceived cultural differences were in fact better explained by differences in gender, age, power relations, age, and socio-economic background.

Traditionally the British system, like its counterparts in other countries, was elite (Hughes, 1995). As recently as 1979, only 12.4 per cent of young British adults (18–19-year-olds) were involved in higher education. Since that time, British higher education has been transformed into a mass system, with an increase of 107 per cent in full-time students and with the number of enrolled 18–19-year-olds reaching 30 per cent. In addition, there has been an increase in part-time, postgraduate, overseas and female students.

Australia has experienced similar changes. Rapid expansion in higher education has ensured first-year, first-degree places for 36 per cent of Australia's 18-year-old high school leavers (IDP Education Australia, 1995). Further, the gender mix is almost exactly the reverse of 20 years ago; for example, in 1994 at the University of Sydney, 56 per cent of students were female, in contrast to the 60 per cent male student population there in 1974 (The University of Sydney Planning Office, 1995).

(d) Students with disabilities

Another change in the student cohort is the number of students who report some form of disability. In the United States, in 1992–3, more than 800,000 students with disabilities were enrolled in institutions of higher education (Henderson, 1995). During the 1992–3 academic year, orthopedic disabilities were the most often reported; other types included health-related disabilities and disabilites in hearing, learning, sight and speech. Sixty per cent of the graduate and professional students with disabilities were over 35; 36 per cent of undergraduates were over 35. Students with disabilities need appropriate accommodations for their learning needs, both in the classroom and in professional placements. These accommodations need to be achieved, whilst respecting the students' rights to privacy and confidentiality. In order to speak to issues of confidentiality in clinical education programmes in the United States, Kornblau (1995) has proposed DIALOGUE, a system to facilitate communication among students with disabilities, their clinical educators and the administrators of their university professional education programmes.

Case Study 9.6 Ensuring successful clinical placements for students with disabilities: A challenge for occupational therapy in the United States

Amy is 'a student with juvenile rheumatoid arthritis, [who] decides not to disclose her disability to her fieldwork supervisor [clinical educator] before beginning her placement. After four weeks on the placement, Amy's knee swells with fluid. She asks her supervisor if she may have the afternoon off to have her knee drained. The supervisor, considering Amy lazy because she always looks for opportunities to sit while she works, refuses' (Kornblau, 1995, p. 140). In the absence of a visible disability and without the student's disclosure, the clinical educator understandably fails to support Amy's accommodations of her disability. When Amy does eventually discuss her disability, the clinical educator complains to the university clinical education co-ordinator that she should have been informed.

(e) Cultural diversity in higher education

Concurrent with structural changes in higher education and changes in the student body has been the internationalization of higher education. Australian universities, like many in the United Kingdom and North America, now have overseas campuses, internationalized curricula and mobile students and staff. Of the 31,000 students enrolled at the University of Sydney in 1994, 11 per cent spoke as their first language Cantonese, Korean, Mandarin or Vietnamese (The University of Sydney Planning Office, 1995). Australia also has seen a significant increase of Aboriginal students within its universities (Maslen, 1995). Five years ago, only about 3,000 Aboriginal students attended Australian universities; the number is now 6,000. As a result of these changes in the student body, special preparation and support programmes for staff and students have been developed in an effort to provide students with high quality, culturally sensitive education and to increase completion rates.

Academic and administrative cohorts also are changing. In the United States, the percentage of people of colour in full-time academic positions increased by 48.6 per cent from 1981 to 1991, compared with a 7.6 per cent increase in white academics (Carter & Wilson, 1995). In the administrative ranks, the percentage of people of colour increased by 59.4 per cent from 1981 to 1991 (Carter & Wilson, 1995).

As cultural and ethnic diversity increases at universities, whether as a result of changes in academic staff, administrators, or students, cultural differences become an area of consideration. Clinical educators will need to enhance their own cross-cultural awareness and competence as they provide opportunities for students to enhance theirs.

(f) Change in approaches to learning and teaching

The increase of mature age or non-traditional learners in the traditional university classroom presents additional challenges. In the United States, individuals usually are categorized as non-traditional students when, as undergraduates, they are aged 25 or older, or if under 25, they did not proceed directly into higher education from secondary school or they interrupted their university experience by leaving and returning. In Australian universities, 30 per cent of first degree students are over the age of 25 years (IDP Education Australia, 1995). Mature age students enter the university rich in experience, often as part-timers and often juggling school, work and family demands. Mature age students can present considerable challenges to clinical educators experienced in teaching only young students (see Chapter 7).

Berquist and Smith (1992) note that non-traditional students are likely to be preparing for professional careers and may be entering the university disillusioned with traditional, fragmented academic ways of responding to complex society issues. These United States educators state, 'the traditional model of the learner in higher education is no longer valid' (p. 25) and suggest the need for educators to provide more 'connectedness' and 'relatedness.' They call for an educational model that is interactive and collaborative, believing that such a model is particularly useful to non-traditional learners. Tarule (1992), also concerned about non-traditional students, discusses classroom dialogue both as a necessary component of adult learning and as an epistemology.

A related problem is arising in Central and Eastern Europe, where academic staff may need to adapt their teaching styles and research methodologies for a new era. As Gotchev (1993) states about the social sciences in Bulgaria: 'University professors must become active researchers, stimulating intellectual inquiry and becoming directly involved with the students'

(p. 50). His argument is that prior to 1989, the 'main trends in social sciences research were explanatory and ideologically oriented' (p. 44) and that this aspect of higher education is one of the transition dilemmas higher education needs to face.

An issue for higher education worldwide is how to present intellectually current material to its students, that is, how to bring about student learning in areas with which current staff have little or no familiarity. Such situations pose numerous challenges for a staff, including issues of staff development.

Case Study 9.7 Utilizing professional community resources within higher education: Professional speech therapists teach a medically related course in the United States

The University of Georgia was faced with the need to offer its speech-language pathology students a course in dysphagia, but none of the academic staff felt sufficiently competent to teach it. Community professionals with expertise in the area were contacted and agreed to team teach a ten-week course, thus providing students with the most current medical information and clinical experience (Brasseur, 1995, p. 10). The programme, though experimental, illustrates a creative response to the curriculum-practice gap.

(g) Change in higher education: The impact of change in the professions

A current feature of higher education is the impact felt from changes within the professions themselves. In many countries, competency-based occupational standards have been introduced into the professions (Gonczi, 1994) (see Chapter 6). In Australia, such standards already are used in assessing overseas applicants for membership in professional associations. These standards also have the potential to significantly influence clinical education. Competency-based occupational standards also are being used by some professions to guide students' clinical education and point-of-graduation assessments. Understanding competency-based education and grounding it in appropriate educational theory is an additional challenge for clinical educators in many fields. See Case Study 9.8.

(h) Change in the goals of professional education

Professional education itself is under scrutiny. One of the ongoing discussions in the United States is the role of a liberal, humanistic education within professional education (Eisenhauer & O'Neil, 1995; Grumet, 1995;

Krieger, 1990). Usually, a student entering a four-year course of study within a health sciences or education field in the United States needs to devote about two years to a liberal arts, general education, or core curriculum that includes coursework in the arts, humanities, natural sciences and social and behavioural sciences. An additional two years of the bachelor's degree will be focused on professional coursework and experiences. The usual model of professional education in the United States is based on the belief that liberal arts education helps develop humanistic concerns, as well as the critical thinking needed for professional practice, for life-long learning and for reflection and action.

Case Study 9.8 Using competency-based occupational standards as a curriculum tool: A collaboration between the speech therapy profession and universities in Australia

When the professional association chose to delegate the assessment of graduates against its Competency-Based Occupational Standards (Australian Association of Speech and Hearing, 1994) to the six universities that have speech therapy programmes, it made practical and educational sense for the universities to integrate the standards into their curricula. Clinical education programme managers from the six universities secured a National Teaching Development Grant and also received funding from the professional association to develop *Indicators of Emerging Competence*, which students at different stages of clinical development and clinical educators could use to structure learning experiences and monitor their clinical development. Academic staff also can use these to structure subject curricula.

A number of self-directed packages that target various elements of competence were written for students. Tutorial packages on the use of the Standards and the Indicators were written for staff and students. All the products of the grant were developed using student and staff consultation and were piloted around the country (Worrall *et al.*, 1996). Students feel they better understand what they are aiming to achieve and how to get there; staff feel they understand how better to facilitate students to achieve professional competence.

Although the United States model is not universally shared, the need to develop critical and humanistic thinking probably is. In the United Kingdom and Australia, professional preparation programmes begin immediately after secondary school and do not have the tradition of a liberal arts curriculum as part of the course of study. Typically, the entering first-year student is 18 to 19. Without the assistance of a liberal arts curriculum, clinical educators in these countries face the challenge of helping young adults develop skills of critical thinking, recognize the provisional nature of knowledge and learn to see human experience from more than one perspective. These educators, as well as their counterparts everywhere, face the challenge of working with young adults still in the process of developing moral and ethical positions (see Chapter 7).

In discussing how best to prepare future professionals in the United States, Krieger (1990), an academic in urban planning, argues the importance of the workshop (studio, clinic) model. He envisions an educational approach that would allow a team of students to take on the full complexity of actual situations and figure out what to do. Krieger notes the importance of educating for leadership, for skills in mediation and for skills that have to do with reframing issues, all skills that regularly are needed in the professional workplace. Such a model of professional education would be interdisciplinary and holistic, as opposed to disciplinary and fragmented.

The whole construct of professional education in the health sciences is also under discussion also as a result of changes in health care delivery, in consumer expectations and in the need for cost containment. The Pew Health Professions Commission in the United States took an indepth look at education in the health professions (Broski, 1992). The Commission's five recommendations 'frame the major themes that would enable allied health to contribute all that it is capable of contributing to our nation's health and health services' (p. 43). The report discusses such issues as curricular reform, unification of academic and clinical experiences, outcome standards for accreditation, service delivery in racially and culturally diverse societies, life-long learning and teamwork.

Clinical educators everywhere are part of a higher education system attempting to renew itself. The movement for reform appears universal and is occurring in the context of increasing diversity in the student, staff and client base. Although these changes provide enormous challenges for clinical educators, they also provide exciting opportunities for innovations in teaching and learning.

The last significant area of change to be considered in this discussion is occurring within professional practice and the professional lives of practitioners themselves.

9.3.3 CHANGE IN PROFESSIONAL PRACTICE

As the demographics of populations change, there also will be changes in who requires services and who delivers them. The nature of services delivered also is subject to change, as is the manner in which they are delivered. These changes will be explored in the following sections.

(a) Change in the profiles of the professions

As both client and student cohorts change, it is to be expected that the practitioner base itself will change. In the United States, in Communication Disorders, this change is happening exceedingly slowly. As Cole (1992) notes, 'A stark contrast exists between the number of certified speech-language pathologists and audiologists from racial/ethnic minority backgrounds and the total racial/ethnic minority population of this nation' (p. 39). Although the number of minority professionals in this particular field continues to increase, it still represents an embarrassingly small figure. From 1980 to 1991, minority membership in the American Speech-Language-Hearing Association rose only from 2 to 4 per cent (Cole, 1992, p. 39)

In Australia the data may be somewhat similar. Although the minority membership of the Australian Association of Speech and Hearing is not known, it is known that 21 per cent of members speak a language other than English. It is not known whether this is as a first or subsequent language. Most speak a European language, with French, German and Italian accounting for 50 per cent of the languages other than English (Australian Association of Speech and Hearing, 1995). Individuals who speak an Asian or South East Asian language constitute only 4.5 per cent of the membership and only a few speak these languages as their first language.

The emerging profile in health professions is a mismatch with the linguistic and cultural profile of the country. For example, D'Cruz and Tham (1993) found that although 14.7 per cent of nursing students in the state of Victoria, Australia, in the years 1988 to 1990 came from non-English-speaking backgrounds, a figure similar to the community figure, the students came from groups other than the major cultural and linguistic subgroups of the community.

(b) Change in professional work practices

Professional practice itself also is changing and professional associations are attempting to offer guidance. The focus of the 1995 National Conference of the Australian Association of Speech and Hearing (AASH) was 'Professional Excellence and Diversity'. Programs and papers presented examples of speech therapists undertaking workplace conflict resolution, government liaison, marketing and public relations work (AASH, 1995). Similarly, the focus of the 1995 Annual Conference on Graduate Education in Communication Sciences and Disorders in the United States was 'restructure' (Bernthal, 1995). An additional example comes from *Asha*, the magazine of the American Speech-Language-Hearing Association, which frequently focuses on the changing roles of health science practitioners in general and speech therapists and audiologists in particular. Recent topics include cost containment, marketing, use of support personnel and a team approach to intervention (Ashby, 1995).

Among the changes is an increased pressure to demonstrate outcome effectiveness. Before functional outcomes of intervention in the health sciences can be described, however, clinical indicators need to be developed. Many professions throughout the world are engaged in this difficult process. Thus, for example, in Communication Disorders in the United States, there is an enhanced emphasis on functional assessment of clients. Daily functional behaviours such as social communication, communication of basic needs, daily planning and reading, writing and number concepts become areas to assess for outcome effectiveness (Frattali, Thompson, Holland, Wohl & Ferketic, 1995). An ongoing challenge in the face of managed accountability is the humanistic value of retaining a focus on the individual and the personal. Clinical educators have a particular responsibility to respond to this challenge as they work with the next generation of practitioners.

Venues for professional service delivery also are changing. Forty years ago, when one of us began her undergraduate coursework in Communication Disorders in the United States, the service delivery sites were primarily public schools. Contrast this to the following listing of 'service locations' by the United Kingdom's College of Speech and Language Therapists (1991): acute hospitals, long-stay institutions, rehabilitation centres, community clinics, specialist out-patient clinics, day centres (including adult training centres, social education centres and resource centres), supported living and group homes, domiciliaries (clients' homes), day nurseries, child development centres, mainstream schools, special schools, language units and nursery schools. The situation is similar in other countries. Clearly, as venues change, the way clinical practicum is provided needs to change. Clinical educators whose work experiences have been limited may find working in new venues particularly challenging.

(c) Change in information technology

Another area of change in professional practice in any field concerns electronic access to people and to information. Whether it is Januszkiewicz (1991) discussing the use of distance education as a desirable area of European cooperation, or Woodard (1995) discussing access to global information networks by Central and Eastern European universities, the expansion of technology is a major phenomenon. Whether the technology involves the use of electronic mail, information storage, improved administrative services, data available on CD-ROM, commercial curricular software, multimedia presentations, or distance learning, clinicians and clinical educators need to increase their sophistication. Information technology already is making a difference in service delivery models, as well as in clinical education approaches.

It perhaps can be assumed that many clinical educators in industrialized countries have replaced typewriters with word processors; it cannot be assumed that they use electronic mail (e-mail) as a major resource for scholarly and collegial communication. It also cannot be assumed that most clinical educators regularly use on-line information resources, whether they be through bibliographic data banks or World Wide Web pages. Nor can it be assumed that most clinical educators are sophisticated in electronic publishing, multimedia databases or multimedia presentations. It probably can be assumed that many students are more sophisticated than their clinical educators in many of the new technologies.

Distance learning as a specific use of technology presents an immediate challenge for clinical educators as universities recruit and train students from rural areas and as professionals in rural areas seek to upgrade their skills. As higher education worldwide responds to issues of financing and access, distance education is destined to play a major role, whether the technologies used are conventional telephone lines, fibre-optic networks, micro-relays, satellite down-links, or compressed video.

Case Study 9.9 Linking health care workers around the world: A computer-based telecommunications system

Through the use of low-earth-orbit satellites, ground stations, and telephone networks, a system trademarked as 'HealthNet' allows health workers primarily in Africa and Asia to be in contact with one another, to hold electronic conferences, to have access to worldwide databases and health care centers, and to receive a number of publications (see SatelLife, n.d.). HealthNet is administered by a non-profit organization founded by Nobel peace prize winner, Dr Bernard Lown in the United States. The telecommunications systems responds to two major health care issues: cost of services and access to information. This system allows, for example, a physician or health care provider in an isolated region to be in contact with experts in a timely manner.

The ability to offer opportunities for distance learning intersects with societal issues of cost containment, consumer expectations and increased access to the programmes of study offered by higher education. Mature age students with families and jobs, who want to become allied health professionals or who want to upgrade their skills and who might live a distance away from a professional programme, may seek to take at least some coursework via distance technologies. Many programmes already are in place (for example, Professional Growth, 1995). A future question may be how to manage supervized practicum through distance learning.

Another issue has to do with computer literacy: What is it and how is it developed? Lyman (1995) states that 'mass communication and information technology are texts for the critical mind, different from, but not the opposite of print' (p. 15). Clinical educators, often not trained in the 'texts' of information technology, have an obligation to help students learn to make critical judgements about the authority of information gained through such texts. Not only do images only simulate reality, some images represent a created reality, not a material reality. Although in principle, this may be no different from the study of visual design or art, the access to such information is very different. How then does the clinical educator assist the student in knowing the 'truth' of such information?

Trying to understand information technologies is like trying to hit a moving target. New developments occur daily and the patterns of change are hard to perceive. Nevertheless, the impact of the new technologies represents a major societal change to which clinical educators must respond.

In this section we have discussed how the changes in the professions and professional practice have an impact on who delivers services, what services are delivered and how those services are delivered. We have noted implications for clinical educators and shared stories of how clinical educators are responding creatively to these changes.

Thus far in this chapter, we have identified three areas of significant change affecting clinical educators and clinical education: changes in population, higher education and professional practice. We turn now to a discussion of three areas we consider to be major challenges facing clinical educators.

9.4 CHALLENGES

Clinical educators need to reflect only briefly to realize that they must design educational programmes that truly prepare students for the future world of work. Because of their unique responsibilities relative to the next generation of professionals, clinical educators should be leaders who are sensitive to the implications of societal and professional changes. If clinical educators fail, the next generation will enter the workforce unprepared for what society presents (and what society expects).

What will clinical education look like in the future? Rather than imagining how clinical education will be different, we have identified three significant areas especially challenging for clinical educators to consider as they respond to change:

- development of cross-cultural awareness and competence
- incorporation of gender factors in education and practice
- recognition of social responsibility brought about through global interconnectivity.

9.4.1 CROSS-CULTURAL AWARENESS AND COMPETENCE

A significant challenge for clinical education worldwide is to educate students to work successfully across cultures, whether the work is in their own backyard or in another country. Hughes (1992), examining multicultural issues in the United States, believes the future rests with people who 'can think and act with informed grace across ethnic, cultural, linguistic lines' (p. 47). Writing about individuals working in the global marketplace, Bikson and Law (1995) note the importance of becoming *competent*, not merely sensitive. Awareness or sensitivity is a first step, but the training cannot stop there. Competencies must be identified and learned.

Case Study 9.10 Threading cultural awareness and cultural competence throughout an institution: An United States university's approach

The University of Texas Medical Branch (UTMB) is located in the island community of Galveston, where one-fifth of the population is Hispanic. More than 50 per cent of the population of the island is non-white. The UTMB offers professional preparation for doctors, nurses, allied health professionals and biomedical scientists. Thorpe and Baker (1995) describe a multi-strand programme aimed at promoting cultural competence in students as well as in the academic and health care staff associated with UTMB. There is an active programme of recruitment and retention of minority and disadvantaged students. Classes in medical and conversational Spanish are offered to all employees. Leaders in each field are trained in prejudice reduction and conflict resolution, and there are networks that promote multicultural awareness and understanding. Many of the health care staff are bilingual, and students are placed with these clinicians for clinical placements in a variety of settings. Objectives for the achievement of cultural competence are written for academic coursework and university teaching staff are active in research that focuses on the health and culture of the Hispanic American population.

(a) Promoting cross-cultural awareness and competence: The roles of professional and government bodies

In the health sciences and education, professional associations and government councils are giving guidance to practitioners as they upgrade both their levels of awareness and their repertoire of skills. In Australia, such initiatives often are derived from the professions' growing recognition of the needs of their diverse client groups, somewhat pre-empting the promulgation of the government's policies. For example, the Australian Association of Speech and Hearing has had a Multicultural Interest Group since the mid-1980s. This national network examines issues of multiculturalism and diversity within the field of Communication Disorders; it regularly holds state-level seminars, collates resources for members and publishes a bulletin.

The nursing professions in Australia and New Zealand have been prominent in highlighting the needs for cross-cultural communication and cultural safety in both the education of health professionals and in service delivery. Australian nurses held their first transcultural nursing conference in 1992, the same year that Kanitsaki (1992) published an introductory teaching package on transcultural nursing for nurse educators. This trend parallels the initiatives of government bodies such as the Transcultural Health Care Council (1991), which published a strategic plan for a transcultural approach to education of health professionals and for service delivery in the Australian state of Victoria.

In the United States, the American Speech-Language-Hearing Association also plays a major leadership role in increasing the awareness of diversity within the client populations served by its membership. Further, the Association considers the management of diversity to be a 'strategic long-term process', that 'requires a culture and systems change' (Goldberg, 1994, p. 45).

Other resources for clinical educators, in addition to their governments and professional associations, include scholarly literature. One such resource is Adler's (1993) work, which is intended for classroom teachers, special educators and speech therapists.

(b) Skills for cross-cultural awareness and competence

There is no one definitive source for understanding the skills needed for cross-cultural work. Lynch (1992), a special education professor, discusses the development of cross-cultural competence within three primary areas: self-awareness, culture-specific understanding and communication (p. 35). She stresses listening to the family's perspective and respecting rather than minimizing cultural differences.

The work of national and international businesses can be a good resource on understanding and meeting this challenge. In order to respond to changing population demographics in globally competitive markets, businesses have had to be responsive to issues of diversity in the workplace (for example, Deane, 1994; Evans, 1993; Howard, 1994). The early stages of diversity work might be considered to be training in awareness and valuing of differences. Currently the focus is shifting to a skill or competency focus (for example, Bikson & Law, 1995; Deane, 1995; Evans & Martinez, 1995). The business world is finding that awareness is not enough; appropriate skill usage is required.

Deane (1995), among others, has identified cross-cultural communication skills that include skills of listening, conflict resolution, negotiation, team work, group process, dialogue and systems thinking. The ability to understand issues from multiple perspectives becomes a major skill, with the concomitant ability to change one's frame of reference. Other key skills include becoming sufficiently knowledgeable about cultures different from one's own in order to give culturally appropriate feedback and becoming sufficiently flexible to accept approaches different from one's own.

Work in intercultural communication is a major resource for both practice and theory. Weiss (1992), for example, discusses four modes of intercultural encounters, citing Yoshikawa's work: the ethnocentric mode, the control mode, the dialectical mode and the dialogical mode. The latter is the one that strives for *inter*dependence, in which the participants work to establish areas of commonality across their differences, while allowing their differences to retain their 'identity-giving significance' (Weiss, 1992, p. 15). This theoretical perspective can be the grounding for developing communication skills that are based in a collaborative, respective stance, as opposed to an ethnocentric, paternalistic, or colonial stance. Such skills include listening, questioning, giving feedback and managing conflict. See Case Studies 9.11 and 9.12.

Case Study 9.11 Developing cross-cultural competence: Occupational therapy education in the United Kingdom

The occupational therapy programme at the University College of Ripon and St John has developed an integrated approach to cultural competence in its students (McDonald & Rowe, 1995), as opposed to having discrete academic units on transcultural practice, a model often adopted elsewhere (Leininger, 1978). The latter approach has been criticized for leading to simplified cultural stereotyping and the perpetuation of notions of difference. The method chosen by McDonald and Rowe integrates a case history approach into all years of the course of study, employs visiting lecturers from minority groups, and runs workshops on topics such as 'valuing the individual' and on issues associated with particular community groups. The students complete assignments and projects that encourage them to reflect on multicultural working environments and transcultural practice.

(c) Cross-cultural awareness and competence: Insights from anthropology

The intersection of health care and anthropology generates ideas useful to clinical educators. Kleinman (1980), a psychiatrist trained in anthropology, notes that health care occurs within three different cultural environments: the popular arena, the folk arena and the professional arena. The popular arena relates to issues of health care within the circle of family and friends and in some societies, the media. The folk arena can include sacred healing, herbalism and particular systems of exercise. The professional arena is comprised of the organized healing professions of a given society. Kleinman believes these arenas to be present across cultures, but with differing content. Thus how an Anglo-Celtic social worker in London understands and experiences professional health care may be very different from how an immigrant Chinese client in London has experienced it. Different societies manage illness differently in each arena; thus when cultures are crossed, mixed, or merged, the possibility for misunderstanding is immense.

Case Study 9.12 Developing cross-cultural competence: An experiential approach in nursing education in Canada

The McMaster University School of Nursing has integrated experiential learning activities designed to teach transcultural nursing principles into its problem-based curriculum. The emphasis is less on culture specific content than on facilitating change from ethnocentrism to awareness of difference, acceptance (or rejection), valuing, and adaptation. Carpio and Majumdar (1992) describe the setting of a climate favourable to acceptance and change, games that introduce students to cross-cultural experiences, the use of simulation to highlight cross-cultural communication issues, and initiatives taken by students to obtain information and understand other cultures.

Another concept from anthropology that can be useful in cross-cultural understanding comes from Hall's (1976, 1983) work on high and low context societies. Briefly put, high context societies are relatively homogeneous and individuals do not need to communicate extensive information verbally. The context (experiences, history, tacit information) is shared by the participants; thus it does not need to be talked about. Low context societies are relatively diverse and the communication partners cannot assume a shared context. Emphasis then is placed on words and oral interaction. Practitioners from low context societies, accustomed to the importance of oral and other forms of verbal communication, interacting with clients from high context societies, are likely to encounter significant communication differences. Lynch (1992) provides an interesting discussion on communication in high and low context cultures.

As noted earlier, changes in populations and in higher education are bringing about a diverse client and student base with whom clinical educators must work. We believe that to provide exemplary clinical services and concurrent learning opportunities for students, clinical educators need to be cross-culturally competent. They must be able to promote cross-cultural awareness and sensitivity in their students. In our case studies, we have provided examples of how some programmes are striving to meet the challenge for cross-cultural competence.

A second challenge within professions worldwide pertains to men, women and gender.

9.4.2 MEN, WOMEN AND GENDER

The prevalence of female practitioners is one of the most noticeable facets of the health sciences and education. In Communication Disorders in the United States, male speech therapists constitute less than 7 per cent of the total association membership (Werven, 1994). In Australia, males comprise only 3.4 per cent of the membership of the Australian Association of Speech and Hearing (Australian Association of Speech and Hearing, 1995). These figures are similar for related fields: in the United States, the physiotherapy workforce is 74.6 per cent women; in occupational therapy it is 94.3 per cent (Montgomery, 1995). In the United States in Communication Disorders, the current percentages are remarkably different from the early days of the profession, when 40 per cent of the original members of the predecessor association were men (Werven, 1994).

(a) Gender stereotyping in the professions

Among the many issues raised by these demographics is gender stereotyping in the professions. How can men be attracted to fields traditionally associated with female behaviours and interests? Might professions want to consider the advantage of humans being nurtured, treated and educated by both men and women (Werven, 1994)? When one sex predominates in a field, the need for dialogue across the sexes and across gender stereotypes is an important consideration (Shapiro, 1994). Gender issues also touch on compensation issues. In many fields men are higher paid than women for similar work and men often are the heads of various units or programmes. A question for clinical educators concerns whether they should be training the next generation of professionals so that they can respond appropriately to various professional inequities and patterns.

(b) Gender and culture based communication differences in educational settings

The practice of co-education of women and men in professional education raises the issue of 'classroom climates', whether the classroom be the traditional university one, clinic or laboratory. In the United States, much has been written about the classroom climate encountered by female students in higher education (for example, Hall & Sandler, 1982; Lewis & Simon, 1986; Sandler & Hall, 1986). In classrooms designed for the young adult male, women experience being 'different' in ways both subtle and overt. In particular, Hall and Sandler (1982) suggest that staff (male and female) may:

- make eye contact more often with male students than with female
- respond non-verbally more to men's questions and comments than to women's
- use a patronizing or impatient tone when responding to women, but not with men
- allow women to be on a group's margins during laboratory demonstrations
- give men more detailed answers to questions
- assume a body posture of interest when listening to men and doing the opposite when listening to women
- interrupt female students and allow male students to do likewise.

The list can be expanded; it also can be extended to minority groups in the classroom.

The changing student cohort in educational settings is a compounding factor in gender communication. Increasingly, clinical educators encounter mature age students and people of colour, representing a variety of racial and ethnic backgrounds. It has become imperative for educators to understand this population of learners and the communication and cultural styles they present (Pearson, Shavlik & Touchton, 1989). Nieves-Squires (1991) believes that cultural and communication differences account for much of the stress, misinterpretation and misunderstanding occurring in the classroom between Hispanic women and non-Hispanic professors. Further, a study currently in progress (Valuable Lessons, 1995) of three United States institutions serving significant numbers of older, returning students and/or women of colour, suggests that certain elements are necessary in order to have an educational climate where these students can flourish. Key elements appear to include extensive support systems, assessment of students' needs, feedback protocols and programmes to enhance self image.

Female and male communication and relationship patterns deserve detailed attention by clinical educators. Issues specifically within supervision, such as relationship maintenance, discourse patterns, status, hierarchy and control, are being examined by writers in various fields (for example, Chernesky, 1986; Langellier & Natalle, 1987; McCready, Shapiro & Kennedy, 1987). Tannen (1990), a United States-based professor of linguistics, has examined male and female styles of communication and concludes 'male–female communication is cross-cultural communication' (p. 42). Clearly an understanding of gender styles can potentially open channels of communication across the gender-culture divide.

(c) Gender based communication styles in therapeutic settings

Male and female communication styles within clinical interactions evoke added complications, beyond those Tannen (1990) reports. In particular, what does a young female speech therapist need to know about male communication patterns as she works with young male head-injured clients (Bourne & Wilks, 1995)? Or with the single male parent of a language-disordered child? Or with the child himself? And conversely, what does the male student need to know about female communication as he provides services to females, especially older females whose numbers in the United States are projected to increase markedly by the year 2010 (Where The Boys Aren't, 1992). Gender-related communication issues become additionally compounded by the increased cultural diversity of the client base.

(d) Feminist and female issues in health professions

Feminism itself offers useful insights for clinical educators. Feminist discourse is providing an opportunity to challenge and change the traditional world view that is androcentric. In her articulation of a 'Feminist Vision for Clinical Education,' Pickering (1992) notes the importance of expanding ways of knowing beyond the traditional, in order to come to a realization that the world of human meaning consists of multiple realities. The assumption is that historically women's realities and ways of knowing have not been part of the traditional canon of most fields. Scholars are formulating feminist visions within their professions. In their application of feminist theory to social work, VanDenBergh and Cooper (1986b, pp 10–25), discuss five major premises of feminist analysis:

- eliminating false dichotomies and artificial separations within the knowledge base and practice of the field
- re-conceptualizing power so that therapeutic strategies would become directed toward the empowerment of clients
- valuing process equally with product, which acknowledges therapy as a learning experience
- renaming and claiming one's background, heritage and life story
- understanding the connection of personal problems with social realities.

These and other social work scholars apply their views to all phases of social work: practice; research; administration; social policy; and education, training and supervision (VanDenBergh & Cooper, 1986a).

The Platform for Action by the Fourth World Conference on Women held in Beijing, China, in September 1995, offers an additional and contemporary view of issues particularly affecting women (United Nations, 1995). The Conference is assumed to be the largest ever held by the United

Nations and the largest on women, with almost 50,000 people in attendance at the Conference and its parallel Non-Governmental Organisations
(NGO) Forum. United Nations members sending representatives totalled
181; in addition, non-members sent observers.

A consideration of the Platform for Action and its 12 areas of concern
makes it clear that the discourse around the needs of women is a worldwide phenomenon. It is also clear that women from the non-industrialized
world are speaking out loudly and strongly on issues that are of significant
and crucial importance relative to the advancement of women.

Because so much of reality, including the way universities educate, the
content taught and the prevailing world view of professional service and
structure, has been influenced predominantly by male experience and a
male-centered perspective, viewing the world from other perspectives
offers the opportunity for interpretations significantly different from traditional ones. Clinical educators, both women and men, should have a
particular interest in gender issues and factors that might illuminate their
relationships with their students, clients and colleagues.

The third challenge we discuss concerns obligations to the larger world.

9.4.3 SOCIAL RESPONSIBILITY AND GLOBAL INTERCONNECTIVITY

Federico Mayor, Director-General of the United Nations Educational,
Social and Cultural Organization (UNESCO) has sought to find ways 'in
which education can be employed to fashion a more tolerant and less vio-
lent world' (James, 1993, p. 17). He is unequivocal in his belief that this is
one of the responsibilities of education. Further, a recent and major
UNESCO report on 'Education for the 21st Century', discusses worldwide
interdependence and globalization and states that education has the 'task
of helping people to understand the world and to understand others'
(Delors *et al.*, 1996; p. 51).

(a) Education for social responsibility

Mayor's views can lead to the question of what is the role of professional
education relative to social responsibility. In the United States, the
assumption in most clinical education programmes probably would be
that social and cultural issues are handled by the humanities faculty when
the students take their general education core. That is, when the students
take their minimal number of courses in literature, science, history, arts
and philosophy, a link somehow will be made to the values of non-vio-
lence, equality and liberty. Educating students to be good citizens is even
less well defined in professional programmes in countries such as Australia, where students traditionally enter the university's professional programme straight out of secondary school, take their whole curriculum

within the professional framework and do not have a humanities or general education curriculum.

Mayor's focus on education relative to world issues is a view shared by the political scientists Rothchild and Groth (1995) in their discussion on domestic and international ethnicity. Following an analysis of ethnic conflict in the world, they indicate that responses 'by modern societies can only be anchored in the appropriate use of educational systems and mass communication media' (pp 81–2).

Other writers express concerns about education and social responsibility. United States educators Prakash and Waks (1985) argue for 'the adoption of the social responsibility conception of educational excellence as our national educational goal' (p. 79). In their articulation of this view, they posit four standards of educational excellence: mental proficiency, disciplinary initiation, self-actualization and social responsibility. Mental proficiency is viewed in its more mechanical dimensions of learning information, skills and problem-solving techniques. Disciplinary initiation moves into conceptual structures, whether they be historical, philosophical, mathematical, psychological or medical. Self-actualization relates to the development of the individual learner, his or her unique mind and personality. Social responsibility moves the education of the learner beyond the individual and into the larger group – local, regional, national, international. It places the student learner in the context of a community.

Can clinical educators adopt all four conceptions of excellence? Do clinical educators tend primarily toward mental proficiency and disciplinary initiation? If clinical educators were to attempt to integrate these four conceptions of excellence, including social responsibility, what might such a curriculum look like? Would there be, as Prakash and Waks (1985) imply, enhanced concern for communication skills that stress listening and empathy, as well as the ability to speak intelligently in public contexts? Following their argument further, would there be assignments in professional education that are shaped by a concern for 'cooperation and group interests' (p. 94)? Would clinical educators use case studies or critical incident discussions that identify ethical and moral issues?

(b) Social responsibility and cross-cultural awareness

Cole (1989), the president of an historic black woman's college in the United States, links social responsibility with cross-cultural awareness and a respect for human diversity. In discussing her hopes for higher education in the year 2000, Cole speaks of a community of scholars that 'would have learned how to discourage the perpetuation of systems of inequality' (p. 28). She writes of fostering a sense of social responsibility in students and of building that value into the curriculum through both coursework and social service projects. She states, 'In short, our institutions of higher education would consist of conscious and informed communities committed to local, national and international service' (p. 28). For her, such a curriculum would include having a student live for a time among people 'not of that student's own race, ethnic group, culture, or class' (p. 28).

What might a socially responsible curriculum for health professionals look like? How might it be developed and implemented? These are questions that all clinical educators need to consider. The challenge is particularly great in 'developing' countries.

Case Study 9.13 Creating alliances: Community involvement in designing a public health curriculum in Tonga

In pursuing the global goal of *Health for All by the Year 2000*, the Kingdom of Tonga sought to develop a public health training programme for its nurses. Traditionally its nurses had been trained in a curative-oriented model aimed at hospital-based practice. Tenn, Sovaleni, Latu, Fotu and Smith (1994) describe the process of working with a panoply of stakeholders to identify the desired objectives, appropriate curricula content, and appropriate curricula design for a public health nursing course. The stakeholders included agencies such as WHO and UNFPA, Tongan government bodies, non-government organizations, practising nurses, student nurses, other health care providers including doctors and village health care workers, agricultural and environmental organizations, and community groups holding traditional beliefs and practices, needs and expectations.

Consultation with the community was extensive and involved contacting people through diverse activities such as church choirs, craft groups, village meetings, men's kava parties, and funerals, which are described as important social events in Tonga (Tenn *et al.*, 1994, p. 144). The authors note that although the participatory process is not a concept embedded in Tongan cultural traditions, its use has lead to appropriation of the new curriculum and to active lobbying for its successful implementation. Evaluation of the curriculum, its implementation, and its outcomes was conducted across stakeholder groups, with positive outcomes.

The question of social responsibility leads to other questions for clinical educators, such as the question of tacit learning relative to the kinds of values that are implicitly inculcated as courses are taught, students are tested and professionals communicate with one another (Astin, 1989). Do clinical educators talk about cooperation while implicitly encouraging competitiveness, speak about team work while encouraging individualism, or discuss cross-cultural awareness while being critical of differences?

(c) Global interconnectivity and professional practice and education

The earlier discussions in this chapter on population diversity, higher education and information technology point to the fact of global interconnectivity, the fact of an increasingly interdependent world. It is probably the case that individuals are coming together and interacting (either face-to-face or via technology) in a way unprecedented in the history of the world, as a result of developments in technology, changes in immigration laws, various political upheavals and the ease of travel.

What does global interconnectivity mean for professional education? At the very least, it means that there is an intersection between what is happening in the world and the need to educate for cross-cultural awareness and competency within the local area. Surely, if one is in Hobart, Tasmania, Australia and has a child of the refugee Hmong peoples in the case load, knowledge about the family's home culture, their reason for immigrating to Australia, salient features of the home language and key facts about the native country can only help with the intervention and educational processes. The same is true when a teacher in the American state of Maine has an Eritrean child in her classroom.

Global interconnectivity leads to considering overseas and cross cultural learning and living. Are professional students encouraged to study overseas or to take a placement in a section of their home country where they would be living out-of-culture? Much can be learned from living out-of-culture, even for a brief time (see Case Study 9.1). In part, one learns that the rest of the world does not necessarily share or even value the cultural assumptions, norms and attitudes that seem so universal at home. This kind of learning has a direct relationship with what one needs to learn to work with clients different from oneself. The professional-in-training needs to learn and re-learn about the existence of multiple perspectives and the provisional nature of knowledge. Living out-of-culture can enhance that learning.

For some people, international involvement relates to a sense of social responsibility and the desire to offer professional assistance (Fain, 1990; Philips, 1990). Whatever the motivation for international work, the literature is replete with examples of professionals working on both short-term and long-term projects in societies where social services are less developed than 'at home'; for example, training a Nepalese medical team to work with cleft palate problems (Crabtree-Kampe, 1993). Those professionals interested in specific resources for international involvement can refer to Wilson (1994) and to Pickering (1994).

Working internationally is not all 'fun and festivals'. Working internationally raises questions of cultural imperialism and colonialism. It becomes imperative, as Pressman and Rudner (1990) point out, for the educational or rehabilitative goals and objectives of the host government and institution to be understood and for professionals in the host country to participate in the intervention strategies under consideration. If the guest professionals assume they can transpose their own goals, objectives, strategies and values, then they are engaging in a particular kind of paternalism and cultural imperialism. Pickering (1994) has written about the importance of professional-as-learner as an alternative model to professional-as-helper or professional-as-adventurer. With this model comes the concept of professionals working with others toward the 'gift of cultural interchange and shared learning' (Pickering, 1996).

An additional dimension of global interconnectivity is learning that within a field, professional practice around the world includes both common and differing elements. In Monahan's (1995 a,b) report of personal accounts of physiotherapy in Australia, Brazil, Germany, Hong Kong, Israel, South Africa and Taiwan, the clinical educator can identify numerous similar issues as well as differing models and regional variations underpining practice. Global work, study and interactions with one's professional colleagues increasingly are options for clinical educators. The dimensions of what this means for themselves, as well as students, is one of the newer issues for clinical educators.

In this chapter we have discussed three areas of change: in populations, higher education and professional practice and identified three sets of issues, among the many possibilities, that provide crucial challenges for clinical educators. We have discussed the challenges that cross-cultural awareness and competence, gender differences and social responsibility and global interconnectivity present for clinical educators. Through the case studies we have provided examples of creative responses by clinical educators and other professionals from around the world. The mosaic that has emerged for us (and we hope for the reader of both this chapter and the other chapters in this book) is truly one of change, challenge *and* creativity.

9.5 CONCLUSION

9.5.1 MARISUE PICKERING

A recent book review quoting Sanford Ungar in his book *Fresh Blood: The New American Immigrants*, states, 'To be American, Mr Ungar says, "is being part of an ever more heterogeneous people" and to take part in a constant redefinition of its fabric' (American immigrants, 1995, p. 93). I am quite taken with the phrase 'redefinition of its fabric', as that seems to me to be what professional and personal life truly is about: we are constantly needing to redefine what we are about. As I write this, I am listening to National Public Radio in the United States and have heard a story about a grocery chain in the state of Texas that has completely redefined itself to meet the shopping needs of low-income people from a variety of immi-grant communities and to do so in a considerate, creative, sensitive and gracious way. Clinical education is not alone in its efforts to change.

Writing my parts of this chapter has allowed me to take a broader per-spective on many of the issues facing my university on a daily basis. It has allowed me to re-conceptualize much of what I experience in the United States and in my recent work assignments in the countries of Bulgaria and Australia. It has been an educational, interesting and energizing exper-ience.

Redefining our professional lives is not easy, but a lot of people are working very hard to do it well and I am convinced we can learn from one another about how to make change a positive experience and how to effect positive change. I also remain convinced that a major guiding principle has to do with treating one another well during the difficult process of change.

9.5.2 LINDY MCALLISTER

As I sit to write the conclusion of this chapter and of the book, I find myself thinking once again of my final year student Sally who last week returned from her experience as a volunteer involved with four local community-based rehabilitation (CBR) workers in establishing an early intervention programme in a 'remote' region of an Asian country. To my amazement, the project was not so 'remote' – we had been able to maintain fax contact with Sally, and, she reported, the Australian paediatrician at the hospital who originally invited her to participate in the project is newly connected to the world by email.

As I listened to Sally's stories and looked at some of her photos, I was struck by how much she had grown as a person and a professional in such a short space of time. I can not imagine an experience more likely to have evoked deep approaches to learning and peer learning as described in this book. Sally drew on all her personal and professional attributes – commu-nication skills, team skills, negotiation skills, cross-cultural awareness, a sense of personal agency, application of knowledge and skills into new and uncertain environments. She was attentive to the cultural differences of dress, food, lifestyle, religion and communication. She dressed in local attire. She learned basic greetings and phrases, for example, colours, num-bers, body parts and 'point to' in the local language. She organized ses-sions and home visits with CBR workers in a way that fitted with the local organization of time and daily activities.

Sally struggled to become cross-culturally competent. She consulted with other international staff who had been in the country for some time as to how to ask for and give feedback on skills without risking loss of face for either party. She learned to negotiate in a tactful and ethical manner, some of the expectations placed on her as visiting 'expert'. She worked with the local CBR workers within a model of consultative supervision, recognizing their expertise.

Listening to Sally's stories, I believe she functioned as an adult learner engaged in that exciting process of life-long learning. Through the provision of clinical education grounded in adult learning approaches, I believe our programme empowered her to use adult learning approaches with the clients and the project team members. I am looking forward to hearing more of her stories about the contexts, challenges and changes – there is a lot to learn!

REFERENCES

Adler, S. (1993). *Multicultural communication skills in the classroom*. Needham Heights, MA: Allyn & Bacon.

Akiwumi, A. (1994). In search of the 21st century nurse for Ghana. *International Nursing Review*, **41** (4), 118–22.

American immigrants: Mixed reception (1995, 4 November). *The Economist*, **337** (7939), 92–3.

Ashby, S. (1995). The renaissance professional: Doing more with less. *Asha*, **37** (6/7), 32–6.

Astin, A. (1989). Curriculum in the year 2000: Perspectives. *Liberal Education*, **75** (1), 26.

Australian Association of Speech and Hearing (1994). *Competency-based occupational standards*. Melbourne: Author.

Australian Association of Speech and Hearing (1995). Professional excellence and divesity, AASH 1995 national conference programme and summaries of papers. Melbourne: Author.

Australian Association of Speech and Hearing (1995, December). Personal communication.

Australian Bureau of Statistics (1993). *Australia's Aboriginal and Torres Strait Islander population: 1991 census of population and housing*. Canberra: Author.

Bergquist, W. & Smith, R. (1992). Research and scholarship: New challenges and strategies for serving nontraditional learners. *Liberal Education*, **78** (4), 20–5.

Bernthal, J. (Ed.) (1995). *Proceedings of the Annual Conference on Graduate Education*. Minneapolis, MN: Council of Graduate Programs in Communication Sciences and Disorders.

Berube, B. (1994, October). *Data collection report on language minority children*. Augusta, ME: State of Maine, Department of Education, Federal Projects for Language Minorities, Bureau of Administrative Services.

Bikson, T. & Law, S. (1995). Toward the borderless career: Corporate hiring in the '90s. *International Educator*, **IV** (2), 12–15, 32–3.

Blacks in America: The other half (1995, 4 November). *The Economist*, **337** (7939), 35.

Brasseur, J. (1995). Council of Graduate Programs in Communication Sciences and Disorders (CGPCSD) Sixteenth Annual Conference. *SUPERvision*, **19** (3), 6–12.

Bourne, W. & Wilks, V. (1995, Spring). A group to retrain male communication skills. *Australian Communication Quarterly*, 24–5.

Boyer, E., Altbach, P. & Whitelaw, M. (1994). *The academic profession: An interna-*

tional perspective. Princeton: The Carnegie Foundation for the Advancement of Teaching.

Broski, D. (Ed.). (1992). Healthy America: Practitioners for 2005 (Special Issue). *Journal of Allied Health,* **21** (4).

Carpio, B. & Majumdar, B. (1992). Experiential learning: An approach to transcultural education for nursing. *Journal of Transcultural Nursing,* **4** (2), 4–11.

Carter, D. & Wilson, R. (1995). *Minorities in higher education: 1994 thirteenth annual status report.* Washington, DC: American Council on Education.

Chernesky, R. (1986). A new model of supervision. In N. Van Den Bergh & L. Cooper (Eds). *Feminist visions for social work* (pp 128–48). Silver Springs, MD: National Association of Social Workers.

The Chronicle of Higher Education Almanac (1995, 1 September). The nation: Students, p. 14. Washington, DC: *The Chronicle of Higher Education.*

Cole, L. (1992). We're serious. *Asha,* **34** (5), 38–9.

Cole, J. (1989). Curriculum in the year 2000: Perspectives. *Liberal Education,* **75** (1), 28.

College of Speech and Language Therapists (1991). Communicating quality: Professional standards for speech and language therapists. London: Author.

Commonwealth Department of Health and Human Services (1995). *Best practice in the health sector: Overview of projects funded in the first round.* Canberra: Author.

Council for Aboriginal Reconciliation: An introduction (1991). Department of Prime Minister and Cabinet, Aboriginal Reconciliation Unit. Canberra: Australian Government Publishing Service.

Crabtree-Kampe, R. (1993). ASHA ABROAD: Cleft lip/palate team in Nepal. *Asha,* **35** (4), 22.

D'Cruz, J. & Tham, G. (1993). *Nursing and nursing education in multicultural Australia.* Brunswick, Victoria, Australia: David Lovell Publishing.

Deane, B. (1994). Diversity means negotiating change. *Cultural Diversity at Work,* **6** (6), 1–6.

Deane, B. (1995). Cultural competencies: Serious business requirements. *Cultural Diversity at Work,* **8** (1), 10.

Delors, J., Al Mufti, I., Amagi, I., Carneiro, R., Chung, F., Geremek, B., Gorham, W., Kornhauser, A., Manley, M., Quero, M., Savane, M., Singh, K., Stavenhagen, R., Suhr, M. & Nanzhao, Z. (1996). Learning: The treasure within. *Report to UNESCO of the International Commission on Education for the Twenty-first Century.* London: HMSO Books.

Eisenhauer, L. & O'Neil, J. (1995). Synthesis and praxis: Liberal education and nursing. *Liberal Education,* **81** (1), 12–17.

European Association for International Education (1995). *The cultures of education, 7th annual EAIE conference programme.* Amsterdam: Author.

Evans, S. (1993). Resolving conflicts with diverse groups. *Cultural Diversity at Work,* **5** (3), 4–5.

Evans, S. & Martinez, M. (1995). Skills-focused diversity training. *Cultural Diversity at Work,* **8** (1), 8–9.

Fain, M. (1990). Opportunities for service in third world countries. *Asha,* **32** (5), 45–7.

Francese, P. (1995). America at mid-decade. *American Demographics,* **17** (2), 23–9.

Frattali, C., Thompson, C., Holland, A., Wohl, C. & Ferketic, M. (1995). The FACS of life ASHA FACS: A functional outcome measure for adults. *Asha,* **37** (4), 40–6.

Gaither, G., Nedwek, B. & Neal, J. (1994). *Measuring up: The promises and pitfalls of performance indicators in higher education.* ASHE-ERIC Higher Education Report No. 5. Washington, DC: The George Washington University, Graduate School of Education and Human Development.

Goldberg, B. (1994). Managing diversity: It's common sense. *Asha,* **36** (6/7), 44–8.

Gonczi, A. (1994). Competency based assessment in the professions in Australia. *Assessment in Education,* **1** (1), 27–44.

Governor's Commission to Promote the Understanding of Diversity in Maine (1994). *Diversity in Maine: Facing hate, feeling hope: Final report of the Governor's Commission to Promote the Understanding of Diversity in Maine.* Augusta, ME: Author.

Gotchev, A. (1993). Education and research in the social sciences: Transition dilemmas in Bulgaria. *East European Politics and Societies,* **7** (1), 43–58.

Grumet, M. (1995). Lofty actions and practical thoughts: Education with purpose. *Liberal Education,* **81** (1), 4–11.

Gundykunst, W. & Kim, Y. (1992). *Communicating with strangers: An approach to intercultural communication.* New York: McGraw Hill.

Hall, E. (1976). *Beyond culture.* Garden City, NY: Anchor Books.

Hall, E. (1983). *The dance of life.* New York: Anchor Books/Doubleday.

Hall, R. & Sandler, B. (1982, February). *The classroom climate: A chilly one for women?* Washington, DC: Association of American Colleges.

Hansen, K. & Bachu, A. (1995, August). *The foreign-born population: 1994.* Current Population Reports, Census Bureau, P20–486. Washington, DC: United States Department of Commerce, Economics and Statistics Administration.

Hartley, S. (1995a). Reports. *ASHA in the world,* **6** (1), 2–3. (Available from International Affairs Association, c/o Margo Wilson, Editor, 8039 E. Cholla St., Scottsdale, AZ 85260, USA)

Hartley, S. (1995b, March). *Report of the study day in London.* (Available from Communication Therapy International, c/o Mrs Sally Hartley, Carlton Green Farm, Saxmundham, Suffolk IP17 2QN, UK)

Hayhoe, R. (1995). An Asian multiversity? Comparative reflections on the transition to mass higher education in East Asia. *Comparative Education Review,* **39** (3), 299–321.

Henderson, C. (1995). *Postsecondary students with disabilities: Where are they enrolled?* ACE Research Brief Series, Vol. 6, No. 6. Washington, DC: American Council on Education.

Hillard, S., Tronolone, V., Mendel, M., Manning, W. & Taylor, M. (1994). Face to FASCE with strangers: The challenge of cultural diversity. *Asha,* **36** (12), 31–3.

Howard, W. (1994). The next step: Building and sustaining relationships. *Cultural Diversity at Work,* **6** (5), 3–4.

Hughes (1992, 3 February). The fraying of America. *Time,* pp 44–9.

Hughes, J. (1995). Financing constraints transform British higher education. *World Education News & Review,* **8** (3), 10–19.

International Development Program Education Australia (1995). *Curriculum development for internationalisation: Australian case studies and stock take.* A study conducted for the OECD, on behalf of the Department of Employment, Education and Training. Canberra: Australian Government Printing Service.

Jager, G. (1994). Community based education in speech pathology and audiology at the University of Durban-Westville in an under served community. *The South African Journal of Communication Disorders,* **41**, 93–102.

James, B. (1993, 17 February). UNESCO panel to ponder the challenge to education of creating a new humanism. *International Herald Tribune*, p. 17.

Januszkiewicz, F. (1991). Polish higher education in a changing Europe: Selected problems and research suggestions. *Higher Education in Europe*, **XVI** (3), 78–86.

Jelsma, J., Cortes-Meldrum, D., Moyo, A. & Powell, G. (1995). The Children's Rehabilitation Unit, Harare, Zimbabwe: An integrated model of rehabilitation. *Pediatric Physical Therapy*, **7** (3), 140–2.

Jones, B. (1992). *House of Representatives Standing Committee for Long Term Strategies, Expectations of Life: Increasing the options*. Canberra: Australian Government Printing Services.

Kamien, M. & Buttfield, I. (1990). Some solutions to the shortage of general practitioners in rural Australia. Part 2: Undergraduate education. *Medical Journal of Australia*, **153**, 107–12.

Kanitsaki, O. (1992). *Transcultural nursing: An introductory teaching package for nurse lecturers and teachers*. Melbourne: La Trobe University.

Kayser, H. (1994). Service delivery issues for multicultural populations. In R. Lubinski & C. Frattali (Eds). *Professional issues in speech-language pathology and audiology* (pp 282–92). San Diego, CA: Singular Publishing Group.

Kleinman, A. (1980). *Patients and healers in the context of culture: An exploration of the borderland between anthropology, medicine, and psychiatry*. Los Angeles, CA: University of California Press.

Koch, C. & Maserang, J. (1994). Population-oriented nursing: Preparing tomorrow's nurses today. *Journal of Nursing Education*, **33** (5), 236–7.

Kornblau, B. (1995). Fieldwork education and students with disabilities: Enter the Americans with Disabilities Act. *The American Journal of Occupational Therapy*, **49**, 139–45.

Krieger, M. (1990). Broadening professional education: On the margins and between the niches. *Liberal Education*, **76** (2), 6–10.

Lack, J. & Templeton, J. (1995). *Bold experiment: A documentary history of Australian immigration since 1945*. Melbourne: Oxford University Press.

Lambert, R. (1995). Foreign student flows and the internationalisation of higher education. In K. Hanson & J. Meyerson (Eds). *International challenges to American colleges and universities* (pp 18–41). Phoenix, AZ: American Council on Education and The Oryx Press.

Langellier, K. & Natalle, E. (1987). Communication, gender perspectives, and the clinical supervisor. In S. Farmer (Ed.), *Clinical Supervision: A Coming of Age, Proceedings of A National Conference on Supervision* (pp 14–37). Las Cruces, NM: New Mexico State University.

Leininger, M. (1978). *Transcultural nursing: Concepts, theories and practices*. New York: Wiley & Sons.

Lewis, M. & Simon, R. (1986). A discourse not intended for her: Learning and teaching within patriarchy. *Harvard Educational Review*, **56** (4), 457–72.

Lipman, T. & Deatrick, J. (1994). Enhancing specialist preparation for the next century. *Journal of Nursing Education*, **33** (2), 53–8.

Lubinski, R. & Masters, M. (1994). Special populations, special settings: New and expanding frontiers. In R. Lubinski & C. Frattali (Eds). *Professional issues in speech-language pathology and audiology* (pp 149–65). San Diego, CA: Singular Publishing Group.

Lyman, P. (1995). What is computer literacy and what is its place in liberal education? *Liberal Education*, **81** (3), 4–15.

Lynch, E. (1992). Developing cross-cultural competence. In E. Lynch & M. Hanson (Eds). *Developing cross-cultural competence: A guide for working with young children and their families* (pp 35–62). Baltimore, MD: Paul H. Brookes Publishing Co.

Marfo, K. & Walker, B. (1986). *Childhood disability in developing countries: Issues in habilitation and special education.* New York: Praeger Publishers.

Maslen, G. (1995, 6 October). Progress for Aborigines. *The Chronicle of Higher Education*, A7–8.

McAllister, L., Eadie, P. & Hays, R. (1992). Promoting rural careers. *Australian Communication Quarterly*, Spring, 6–7.

McAllister, L., Masel, C., Tudehope, D., O'Callaghan, M., Mohay, H. & Rogers, Y. (1993a). Speech and language outcomes three years after neonatal intensive care. *European Journal of Disorders of Communication*, 28, 369–82.

McAllister, L., Masel, C., Tudehope, D., O'Callaghan, M., Mohay, H. & Rogers, Y. (1993b). Speech and language outcomes in preschool-aged survivors of neonatal intensive care. *European Journal of Disorders of Communication*, 28, 383–94.

McCready, V., Shapiro, D. & Kennedy, K. (1987). Identifying hidden dynamics in supervision: Four scenarios. In M. Crago & M. Pickering (Eds), *Supervision in human communication disorders: Perspectives on a process* (pp 169–201). Boston, MA: Little, Brown & Company, A College-Hill Publication.

McDonald, R. & Rowe, N. (1995). Minority ethnic groups and occupational therapy, Part 2: Transcultural occupational therapy, a curriculum for today's therapist. *British Journal of Occupational Therapy*, 58 (7) 286–90.

McKenna, K. (1993). Quality of life: A question of functional outcomes or the fulfilment of life plans. *The Australian Occupational Therapy Journal*, 40, 33–5.

Millward, C. (1995). Family networks in rural and urban settings. *Family Matters*, 41, Winter, 10–14.

Mogey, N. (1995). Teaching IT in OT: An introduction to therapeutic uses. *British Journal of Occupational Therapy*, 58 (6), 250–2.

Monahan, B. (1995a). A look overseas. *Magazine of Physical Therapy*, 3 (4), 30–1.

Monahan, B. (1995b). Postcards from abroad. *Magazine of Physical Therapy*, 3 (4), 32–42.

Montgomery, J. (1995). The salary gap remains. *Asha*, 37, 7.

Murphy, B., McEwen, E. & Hays, R. (1995). The University of Sydney Rural Careers Project: A nursing perspective. *Australian Journal of Rural Health*, 3, 20–4.

Native Title Act 1993: What it does and how it works (1994). Department of Prime Minister and Cabinet. Canberra: The Department.

Nieves-Squires, S. (1991). *Hispanic women: Making their presence on campus less tenuous.* Washington, DC: Association of American Colleges.

Office of Multicultural Affairs (1989). *A national agenda for a multicultural Australia.* Canberra: Australian Government Printing Service.

Pan American Health Organisation (1994). *Health Conditions in the Americas.* Washington, DC: World Health Organisation.

Pannbacker, M., Middleton, G. & Click, P. (1995). Professional development for older audiologists and speech-language pathologists. *Asha*, 37 (8), 26-8.

Pearson, C., Shavlik, D. & Touchton, J. (Eds) (1989). *Educating the majority: Women challenge tradition in higher education.* New York: Collier Macmillan Publishers.

Pew Higher Education Roundtable (1995, July). A calling to account. *Policy Per-*

spectives, **6** (2). (Available from Institute for Research on Higher Education, 4200 Pine Street, 5A, Philadelphia, PA, USA)

Philips, B. (1990). Our international responsibility. *Asha*, **32** (5), 51.

Pickering, M. (1992). A feminist vision for clinical education. In S. Dowling (Ed.), *Total Quality Supervision: Effecting Optimal Performance, Proceedings of 1992 National Conference on Supervision* (pp 41–5). Houston, TX: University of Houston.

Pickering, M. (1994). The unexpected, the amazing, and the elusive: Applying international perspectives to clinical education. In M. Bruce (Ed.), *Proceedings of the 1994 International and Interdisciplinary Conference on Clinical Supervision: Toward the 21st Century* (pp 68–81). Burlington, VT: University of Vermont.

Pickering, M. (1996, 25 October). Reflections on celebration of the 5th anniversary of the American University in Bulgaria. Strouma, pp 7, 10. (Printed in Bulgaria, in Bulgarian language. English version from author, University of Maine, Orono, ME, USA)

Prakash, M. & Waks, L. (1985). Four conceptions of excellence. *Teachers College Record*, **87** (1), 79–101.

Pressman, D. & Rudner, M. (1990). International service delivery. *Asha*, **32** (5), 48–9.

Professional Growth … By Degrees (1995). *Asha*, **37** (3), 11–12.

Rinehart, N. (1995). Picking up the pieces: Reassembling the universities of the former German Democratic Republic. *International Educator*, **V** (1), 15–18.

Rothchild, D. & Groth, A. (1995). Pathological dimensions of domestic and international ethnicity. *Political Science Quarterly*, **110** (1), 69–82.

Rowland, D. (1991). *Ageing in Australia*. Melbourne: Longman Cheshire.

Sandler, B. & Hall, R. (1986, October). *The campus climate revisited: Chilly for women faculty, administrators, and graduate students*. Washington, DC: Association of American Colleges.

SatelLife (n.d.). SatelLife [Brochure]. Cambridge, MA: Author. (Available at 126 Rogers St.).

Sawadogo, G. (1994). The future missions and roles of the African universities. *World Education News & Reviews*, **8** (1), 1, 20–3.

Sax, S. (1993). *Ageing and public policy in Australia*. Sydney: Allen & Unwin.

Shadden, B. & Warnick, P. (1994). Multicultural aspects of aging. *Asha*, **36** (4), 45–6.

Shapiro, D. (1994). Tender gender issues. *Asha*, **36** (11), 46–9.

Siegloff, L. (1995). The nurse practitioner project, Wilcannia: Moving from anecdotes to evidence. *Australian Journal of Rural Health*, **3**, 114–21.

Statistics Canada (1993). *Canada Year Book 1994*. Ottawa: Author.

Tannen, D. (1990). *You just don't understand: Women and men in conversation*. New York: William Morrow & Co., Inc.

Tarule, J. (1992). Dialogue and adult learning. *Liberal Education*, **78** (4), 12–19.

Tenn, L., Sovaleni, P., Latu, R., Fotu, A. & Smith, J. (1994). Getting the community involved in developing a PHC curriculum in Tonga. *International Nursing Review*, **41** (5), 141–7.

The University of Sydney Planning Office (1995, 11 September). Personal communication.

Thorpe, D. & Baker, C. (1995). Addressing 'cultural competence' in health care education. *Pediatric Physical Therapy*, **7** (3), 143–4.

Transcultural Health Care Council (1991). *Towards a transcultural approach to the education of health professionals and to health care delivery in Victoria: Proposal for a strategic plan*. Melbourne: Author.

Author index

United Nations Educational, Scientific and Cultural Organisation (1995). *Policy paper for change and development in higher education.* Paris: Author.

United Nations (1995, October). *Women: From Beijing, a platform for action and a clear mandate for women's progress.* DPI/1749/Wom.—95–30876. New York: United Nations Department of Public Information.

VanDenBergh, N. & Cooper, L. (1986a). Introduction. In N. VanDenBergh & L. Cooper (Eds). *Feminist visions for social work* (pp 1–28). Silver Springs, MD: National Association of Social Workers.

VanDenBergh, N. & Cooper, L. (Eds) (1986b). *Feminist visions for social work.* Silver Springs, MD: National Association of Social Workers.

Valuable Lessons From Women's Colleges (1995, Summer). *On Campus with Women,* **24** (5), 3. (Available from Association of American Colleges and Universities, 1818 R Street, NW, Washington, DC, USA, 20009)

Weiss, T. (1992). *On the margins.* Amherst, MA: University of Massachusetts Press.

Werven, G. (1994). Perspectives on the male speech-language pathologist. *Asha,* **36** (11), 42–5.

Where the boys aren't (1992). *American Demographics Desk Reference Series, No. 4: American Workers,* pp 8–10, 14.

Wilson, M. (1994). International perspectives. In R. Lubinski & C. Frattali (Eds). *Professional issues in speech-language pathology and audiology* (pp 75–88). San Diego, CA: Singular Publishing Group.

Wingspread Group on Higher Education (1993). *An American imperative: Higher expectations for higher education.* Racine, WI: The Johnson Foundation, Inc.

Woodard, C. (1995, 9 June). Internet international. *The Chronicle of Higher Education,* A21.

Worrall, L., McAllister, L., Mortensen, L., Franke, M., Dann, N., Russell, A., McAllister, S., Barrie, S., Robertson, C. & Dawson, V. (1996). *Developing professional competency – Self-directed learning modules for speech pathology students.* Queensland: Department of Speech Pathology and Audiology, University of Queensland, Australia.

Subject index